United States Skin Disease Needs Assessment

Guest Editor

ROBERT P. DELLAVALLE, MD, PhD, MSPH

DERMATOLOGIC CLINICS

www.derm.theclinics.com

Consulting Editor

BRUCE H. THIERS, MD

January 2012 • Volume 30 • Number 1

SAUNDERS an imprint of ELSEVIER, Inc.

W.B. SAUNDERS COMPANY
A Division of Elsevier Inc.

1600 John F. Kennedy Boulevard • Suite 1800 • Philadelphia, PA 19103-2899

http://www.theclinics.com

DERMATOLOGIC CLINICS Volume 30, Number 1
January 2012 ISSN 0733-8635, ISBN-13: 978-1-4557-3851-9

Editor: Stephanie Donley

Dermatologic Clinics (ISSN 0733-8635) is published quarterly by Elsevier Inc., 360 Park Avenue South, New York, NY 10010-1710. Months of publication are January, April, July, and October. Business and editorial offices: 1600 John F. Kennedy Blvd., Suite 1800, Philadelphia, PA 19103-2899. Customer service office: 11830 Westline Drive, St. Louis, MO 63146. Periodicals postage paid at New York, NY, and additional mailing offices. Subscription prices are USD 346.00 per year for US individuals, USD 512.00 per year for US institutions, USD 404.00 per year for Canadian individuals, USD 613.00 per year for Canadian institutions, USD 473.00 per year for international individuals, USD 613.00 per year for international institutions, USD 161.00 per year for US students/residents, and USD 233.00 per year for Canadian and international students/residents. International air speed delivery is included in all *Clinics* subscription prices. All prices are subject to change without notice. **POSTMASTER:** Send address changes to *Dermatologic Clinics*, Elsevier Health Sciences Division, Subscription Customer Service, 3251 Riverport Lane, Maryland Heights, MO 63043. **Customer Service: 1-800-654-2452 (U.S. and Canada); 314-447-8871 (outside U.S. and Canada). Fax: 314-447-8029. E-mail: journalscustomerservice-usa@elsevier.com (for print support); journalsonlinesupport-usa@elsevier.com (for online support).**

Reprints. For copies of 100 or more, of articles in this publication, please contact the Commercial Reprints Department, Elsevier Inc., 360 Park Avenue South, New York, New York 10010-1710. Tel.: (212) 633-3813; Fax: (212) 462-1935; Email: repritns@elsevier.com.

The *Dermatologic Clinics* is covered in *MEDLINE/PubMed (Index Medicus)*, *Current Contents/Clinical Medicine*, *Excerpta Medica, Chemical Abstracts,* and *ISI/BIOMED*.

Printed and bound by CPI Group (UK) Ltd, Croydon, CR0 4YY
Transferred to Digital Print 2012

Contributors

CONSULTING EDITOR

BRUCE H. THIERS, MD
Professor and Chairman, Department of
Dermatology and Dermatologic Surgery,
Medical University of South Carolina,
Charleston, South Carolina

GUEST EDITOR

ROBERT P. DELLAVALLE, MD, PhD, MSPH
Chief, Dermatology Service, Denver
Department of Veterans Affairs Medical
Center; Associate Professor of Dermatology,
University of Colorado School of Medicine;
Associate Professor of Epidemiology,
Colorado School of Public Health, Denver,
Colorado

AUTHORS

CHRISTINE AHN, BA
Department of Dermatology, Center for
Dermatology Research, Wake Forest School
of Medicine, Winston-Salem, North Carolina

MURAD ALAM, MD, MSCI
Departments of Dermatology, Otolaryngology-
Head and Neck Surgery and Surgery,
Northwestern University Feinberg School of
Medicine, Chicago, Illinois

APRIL W. ARMSTRONG, MD, MPH
Assistant Professor of Dermatology; Director,
Dermatology Clinical Research Unit; Director,
Teledermatology Program, Department of
Dermatology, University of California Davis
Health System, University of California Davis
School of Medicine, Sacramento, California

MARYAM M. ASGARI, MD, MPH
Division of Research, Kaiser Permanente
Northern California, Oakland; Department of
Dermatology, University of California at San
Francisco, San Francisco, California

NANCY J. BURNSIDE, MD
Alpert Medical School of Brown University;
Providence Veterans Affairs Medical Center,
Providence, Rhode Island

KESHA J. BUSTER, MD
Department of Dermatology, University
of Alabama at Birmingham, Birmingham,
Alabama

MICHAEL W. CASHMAN, MD
School of Medicine and Health Sciences,
George Washington University,
Washington, DC

LILY S. CHENG, BS
Department of Dermatology, University
of California Davis School of Medicine,
Sacramento, California

TUSHAR S. DABADE, MD
Department of Dermatology, Center for
Dermatology Research, Wake Forest School
of Medicine, Winston-Salem, North Carolina

SCOTT A. DAVIS, MA
Department of Dermatology, Center for
Dermatology Research, Wake Forest School
of Medicine, Winston-Salem, North Carolina

ANNELISE L. DAWSON, BA
Department of Dermatology, University
of Colorado Denver, Aurora, Colorado

ROBERT P. DELLAVALLE, MD, PhD, MSPH
Chief, Dermatology Service, Denver
Department of Veterans Affairs Medical
Center; Associate Professor of Dermatology,
University of Colorado School of Medicine;
Associate Professor of Epidemiology,
Colorado School of Public Health, Denver,
Colorado

CORY A. DUNNICK, MD
Associate Professor, Department of
Dermatology, University of Colorado Denver,
Aurora, Colorado

ALISON EHRLICH, MD, MHS
Clinical Professor of Dermatology, School of
Medicine and Health Sciences, George
Washington University; Director of
Dermatology Clinical Research, Department of
Dermatology, George Washington University
Medical Faculty Associates, Washington, DC

CRAIG A. ELMETS, MD
Department of Dermatology, University
of Alabama at Birmingham, Birmingham,
Alabama

DIRK M. ELSTON, MD
Department of Dermatology, Geisinger
Medical Center, Danville, Pennsylvania;
Managing Director, Ackerman Academy
of Dermatopathology, New York, New York

STEVEN R. FELDMAN, MD, PhD
Departments of Dermatology, Pathology,
Public Health Sciences, Center for
Dermatology Research, Wake Forest School
of Medicine, Winston-Salem, North Carolina

ALAN B. FLEISCHER Jr, MD
Department of Dermatology, Center for
Dermatology Research, Wake Forest School
of Medicine, Winston-Salem, North Carolina

RYAN GAMBLE, MD
Department of Dermatology Research Labs,
University of Colorado School of Medicine,
Aurora, Colorado

MARIUS LAURENTIU HAIDUCU, BSc
Department of Dermatology and Skin Science,
University of British Columbia; Vancouver
Coastal Health Research Institute, Vancouver,
British Columbia, Canada

LAURA HUFF, MD
Department of Dermatology Research Labs,
University of Colorado School of Medicine,
Aurora, Colorado

SUNIL KALIA, MD, MHSc, FRCPC, FAAD
Department of Dermatology and Skin Science,
University of British Columbia; Vancouver
Coastal Health Research Institute, Vancouver,
British Columbia, Canada

RANDIE H. KIM, MD, PhD
Department of Dermatology, University of
California Health System, Sacramento,
California

SIRI KNUTSEN-LARSON, MD
Dermatology Resident Physician, PGY-2,
Department of Dermatology, University of
Colorado Denver, Aurora, Colorado

JENNA LESTER, BA
Alpert Medical School of Brown University,
Providence, Rhode Island

KAI LI, BS
Department of Dermatology, University of
California Davis Health System, University
of California Davis, Sacramento, California

ALINA MARKOVA, BA
Alpert Medical School of Brown University,
Providence, Rhode Island

LAUREN MCLAUGHLIN, BS
Rocky Vista University College of Osteopathic
Medicine, Parker, Colorado

ELIOT N. MOSTOW, MD, MPH
Department of Dermatology, Case Western
Reserve University School of Medicine,
Cleveland; Department of Dermatology,
Northeast Ohio Medical University,
Rootstown, Ohio

JONATHAN M. OLSON, MD
Division of Dermatology, Department of
Medicine, University of Washington School
of Medicine, Seattle, Washington

BALVINDER REHAL, BS
Medical Student, Department of Dermatology,
University of California Davis Health System,
University of California Davis, Sacramento,
California

PATRICIA A. REUTEMANN, MD
School of Medicine and Health Sciences,
George Washington University,
Washington, DC

ERICA I. STEVENS, BS
University of Alabama at Birmingham School
of Medicine, Birmingham, Alabama

WILLIAM TUONG, BA
Department of Dermatology, University
of California Davis School of Medicine,
Sacramento, California

MICHAEL XIONG, BA
Alpert Medical School of Brown University,
Providence, Rhode Island

Contents

Preface xiii

Robert P. Dellavalle

Dedication xv

Introduction: US Dermatologic Health Care Needs Assessment 1

Laura Huff, Lauren McLaughlin, Ryan Gamble, and Robert P. Dellavalle

The health care needs assessment (HCNA) addressed in this issue of *Dermatologic Clinics* is designed to aid practitioners and policy makers by providing current, evidence-based research that can be used to guide United States' dermatologic care. The topics covered in this skin disease HCNA include those that are considered common dermatology care needs in society and those severe enough to create a burden on the medical system. Disease discussions address epidemiology, costs to society and patients, prevention, treatment, gaps in management, and future recommendations.

The Burden of Skin Disease in the United States and Canada 5

Sunil Kalia and Marius Laurentiu Haiducu

The burden of skin disease is a crucial indicator of the impact of skin disease in the general population. Despite many documented attempts in the literature to quantify independent parameters of skin disease burden, strides towards more comprehensive estimations have mainly arisen in the last decade. Utilizing the World Health Organization breakdown of disease burden, the literature was surveyed and summarized in respect to the classification, epidemiology, quality of life, and costs associated with skin disease.

Services Available and Their Effectiveness 19

Christine Ahn, Scott A. Davis, Tushar S. Dabade, Alan B. Fleischer Jr, and Steven R. Feldman

This article describes the range of services available for patients with skin disease in the United States. Within the structure of health care systems, 4 levels of care are characterized and discussed: self-care and management, generalist care, specialist care, and subspecialist care. Within each level, this article discusses the profiles of individuals involved in delivering medical care, the location or setting in which these services are provided, the capacity and specific activities of care providers, and current literature on the efficacy of these different levels of care.

Models of Care and Organization of Services 39

Alina Markova, Michael Xiong, Jenna Lester, and Nancy J. Burnside

This article examines the overall organization of services and delivery of health care in the United States. Health maintenance organization, fee-for-service, preferred provider organizations, and the Veterans Health Administration are discussed, with a focus on structure, outcomes, and areas for improvement. An overview of wait times, malpractice, telemedicine, and the growing population of physician extenders in dermatology is also provided.

Dermatologic Health Disparities   53

Kesha J. Buster, Erica I. Stevens, and Craig A. Elmets

Although significant data highlight the extent of health disparities, data regarding dermatologic health disparities are limited. Ethnic minorities, people of low socioeconomic status, the less educated, elderly, and uninsured have poorer melanoma and nonmelanoma skin cancer outcomes. Atopic dermatitis is more prevalent among ethnic minorities, but whether morbidity is also increased in these populations is unclear. Given the current dermatology workforce shortage, increased patient load from health care reform may have an adverse effect on access to dermatologic care. Additional concerns include status of dermatologic training, insufficient research involving ethnic minorities, and lack of investigation of dermatologic health disparities.

A Review of Health Outcomes in Patients with Psoriasis   61

Kai Li and April W. Armstrong

Psoriasis, a chronic inflammatory skin condition, is a complex disease in terms of its significant comorbidities and impact on patients' quality of life. The objective of this article is to elucidate the health outcomes of the disease, including its economic and psychosocial burden on the patient. Current treatments options and the economic considerations of treatment costs are reviewed. Psoriasis is a multidimensional disease, so patients benefit from having a multidisciplinary team of dermatologists and other physicians for management of it and of associated comorbid conditions.

Health Outcomes in Atopic Dermatitis   73

Balvinder Rehal and April W. Armstrong

Atopic dermatitis is a chronic inflammatory skin disease that disrupts the daily work and social lives of patients. Treatment of atopic dermatitis makes use of a variety of therapies, from medications to nutritional supplements to psychotherapy. Health outcomes research evaluates the efficacy, safety, and impact on health-related quality of life of these therapies.

**Contact Dermatitis in the United States: Epidemiology, Economic Impact, and
Workplace Prevention**   87

Michael W. Cashman, Patricia A. Reutemann, and Alison Ehrlich

Contact dermatitis in the United States poses a significant public health concern. This article provides a definition of contact dermatitis and its associated risk factors. The authors discuss the epidemiology of occupational contact dermatitis including its incidence and prevalence, and describe how estimates are calculated in the United States. The burden of disease on the individual, and its economic impact and cost to society, are also elucidated. A review of preventive measures to help reduce contact dermatitis in the workplace and an additional section on patch testing concludes the article.

Acne Vulgaris: Pathogenesis, Treatment, and Needs Assessment   99

Siri Knutsen-Larson, Annelise L. Dawson, Cory A. Dunnick, and Robert P. Dellavalle

Acne vulgaris is a common skin condition with substantial cutaneous and psychologic disease burden. Studies suggest that the emotional impact of acne is comparable to that experienced by patients with systemic diseases, like diabetes and epilepsy. In conjunction with the considerable personal burden experienced by patients with acne, acne vulgaris also accounts for substantial societal and health care burden. The pathogenesis and existing treatment strategies for acne are complex. This article discusses the epidemiology, pathogenesis, and treatment of acne vulgaris. The burden of disease in the United States and future directions in the management of acne are also addressed.

US Skin Disease Assessment: Ulcer and Wound Care   107

Alina Markova and Eliot N. Mostow

Chronic ulcers are a growing cause of patient morbidity and contribute significantly to the cost of health care in the United States. The most common etiologies of chronic ulcers include venous leg ulcers (VLUs), pressure ulcers (PrUs), diabetic neuropathic foot ulcers (DFUs), and leg ulcers of arterial insufficiency. Chronic wounds account for an estimated $6 to $15 billion annually in US health care costs; however, it is difficult to get accurate measurements on this, because these patients are often seen in a variety of settings or simply fail to access the health care system.

Melanoma: Epidemiology, Diagnosis, Treatment, and Outcomes   113

William Tuong, Lily S. Cheng, and April W. Armstrong

Melanoma is a skin cancer that arises from the malignant transformation of melanocytes. Although it is typically considered a pigmented lesion, the clinical presentation of melanoma can vary greatly. With increased efforts in screening and detection of early-stage melanoma, researchers and clinicians hope to improve clinical outcomes for patients with melanoma. Novel immunotherapies directed at specific molecular targets in the pathogenesis of melanoma usher in a new era of treatment of advanced melanoma.

Nonmelanoma Skin Cancer   125

Randie H. Kim and April W. Armstrong

Nonmelanoma skin cancers (NMSCs) represent the most common cancer in the United States, accounting for more than 2 million cases per year. Despite the magnitude of health burden on the US population, there remain many questions regarding the epidemiology, health outcomes, and treatments of NMSCs. This article highlights these areas of clinical and research need. The article focuses on the recent epidemiologic trends as well as health outcomes of NMSCs in the United States. In addition, current national guidelines, available treatments and care pathways, and clinical trials are discussed.

Infectious Skin Diseases: A Review and Needs Assessment   141

Annelise L. Dawson, Robert P. Dellavalle, and Dirk M. Elston

Infectious skin diseases pose considerable treatment challenges, especially given the recent appearance of several highly virulent pathogens as well as the rising number of immunocompromised patients in the United States. This article discusses common bacterial, fungal, and viral skin infections with an emphasis on cellulitis, dermatophyte infections, and herpes simplex viral infections. Disease pathogenesis, treatment, and cost of treatment are addressed with an emphasis on therapeutic needs and future research directions. Common priorities for all infectious skin disease categories include increased disease surveillance, study of existing treatments, and efforts in drug development.

Needs Assessment for General Dermatologic Surgery   153

Jonathan M. Olson, Murad Alam, and Maryam M. Asgari

This article reviews current recommendations, strength of evidence, and areas in need of further research in the surgical treatment of melanoma and nonmelanoma skin cancers, as well as other select cutaneous neoplasms. Cryosurgery, electrosurgery, photodynamic therapy, and surgical excision are discussed. Local anesthesia, suturing technique, postsurgical dressings, and optimization of scarring are briefly reviewed. In general, large, high-quality, randomized controlled trials on which to base recommendations are lacking.

Needs Assessment for Mohs Micrographic Surgery   167

Maryam M. Asgari, Jonathan M. Olson, and Murad Alam

Mohs micrographic surgery (MMS) is a unique technique that can offer the highest cure rates and maximum tissue conservation in the management of specific primary and recurrent skin cancers. However, there are many areas of controversy that surround MMS, including appropriate indications for its use, technical quandaries, and outcomes. Recent efforts in these areas need to be assessed to identify research gaps in MMS to help fuel further work. The usefulness of MMS and its methods for delivery need more stringent, evidence-based, rigorous study.

Needs Assessment for Cosmetic Dermatologic Surgery   177

Murad Alam, Jonathan M. Olson, and Maryam M. Asgari

Cosmetic procedures have been an integral part of dermatologic surgery for over half a century, with a more recent proliferation of devices to improve skin color and texture and modify subcutaneous fat. Overall, cosmetic dermatologic procedures are extremely safe. However, detailed information about safety and effectiveness, and especially comparative effectiveness, is not available for many procedures. There are few randomized control trials of comparative effectiveness of different procedures for similar indications. Key comparative effectiveness studies are briefly reviewed, and areas of substantial deficiency in such research are highlighted.

Conclusions and Recommendations: United States Dermatologic Health Care Need Assessment   189

Laura Huff, Lauren McLaughlin, Ryan Gamble, and Robert P. Dellavalle

This United States skin disease health care needs assessment (HCNA) focuses on the most common and severe skin conditions. The purpose of this article is to highlight these skin conditions in a concise manner for efficient use by policy makers. Brief summaries of each article in this issue of *Dermatologic Clinics* are provided along with recommendations for better addressing dermatologic care needs.

Index   195

Dermatologic Clinics

FORTHCOMING ISSUES

April 2012

Quality of Life Issues in Dermatology
Suephy Chen, MD,
Guest Editor

July 2012

Melanoma and Pigmented Lesions
Darrell S. Rigel, MD, and Julie E. Russak, MD,
Guest Editors

October 2012

What's New in Dermatopathology
Tammie Ferringer, MD,
Guest Editor

RECENT ISSUES

October 2011

**Autoimmune Blistering Diseases:
Part II – Diagnosis and Management**
Dédée F. Murrell, MA, BMBCh, FAAD,
MD, FACD, *Guest Editor*

July 2011

**Autoimmune Blistering Diseases:
Part I – Pathogenesis and Clinical Features**
Dédée F. Murrell, MA, BMBCh, FAAD,
MD, FACD, *Guest Editor*

April 2011

Mohs Surgery
Allison T. Vidimos, RPh, MD,
Christine Poblete-Lopez, MD,
and Christopher C. Gasbarre, DO,
Guest Editors

Preface

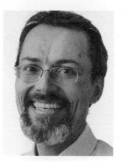

Robert P. Dellavalle, MD, PhD, MSPH
Guest Editor

This edition of the *Dermatologic Clinics* takes a stab at providing the first US dermatology health care needs assessment. This work follows the delineation of the US burden of skin disease[1] and discussion of national clinical dermatology research priorities,[2] while closely following the blueprint set out by the recent dermatology needs assessment of the United Kingdom.[3]

I thank Bruce Theirs for asking me to edit this issue. As I did four years ago for my first *Dermatologic Clinics* issue on dermatoepidemiology and public health, I solicited articles from colleagues on the dermatoepidemiology email list maintained by Martin Weinstock at Brown University (Providence, RI). Members of the American Academy of Dermatology's Epidemiology Expert Resource Group also volunteered articles. Cory Dunnick, Ryan Gamble, Annelise Dawson, Brian Petersen, and Jeffrey Dunn served as reviewers.

This issue also continues the use of podcasts initiated in my previous *Dermatologic Clinics* issue.[4] I thank Stephanie Donley for her professional editorial assistance. And, once again, I thank my wife and children for accommodating the effort this project displaced from our time together.

Robert P. Dellavalle, MD, PhD, MSPH
Dermatology Service
Denver Department of Veterans
Affairs Medical Center
University of Colorado School of Medicine
Colorado School of Public Health
1055 Clermont Street, Mail Code #165
Denver, CO 80220, USA

E-mail address:
Robert.Dellavalle@ucdenver.edu

REFERENCES

1. The burden of skin diseases. The Lewin Group, Inc; 2005. Available at: http://www.lewin.com/content/publications/april2005skindisease.pdf. Accessed June 13, 2011.
2. Katz SI, Carter RH, Serrate-Sztein SA. Skin Diseases Clinical Trials Roundtable Summary: 2009. Available at: http://www.niams.nih.gov/News_and_Events/Meetings_and_Events/Roundtables/2009/skin_diseases.asp. Accessed June 13, 2011.
3. Schofield JK, Grindley D, Williams HC. Skin conditions in the UK: a health care needs assessment. Centre of Evidenced-based Dermatology, University of Nottingham; 2009. Available at: http://www.nottingham.ac.uk/scs/documents/documentsdivisions/documentsdermatology/hcnaskinconditionsuk2009.pdf. Accessed June 13, 2011.
4. Dellavalle RP. Dermatologic Epidemiology and Public Health. 2009;27(2):99–218. Available at: http://www.derm.theclinics.com/content/podcast. Assessed June 13, 2011.

Dermatol Clin 30 (2012) xiii
doi:10.1016/j.det.2011.09.006
0733-8635/12/$ – see front matter © 2012 Elsevier Inc. All rights reserved.

derm.theclinics.com

Dedication

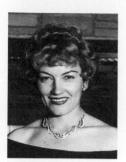

Mabel C. Dellavalle

I dedicate this issue to my mother Mabel C. Dellavalle who died during the production of this issue; I love you and miss you mom.

Dermatol Clin 30 (2012) xv
doi:10.1016/j.det.2011.09.007
0733-8635/12/$ – see front matter

Introduction: US Dermatologic Health Care Needs Assessment

Laura Huff, MD[a], Lauren McLaughlin, BS[b],
Ryan Gamble, MD[a], Robert P. Dellavalle, MD, PhD, MSPH[c],*

KEYWORDS

- Health care needs • Skin disease • Supply • Demand
- Reform

HEALTH CARE NEEDS ASSESSMENT

A health care needs assessment (HCNA) attempts to answer these 3 questions: (1) What is the burden of a specific disease in a population? (2) What impact does this disease burden have on quality of life, the economy, and the health care system as a whole? and (3) How can a health care system best address this burden to reduce the impact of the disease? An HCNA attempts to accurately evaluate the needs of a population and provide a strategy to address the needs with an evidence-based approach. In the United States, with health care spending the heated subject of national political reform, an HCNA is of utmost importance. This is a formal evaluation of dermatologic healthcare needs in the United States and its findings should be used as a tool to guide the provision of health care.

SKIN DISEASE

The HCNA presented in this issue is specific to skin disease. In the United States, 1 of every 3 people is affected by a skin condition at any point in time.[1] Skin disease was listed as a "top 15

medical condition" for its increase in prevalence and health care spending from 1987 to 2000.[2] It accounted for more than $37 billion per year in medical costs and lost productivity in 2004.[3] There are more than 3000 dermatologic diseases encompassing skin, hair, nails, sweat glands, sebaceous glands, and mucosal surfaces.[3]

The skin protects the rest of the body from the environment, especially UV radiation, temperature fluctuations, infections, infestations, and irritants. The skin also has the capability to synthesize vitamin D, which is an emerging interest in medicine. Skin diseases cause a variety of problems, including burning, itching, pain, physical disfigurement, scarring, and emotional distress. When the skin is seriously affected, the devastating results can cause systemic disease, such as cancer metastasis, sepsis, other organ damage, and death. The interaction between skin disease and systemic disease goes both ways. Because the skin is the outermost organ, it provides a window to what is occurring elsewhere in the body. Because many systemic diseases have dermatologic manifestations, thorough physical examinations of the skin may reveal hidden systemic diseases, leading to earlier treatment and improved health.

Funding/Support: None.
[a] Department of Dermatology Research Labs, University of Colorado School of Medicine, Mail Stop F-8127, PO Box 6511, Aurora, CO 80045, USA
[b] Rocky Vista University College of Osteopathic Medicine, 8401 South Chambers Road, Parker, CO 80134, USA
[c] Dermatology Service, Denver Department of Veterans Affairs Medical Center, University of Colorado School of Medicine, Colorado School of Public Health, 1055 Clermont Street, Mail Code #165, Denver, CO 80220, USA
* Corresponding author.
E-mail address: robert.dellavalle@ucdenver.edu

Dermatol Clin 30 (2012) 1–3
doi:10.1016/j.det.2011.09.002
0733-8635/12/$ – see front matter Published by Elsevier Inc.

The skin is also the most visible organ, making the social impact of skin disease arguably the greatest of all organ systems. Although a person's health problems are often kept private and confidential, a skin disease is exposed to all passersby. Skin diseases, such as acne, psoriasis, eczema, warts, and skin cancer, can be devastating to a person's self-image. Affected persons may express feelings of embarrassment, shame, isolation, fear, and poor self-confidence.

HEALTH CARE NEED

To conduct an HCNA one must define what constitutes a health care need. In dermatology, the line is often blurred between a genuine health care need and a health care want. A health care need has been defined as and ability at the population level to benefit from health care.[4] Because a cosmetic procedure can often benefit a person but does not necessarily address a need, this definition has been revised incorporating the concepts of supply and demand.[5] Need overlaps both supply and demand but is not defined by one or the other. **Fig. 1** depicts 2009 provisions for skin disease in the United Kingdom and its relationship to need, supply, and demand; provisions addressed more demands than needs or supply.

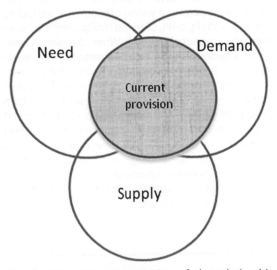

Fig. 1. Schematic representation of the relationship between need, supply, and demand for health care for skin disease in the UK in 2009. (*Data from* Schofield JK, Grindley D, Williams HC. Skin conditions in the UK: a health care needs assessment. University of Nottingham: Centre of Evidenced Based Dermatology. Available at: http://www.nottingham.ac.uk/scs/documents/documentsdivisions/documentsdermatology/hcnaskinconditionsuk2009.pdf.)

In the United States, health care need is largely defined by the large health care payment system, Medicare. Medicare only allows payment for health care that is "reasonable and necessary," which is defined as "reasonable and necessary for the diagnosis or treatment of illness or injury or to improve the functioning of a malformed body member," or is listed as an exception elsewhere in the statutes.[6]

With skin disease, it can be difficult to define illness or a malformed body member. Most persons would agree that melanoma, psoriasis, acne, and eczema are illnesses. Is a wart an illness? How about an irritated seborrheic keratosis? Unwanted hair? The UK HCNA suggests that social attitudes and societal values really determine when a skin condition is considered illness, with treatment being a health care need, or simply an unfortunate variant of normal, with treatment being a health care want.[4] Because subtle skin conditions can point to underlying disease, the need for evaluation by experienced practitioners may be broader than the need for treatment.

WHAT TO EXPECT IN THIS US SKIN DISEASE NEEDS ASSESSMENT

For this skin disease HCNA, widespread skin conditions are included that are accepted as health care needs by society as well as by the Medicare payment system. Common and severe skin diseases receive emphasis due to their greater burden on society. Readers are also provided with an article addressing cosmetic dermatology because of the high health care demand in society for these services. The articles in this issue provide a thorough discussion of skin disease in the United States and highlight major skin diseases separately. Chapters address epidemiology, cost to society, cost to patient, prevention, treatment, gaps in management, and future recommendations. This edition of *Dermatologic Clinics* begins to provide practitioners and policy makers an up-to-date, evidence-based tool for guiding dermatologic care in the United States.

List of Acronyms	
HCNA	Health Care Needs Assessment
UV	Ultraviolet
UK	United Kingdom

REFERENCES

1. Johnson ML. Defining the burden of skin disease in the United States—a historical perspective. J Investig Dermatol Symp Proc 2004;9:108–10. DOI:10.1046/j.1087-0024.2003.09117.x.
2. Thorpe KE, Florence CS, Joski P. Which medical conditions account for the rise in health care spending? Health Aff (Millwood) 2004;(Suppl Web). W4-437–45. doi:hlthaff.w4.437 [pii].
3. The Lewin Group, I. (2005). The burden of skin diseases. Available at: http://www.lewin.com/content/publications/april2005skindisease.pdf. Accessed September 23, 2011.
4. Schofield, JK, Grindley, D, Williams, HC. (n.d.). Skin conditions in the UK: a health care needs assessment. University of Nottingham: Centre of Evidenced Based Dermatology. Available at: http://www.nottingham.ac.uk/scs/documents/documentsdivisions/documents dermatology/hcnaskinconditionsuk2009.pdf. Accessed September 23, 2011.
5. Williams HC. (n.d.). Dermatology. In: Stevens A, Raftery J, editors. Health Care Needs Assessment (ST - Dermatology). Oxford (United Kingdom): Radcliffe Medical Press; 2007. p. 261–348.
6. Laws, S. S. O. C. of the S. S. (ED.). (n.d.). Sec. 1862. [42 U.S.C. 1395y]. Available at: http://www.ssa.gov/OP_Home/ssact/title18/1862.htm#ft580. Accessed September 23, 2011.

The Burden of Skin Disease in the United States and Canada

Sunil Kalia, MD, MHSc, FRCPC[a,b],*
Marius Laurentiu Haiducu, BSc[a,b]

KEYWORDS

- Skin disease • Disease burden • Skin disease classification
- Health care costs

Skin conditions are frequently cited among the most common health problems in the United States and Canada,[1–3] and US collective prevalence estimates surpass those of obesity, hypertension, and cancer.[1] Yet, the national burden of skin disease has avoided accurate estimation for decades. Studies that have sought to estimate it have relied on endpoints of health, social, and economic consequences of disease but such parameters have not displayed consistent measurement. Morbidity and mortality from skin conditions are both expected to increase, and prevalence and health care spending related to skin disease are considered among the fastest growing of any medical condition.[1,4,5] As such, accurate assessments of the skin disease burden become essential for efficient allocation of research and health care resources as well as for public awareness and intervention. Guided by the World Health Organization (WHO) breakdown of disease burden into components of epidemiology (incidence, prevalence, and mortality), costs, and quality of life (QOL) impact,[6] the literature was surveyed in an attempt to quantify these parameters of skin disease in the United States and Canada.

SKIN DISEASE CLASSIFICATION

There are more than 3000 defined varieties of skin disease described in the medical literature, and symptomatology may range from physical discomfort to psychological and emotional toil to death.[7] Given the great diversity of diagnostic possibilities, principles for skin disease nomenclature have become equally expansive, and categorization can be based on symptoms, physical appearance, anatomic distribution, pathologic or histologic examination, immunologic staining pattern, causative agent or resultant disability, and genetic derivation of the disease.[8,9] In addition, many general terms, such as *eczema* and *dermatitis*, are ambiguous in their diagnostic intent because they may encompass a diverse array of pathologies and may be differently interpreted by various specialists.[10,11] Thus, part of the difficulty in acquiring an overall impression of national disease burden has derived from the inconsistent assumptions and limitations that researchers apply when investigating skin disease.

Various investigatory bodies have established their own interpretations skin disease, ranging from the narrow consideration of only conditions treated by dermatologists to all-inclusive appreciation of any disease or condition that affects the skin.[10,12–14] The latter, broad definition scheme is well-suited to capture morbidity and mortality from skin conditions that never bring patients into contact with the medical system, yet it also necessitates more elaborate classification systems of skin disease. Both Canada and the United States make use of the *International*

[a] Department of Dermatology and Skin Science, University of British Columbia, 835 West 10th Avenue, Vancouver, BC, Canada V5Z 4E8
[b] Vancouver Coastal Health Research Institute, 835 West 10th Avenue, Vancouver, BC, Canada V5Z 4E8
* Corresponding author. 835 West 10th Avenue, Vancouver, BC, Canada V5Z 4E8.
E-mail address: sunil.kalia@vch.ca

Dermatol Clin 30 (2012) 5–18
doi:10.1016/j.det.2011.09.004
0733-8635/12/$ – see front matter © 2012 Elsevier Inc. All rights reserved.

derm.theclinics.com

Classification for Diseases (ICD), Ninth Revision, coding scheme to classify skin disease; many past studies attempting to quantify disease burden have relied on this system. The diagnostic codes frequently group together distinct diagnoses and these fail to incorporate skin infections and skin tumors, which together make up a significant portion of dermatologic case loads. Newer iterations, such as ICD-10, fail to address such shortcomings of previous versions. Thus, many early studies that relied on these classification schemes cannot be used to accurately determine trends in burden of skin disease.[7,8,15]

Although past ICD systems have been disappointing, the eleventh iteration, which is set to enter general use in 2015, is proving to mitigate previous inadequacies. Through the joint effort between different national dermatology organizations and the International League of Dermatological Societies, dermatology has become the first specialty to have substantial revisions accepted by the WHO into the ICD-11 draft, and the changes demonstrate strides toward more comprehensive accounts of skin disease for the first time since 1948. With the use of an electronic platform, listed diseases will be elaborated on with textual definitions, diagnostic criteria, etiology, and targeted body sites. Nomenclature preferences will also shift away from eponyms, which are frequent within the field of dermatology, toward categorizations based on pathophysiology. Both the expansion from 4-digit to 6-digit coding schemes and the elaboration of hierarchical patterns to allow for one category to be in multiple locations add to the specificity of a diagnosis. Moreover, diagnostic subcategories will be available to better capture various disease subtypes, such as those of basal cell and squamous cell carcinoma.[8,16] Such a broadened diagnostic scope renders ICD-11 more suitable for statistical investigations.

EPIDEMIOLOGY
Prevalence and Incidence of Skin Disease

The United States
Although conducted between 1971 and 1974, the first US Health and Nutrition Examination Survey (HANES) remains one of the most comprehensive reports on skin pathology and health-seeking behavior. With 20,749 subjects evaluated from 65 samplings of individuals aged 1 to 74, this large-scale study determined that, on dermatologist consultation, approximately 1 in 3 Americans (312.4 per 1000 population or 60 million individuals at the time of the study) had at least one skin condition that merited medical examination.[17,19]

The changing demographic vista of the United States and advancements in technology and medical care, however, render extrapolations from such outdated studies insufficient to predict current disease burdens.[18]

Recent literature reviews have identified 21 databases with information relating to US skin disease prevalence or incidence.[15] Many of these data sources, however, have methodologic inadequacies. For example, a 1999–2000 analysis of office visits to dermatologists in the United States determined that acne and actinic keratosis represented the two most common presentations, with both conditions resulting in 5.2 million visits and 15% of total visits per year (benign growths were only slightly behind in visit count at 4.6 million and 14% of total visits per year).[4] The storage of such data through ICD-9, Clinical Modification, diagnostic codes, however, results in an inability to separate new from recurrent or chronic disease within the given time frame. Only 8 databases do not use this coding scheme and thus have the potential to distinguish incidence from prevalence. Of these 8 databases, 6 relied on surveys to collect patient information: the Bureau of Labor Statistics (Annual Survey of Occupational Injuries and Illnesses); the Medical Expenditure Panel Survey, Household Component; the National Health and Nutrition Examination Survey (NHANES); the National Health Interview Survey; the National Home and Hospice Care Survey; and the National Nursing Home Survey. Most of these surveys contain self-reported measurements and are, therefore, limited in accuracy by the layperson's ability to recognize and categorize skin disease. Furthermore, because the surveys have differences in their sample populations and in the classification systems for skin disease that they rely on, the accuracy of prevalence and incidence measurements cannot be expected to remain consistent among the different databases. The Surveillance, Epidemiology and End Results (SEER) Program is considered one of the most reliable databases for skin cancer incidence and prevalence and may be used in combination with other data sources in an attempt to provide the most current and accurate estimate of skin disease impact on the population.[7,15]

Database storage modalities, as discussed previously, often impede the calculation of incidence rates, even when considering specific skin conditions individually. Enough literature has been published, however, on the most common US skin diseases in order for recent studies to provide estimates of their prevalence, primarily through databases created by the National Center for Health Statistics. **Table 1** lists the 10 most common skin conditions in the United States

Table 1
The most common skin conditions in the United States, 2004

Disease	Herpes Simplex and Herpes Zoster	Solar Radiation Damage	Seborrheic Keratosis	Contact Dermatitis	Hair and Nail Disorders	Human Papilloma Virus/Warts	Acne (Cystic and Vulgaris)	Actinic Keratosis	Benign Neoplasms/Keloid	Atopic Dermatitis
Prevalence (millions)	165	123.1	83.8	72.3	70.5	58.5	50.2	39.5	29.4	15.2
Inpatient hospital stays	119,929	1275	7826	49,643	21,549	12,769	8970	7611	26,284	48,146
Outpatient hospital visits	328,441	—	124,557	935,018	243,831	338,328	221,478	36,098	162,280	1,055,187
Emergency room visits	254,006	—	2909	691,459	141,358	37,430	3433	14,918	8689	603,467
Physician office visits	3,020,111	—	1,025,759	9,218,267	3,268,227	5,158,070	6,979,848	8,240,040	6,788,358	9,944,576

Quantifications of disease-specific inpatient, outpatient, emergency room, and physician office visits derived from the Lewin Group's *The Burden of Skin Diseases 2005*.[7] All numeric estimates correlate to a 1-year time period.

Data from Bickers DR, Lim HW, Margolis D, et al. The burden of skin diseases: 2004 a joint project of the American Academy of Dermatology Association and the Society for Investigative Dermatology. J Am Acad Dermatol 2006;55(3):490–500.

in 2004, along with an interpretation of their frequency of presentation to the hospital and community physician's office.

Canada

No current literature was identified as attempting to offer a holistic appreciation of the national skin disease burden in Canada. The lack of such investigations likely stems from the dearth of epidemiologic analysis of common skin conditions. Although some studies have attempted in recent years to provide insight into incidence or prevalence rates of specific diseases, such as psoriasis,[19] atopic dermatitis,[20] anogenital warts,[21,22] and epidermolysis bullosa,[23] investigations into many other skin disease rates are needed before such data can be compiled to offer an impression on the overall burden of skin disease. An impression of the most common skin diseases in Canada, as well as their prevalence and incidence, may be obtained through examination of the ICD-9 billing code charges to the Medical Service Plan. Such an approach, however, offers the same limitations as described for US studies, because new cases of disease are mixed with chronic conditions and many skin diseases that are treated without a medical intervention or that are never medically investigated would be underestimated in their national significance.

Mortality of Skin Disease

The United States

Investigative interest in nationally quantifying casualties of skin disease dates back to the 1971–1974 HANES study, in which mortality rates were of primary focus. However, with continuing insights on psychosocial aspects of skin conditions such as acne,[24,25] and with recent attempts to estimate the more significant costs of skin disease morbidity and impact on individual and societal function,[17] it is easy for the fatality rates associated with various skin conditions to be overlooked. Many skin disorders, including bullous diseases, psoriasis, herpes simplex and herpes zoster, lupus erythematosus, and skin ulcers and wounds, can cause death of patients, but mortality rates in the United States are low.[1] Death from skin cancers, however, including melanoma, nonmelanoma skin cancer (NMSC), and cutaneous lymphoma, is significant because skin cancer in the United States remains the most common cancer diagnosis. Estimates for the US in 2011 indicate that 3 million diagnoses of skin cancer will be made and that over 11,000 individuals will succumb to the disease.[26,27] Melanoma, which constitutes less than 5% of all skin cancer but contributes to the majority of the casualty toll,

has been steadily increasing in incidence by 2.9% per year in the United States between 1986 and 2006.[28] Incidence rates have almost tripled from 8.02 per 100,000 in 1975 to 21.48 per 100,000 in 2007.[29] When dissecting the impact on specific age groups, however, it can be seen that melanoma is slowly becoming a burden of the aged. Among white individuals over age 50, men have experienced an increase in death rate from melanoma by 1.1% per year since 1989 whereas the rate for women in the same age category has remained relatively constant since 1990. In those under 50, however, the death rate from melanoma has been decreasing by 3.0% per year for men since 1991 and by 2.2% per year for women since 1984. Five-year survival with the disease between 1999 and 2006 was estimated at 93%, a steady increase from previous measurements that will likely continue in an upward direction as diagnostic and therapeutic techniques improve.[27] Not surprisingly, skin cancer is the skin condition associated with the highest monetary loss due to premature death (Table 2), a detriment that ripples to affect not only the patient but dependents and society as well.

Evaluation of trends in NMSC rates is more challenging because cancer registries in the United States do not require data on these diagnoses to be reported.[27] In 2006, it was estimated that the incidence of NMSC in the United States was approximately 3.5 million.[30] Estimates of deaths from NMSC in the United States currently hover at approximately 2000 annually. Longitudinal studies during the past 15 years, however, have nearly unanimously determined the incidence of NMSC to be increasing, sometimes as rapidly as 7% per annum.[31] With the increasing longevity of transplant recipients and higher NMSC incidence, death rate estimates will likely soon rise.

Canada

Skin disease mortality rates follow similar trends in Canada, with the cause of death from diseases of the skin and subcutaneous tissue rising from 307 in 2000 to 346 in 2007 based on ICD-9 coding data[32] which is noninclusive for skin cancer deaths and certain fungal infections. As in the United States, skin cancer is both the most common cancer diagnosis and the major contributor to death from skin disease. Of the estimated 177,800 cancer diagnoses in 2011, 74,100 are expected to be of NMSC and 270 conditions will prove fatal. These quantifications are estimated based on only three cancer registries that track NMSC in Canada via histologic confirmation and are, therefore, likely to underestimate the actual incidence and mortality of NMSC.[2,33]

Table 2
Ranking skin disease cost and impact on QOL in the United States, 2004

Skin Disease Ranking	Direct Medical Cost, $ Millions	Indirect Medical Cost, $ Millions	Future Earnings Lost due to Premature Death, $ Millions	Willingness-to-Pay, $ Billions	Lowest Mean Utility Measurements
1	9712 Skin ulcers and wounds	2852 Melanoma	2826 Melanoma	17.0 Hair and nail Disorders	0.640 Bullous diseases
2	2500 Acne (cystic and vulgaris)	2239 Skin ulcers and wounds	1813.5 Skin ulcers and wounds	12.0 Acne	0.706 Condyloma
3	1704 Herpes simplex and herpes zoster	961 Skin cancer, nonmelanoma	893.2 Skin cancer, nonmelanoma	6.7 Seborrheic keratosis	0.820 Lymphoma
4	1671 Cutaneous fungal infections	619 Acne (cystic and vulgaris)	235.5 Cutaneous lymphoma	2.6 Atopic dermatitis	0.867 Mycosis fungoides
5	1625 Contact dermatitis	619 Atopic dermatitis	132.1 Lupus erythematosus	2.5 Human papillomavirus	0.923 Ulcers

Values are comparable to those obtained by the Lewin Group's *The Burden of Skin Disease 2005*, with two notable exceptions: (1) herpes simplex and herpes zoster, estimated at $1375 in direct costs, rank lower than cutaneous fungal infections, cutaneous fungal infections, atopic dermatitis, nonmelanoma skin cancer, and contact dermatitis, in that order, and (2) atopic dermatitis and acne take the fourth and fifth ranks, respectively, with cutaneous lymphoma estimated to have $37 million in indirect costs.

Numeric values for direct and indirect cost, future earning loss, and WTP are obtained from Bickers DR, Lim HW, Margolis D, et al. The burden of skin diseases: 2004 a joint project of the American Academy of Dermatology Association and the Society for Investigative Dermatology. J Am Acad Dermatol 2006;55(3):490–500; permission obtained from Elsevier (license number 2716011325053). *Mean utility measurements are obtained from* Chen SC, Bayoumi AM, Soon SL, et al. A catalog of dermatology utilities: a measure of the burden of skin diseases. J Investig Dermatol Symp Proc 2004;9(2): 160–8.

In 2011, the incidence of melanoma is expected to approach 5500 and the number of expected deaths is 950; the 5-year survival rate is estimated at 90%. From 1995 to 2005, the incidence rate has varied from 10.11 per 100,000 to 11.47 per 100,000, respectively.[2,34] **Fig. 1** provides a more comprehensive overview of melanoma incidence trends.

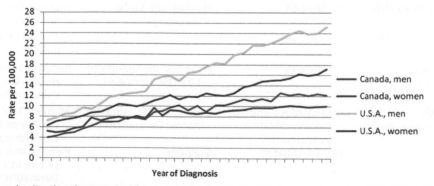

Fig. 1. Age-standardized melanoma incidence rates in the United States and Canada, 1973–2004. (*Canadian data were collected from* the Government of Canada PHAOC. Melanoma skin cancer facts and figures—Public Health Agency Canada. Available at: http://www.phac-aspc.gc.ca/cd-mc/cancer/melanoma_skin_cancer_figures-cancer_peau_melanome_figures-eng.php. Accessed June 26, 2011.[81] *Data from the United States are based on quantifications from* the SEER Program and the SEER Cancer Statistics Review 1975–2008. Available at: http://seer.cancer.gov/csr/1975_2008/index.html.[82])

QUALITY OF LIFE

Traditionally, the impact of skin disease on quality of life has been downplayed because, from a physical perspective, few skin diseases are life threatening or severely debilitating.[18,35] With recent strides in acknowledging the importance of a patient's holistic health, however, QOL has fallen under the richer definition of "physical health, psychological status, level of independence, social relations, beliefs and relationships to the environment."[36] As such, both acute and chronic skin conditions can have a negative impact on QOL in previously unconsidered ways because they may lessen psychological well-being, change behavior such that social functioning and daily activities are impacted, and affect education or employment prospects.[25,37–40]

Although QOL can be influenced by many external factors, such as financial security, marital status, professional career, and the physical and social environment, the impact of overall health on QOL is of prime interest for burden of disease measurements.[41] Extensive literature searches from prior studies have identified 20 health status measures that are derived from US population studies (**Table 3**). These formulations explore QOL in generic, skin-specific, or disease-specific forms. Although many are limited to the adult population, with few able to determine childhood or family impact of the disease,[15] health status instruments are able to interpret, in great detail, the multidimensional health of a patient, including physical, functional, psychological, and social components, as well as the response of each of these variables to medical interventions.[42] Among the most frequently used and most extensively validated generic QOL interpretation instruments are the Short Form 36 Health Survey[43] and the US adaptation of the General Health Questionnaire.[44] Focus, however, is directed toward skin-specific measures of QOL, such as the UK-developed Dermatology Life Quality Index (DLQI). Published in 1994[45] and validated for dermatology patients above age 16, the DLQI incorporates patient factors, such as symptoms and feelings, daily activity, personal relationships, and treatment side effects, into a 10-item questionnaire that is easy to administer. The DLQI has been used in 33 different specific skin conditions and 32 different countries. It is the most frequently used measure in randomized controlled trial investigations in dermatology and has been used in the endpoint measurement of topical and systemic drug efficacy, health service quality, and 14 therapeutic interventions.[46,47] Furthermore, limitations of the DLQI, such as the paucity of emotional aspect consideration,[48,49] may be circumvented by using the measurement in concert with tests that have the desired emotional focus, such as the mental component of the Short Form 36.[41] Skindex, available in 29-item or 16-item administrations, was developed in the United States and represents another modality to capture patient emotions, along with symptoms and functioning while possessing the skin condition.[15,50] Some

---

Table 3
QOL instruments developed from US populations

Generic	Skin Specific	Disease Specific	
Short Form 36 Health Survey[43]	Skindex-61[50]	Psoriasis Life Stress Inventory[51]	Diabetic Foot Ulcer Scale–Short Form[83]
Sickness Impact Profile[84]	Skindex-29[85]		Facial Skin Cancer Index[86]
General Health Questionnaire[87]	Skindex-16[88]	Acne-Specific Quality of Life Questionnaire[52]	Recurrent Genital Herpes Quality of Life Questionnaire[89]
Child Health Questionnaire–Parent Form 50[b,90]	Dermatology-specific Quality of Life instrument[91] HIV-DERMDEX[93]	Quality of Life Index for Atopic Dermatitis[92] Scalpdex[94]	26-Item ITP–Child Quality-of-Life Questionnaire[b,57] Parents' Index of Quality of Life in Atopic Dermatitis[a,95]
		Melasma Quality of Life Scale[96]	26-Item ITP–Parental Burden Quality-of-Life Questionnaire[a,57]

[a] Family focused instruments.
[b] Child-focused instruments.

studies recommend Skindex-29 as the instrument of choice in dermatology because it offers better conceptual validity, retest reliability, and development testing; less item bias; and no issues of floor and ceiling effects in the measurement model compared with the DLQI.[41] Tailored, disease-specific calculations, such as the US population-based Psoriasis Life Stress Inventory[51] and the Acne-Specific Quality of Life Questionnaire,[52] although lacking in applicability across diverse disease populations, have the benefit of increased sensitivity to the particularities and subtleties of the disease they do measure and thus may more fully capture QOL impact.[15,53]

Health status measures developed from Canadian populations have focused on child-specific and family-specific QOL estimations.[15] Having had cross-cultural validations and adaptations, the Childhood Health Assessment Questionnaire has been the most frequently used generic QOL instrument for children and has been primarily used to focus on populations with juvenile idiopathic inflammatory myopathy, juvenile dermatomysitis, and juvenile rheumatoid arthritis.[15,54–56] The Immune Thrombocytopenic Purpura (ITP) Quality-of-Life Questionnaire and the ITP–Parental Burden Quality-of-Life Questionnaire represent skin-disease specific estimations of childhood and family QOL impact, respectively,[15,57] but such methods and others of a similar nature are not in widespread use.

The alternative to the health status models involves individualizing QOL through a consideration of the degree of a patient's desire for particular health outcomes. Although not offering as much detail into QOL, methods of accounting for patient preferences and values allow analysis across multiple diseases and populations, facilitating data comparisons.[42] Furthermore, patient-preference measures permit the incorporation of QOL outcomes into cost-effectiveness analysis. They can also enhance the detection of public issues unique to particular diseases.[58,59] Such detection is of significance in skin disease because chronicity, physical noticeability, and resistance to treatment can often combine to dramatically affect sense of appearance and self-esteem in ways that a physician cannot predict.[40,60,61] Both the willingness-to-pay (WTP) and health utilities models embody the patient-centered approach.

WTP is a measure of perceived value because it offers insight into the maximum amount an individual is willing to pay for a given product or service, which, in dermatology, is a therapy that may improve or resolve the person's skin condition.[62] The model has been applied to a diverse array of skin conditions in US and UK studies.[62–67]

Due to persistent symptomatology and psychosocial impacts, it is perhaps not surprising that monthly WTP values for acne ($169) and psoriasis ($158–$259) surpass those of asymptomatic yet serious health conditions, such as hypertension ($102–$158) and high cholesterol ($69), and even fall within the range of other activity-limiting yet more fatal conditions, such as angina ($108–$191).[62] Such monetary portrayals of a patient's longing for disease-free life can be used in intangible cost estimations of burden of disease,[1] as shown in **Table 4**. Although the selected endpoint for these estimations was symptom relief, the health end target may be varied and thus insight may be gained into which medical interventions may offer patients the most satisfaction. For example, WTP investigations in US psoriasis populations have found that patients value physical comfort and social comfort above the ability to sleep or concentrate.[64]

The health utilities model is another well-established measure of QOL that quantifies a patient's desire to achieve a certain health outcome. The utility score that is given ranges from 0 to 1, with a value close to 1 indicating that living with the condition is almost identical to being in perfect health and a value close to 0 indicating that the detriments the condition brings to the individual are similar to physical death.[42,68] Studies using the utilities model have found that individuals are willing to give up more life years to be rid of condyloma or mycosis fungoides than potentially fatal diagnoses, such as HIV and breast cancer.[42] Skin conditions associated with the lowest utilities are listed in **Table 2** along with collective estimations of the highest WTP values when considering all individuals affected by a condition and an endpoint of symptom relief.

COSTS OF SKIN DISEASE

The final component of the WHO burden of disease measurement framework is financial cost. The cost of a disease is a concept that is broad in scope and it may be considered as the direct costs of treating the disease in either the hospital or the home, the indirect costs to the individual and to society resulting from disability and employment limitations, and the intangible costs of psychological and emotional unease. Such contributions to overall cost are difficult to quantify, and even seemingly objective measures, such as costs of treatment, may be complicated by the lack of firm establishment as to what interventions fall into the category. Conditions affecting solely the skin, those of skin origin but affecting other organ systems or vice versa, and skin

Table 4
Costs associated with the most common skin conditions in the United States, 2004

Disease	Herpes Simplex and Herpes Zoster	Solar Radiation Damage	Seborrheic Keratosis	Contact Dermatitis	Hair and Nail Disorders	Human Papilloma Virus/Warts	Acne (Cystic and Vulgaris)	Actinic Keratosis	Benign Neoplasms/Keloid	Atopic Dermatitis
Hospital inpatient, millions	106	0.8	0.4	8	10	4	0.1	0.8	114	6
Hospital outpatient, millions	29	7	510	93	23	52	30	27	120	108
Hospital emergency department, millions	41	7	N/A	120	23	7	3	N/A	2	105
Office visits, millions	174	55	575	657	412	671	398	766	1156	636
Prescription drugs, millions	1354	27	6	747	231	205	1740	73	11	154

Number of prescriptions, thousands	6064	325	1207	12,514	2069	3367	10,407	1950	183	18,857
Direct cost, millions	1704	434	1092	1625	783	939	2500	867	1402	1009
Lost workdays, millions	99.5	12.7	70.7	294.6	86.1	146.9	307.7	95.7	135.2	182.6
Restricted activity days, millions	61.3	9.9	24.4	172.3	61.2	46.8	153.9	48.9	66.5	188.1
Caregiver lost workdays, millions	26.7	10.0	17.7	98.9	28.1	20.7	157.0	27.7	72.1	248.5
Indirect cost, millions	261	33	113	566	175	214	619	172	281	619
Intangible cost, millions	1400	990	6700	1900	17000	2500	12000	2400	1600	2600

Results are comparable to the Lewin Group's *The Burden of Skin Diseases 2005.* Quantification of disease-specific prescriptions relied on the Lewin Group study.
Data from Bickers DR, Lim HW, Margolis D, et al. The burden of skin diseases: 2004 a joint project of the American Academy of Dermatology Association and the Society for Investigative Dermatology. J Am Acad Dermatol 2006;55(3):490–500.

conditions that emerge through the process of a medical intervention can all have an impact on cost estimation by their inclusion or exclusion from calculations. Even in evaluations of similar data sets, certain degrees of investigator subjectivity come into play when determining the treatment costs and disabilities attributable to a specific skin condition as opposed to a comorbidity.[1,7]

Direct and Indirect Costs

Not surprisingly, studies of the cost of skin disease have been inconsistent in the limitations applied to the calculations, complicating attempts to interpret trends or reproducibility across data sets. Recent literature reviews have uncovered 46 studies attempting to estimate some element of US skin disease cost. Of these, only 5 provided an estimation of national cost for all major skin disease, whereas the others looked at specific disease expenditures.[15] In both approaches, however, computational strategies and sources differed, resulting in variations among the calculated values. For example, of the 2 studies published in 1997 attempting to estimate national skin disease cost, Cohen and Krauss[69] determined total direct cost of skin disease at $8.7 billion whereas Dehkharghani and colleagues[70] obtained a total direct cost value of $34.3 billion. Furthermore, many calculations underestimate holistic cost of skin disease, because few studies showed adequate consideration of societal impact and cost of disease outside of the medical system. The 2005 Lewin Group study[7] currently provides a recent and comprehensive estimate of total national skin disease costs in the United States at $37.2 billion ($27 billion in direct costs and $10.2 billion in indirect costs). The direct cost category can be broken down into its constituents of inpatient care ($8.4 billion), ambulatory care ($9.5 billion), and prescription and over-the-counter (OTC) products ($8.7 billion). Indirect costs, which are a reflection of functional limitations and productivity loses, can be more specifically separated into lost future earnings due to premature death ($6.1 billion), number of lost workdays of both the individual and any caregiver ($2.9 billion), and days of restricted activity ($1.2 billion). **Table 4** associates the 10 most common skin diseases in the United States based on 2004 data with these categorical cost quantifications. Skin ulcers and wounds, with an estimated annual prevalence of 4.8 million,[1] do not rank among the 10 most common skin conditions and thus are not listed in **Table 4**. As indicated

in **Table 2**, however, they are associated with the highest direct and second-highest indirect costs of all skin conditions that were investigated.

Although direct cost estimates by Dehkharghani and colleagues and the Lewin Group are similar, different assumptions and methodologies were applied. Dehkharghani and colleagues, although accounting for a greater array of skin diseases in their study, used generalizations in their calculations of inpatient and ambulatory costs. On determining an average daily monetary cost for inpatient admissions and the total national ambulatory care costs, respectively, they multiplied these values by the fraction of patient cases that were attributable to skin conditions, assuming that procedural costs (medical, surgical, and laboratory) would be the same for all types of skin disease. Furthermore, the OTC cost estimations by Dehkarghani and colleagues were more inclusive,[70] and many products (eg, antiperspirants, feminine hygiene, first aid, baby care) cannot be reliably attributed to specific skin conditions as opposed to other medical issues or daily use. The Lewin Group study chose to be selective in the number of skin conditions they considered, choosing 21 based on disease contribution to health and economic burden as determined by literature searches. For each disease under consideration, national data sets (health care use, procedural and facility costs, and so forth) were gathered individually and later combined to give an overall impression of skin disease burden. Furthermore, the Lewin Group expanded indirect cost interpretations by considering, in addition to decreased productivity, the lost future earning potential resulting from premature death.[7]

Cost estimations of the burden of skin disease in Canada are scarce. Various studies have offered direct cost interpretations of specific disease burdens, including systemic sclerosis,[71] atopic dermatitis,[20] and genital warts,[22] whereas others have offered extensive insight into costs from QOL impingements from conditions such as psoriasis.[72–74] In all, further investigations into direct, indirect, and intangible skin disease costs are needed to better understand the impact on individuals and on society.

Workplace Skin Disease and Contribution to National Burden

Approximately $1 billion of the burden of skin disease cost is estimated to be due to workplace skin disease, which accounts for 15% to 20% of all US occupational disease reports. With an incidence of 3.4 per 10,000 full-time workers in

2009,[75] workplace skin disease has diverse manifestations, including contact dermatitis, immune-mediated responses, and direct skin damage through corrosion. Furthermore, toxicity from systemic absorption of cutaneous toxins may have chronic impacts on worker health and functional capacity, indirectly increasing the burden associated with skin disease.[76–78] Although many chemicals that sensitize or harm the skin are known, the National Institute for Occupational Safety and Health states that precautionary measures for skin contact are often overshadowed by desires to protect the inhalational route of entry.[76] Yet, occupational skin disease is among the most frequently reported exposures, occurring almost twice as often as respiratory conditions.[75] Contact dermatitis represents 70% to 90% of such manifestations and is significant because it ranks as the fourth most common skin condition, with 72.3 million people affected in the United States and $2.2 billion expenditures in direct and indirect costs in 2004 (**Table 4**). Improved contact avoidance may be achieved through better safety labelling and inspection in the workplace. Legislation in Canada, such as the Canadian Workplace Hazardous Materials Information System, requires employers to familiarize their workers with any toxicities relating to workplace chemicals as well as techniques for safely working with such substances.[79] Similar occupational requirements, supplemented with other precautions, such as chemical protective clothing,[80] may represent strategies to mitigate skin disease burden in future years.

General Skin-Care Products and Intangible Costs

Other studies have reported greater annual cost estimations for skin disease burden. For example, OTC products that are not disease specific, such as lip remedies, foot preparations, and multipurpose skin cream, can elevate medication costs for an individual attempting to treat a skin condition. Annual expenditures in the United States on such products are $330.9 million, $383.1 million, and $101.1 million, respectively, and are among the highest of all OTC skin product sales.[7] By factoring in a monetary equivalent of QOL impact (intangible cost of emotional and psychological detriments) using measures, such as the WTP for symptom relief model, the total annual economic burden of skin disease rises to $96 billion.[1] Such an approach is significant for diseases, such as hair and nail disorders, which, despite their little contribution to direct medical costs, have the highest emotional and psychological effects on QOL.[1]

List of Acronyms	
DLQI	Dermatology Life Quality Index
Hanes	US Health and Nutrition Examination Survey
ICD	International Classification of Diseases
NMSC	Non-melanoma skin cancer
QOL	Quality of life
SEER	Surveillance, Epidemiology, and End Results
WHO	World Health Organization
WTP	Willingness-to-pay

SUMMARY

The literature was surveyed in an attempt to quantify the skin disease burden at both a disease-specific and national level in the United States and Canada. The extensive research on the impacts of skin disease in the United States has enabled estimations of national disease burden with thorough assessments of the contributing factors. With an estimated $96 billion burden in direct, indirect, and intangible costs in the United States,[1] skin disease has an impact on millions of individuals and causes a significant toll on health care resources, individual physical and psychosocial health, and societal productivity. Although no estimates have yet been made on the national burden of skin disease in Canada, investigations continue as knowledge of the holistic effects of skin disease is broadened and, more importantly, interventions are established to enhance patient and societal well-being.

REFERENCES

1. Bickers DR, Lim HW, Margolis D, et al. The burden of skin diseases: 2004 a joint project of the American Academy of Dermatology Association and the Society for Investigative Dermatology. J Am Acad Dermatol 2006;55(3):490–500.
2. Canadian Cancer Statistics 2011. Available at: http://www.cancer.ca/~/media/CCS/Canada%20wide/Files%20List/English%20files%20heading/PDF%20-%20Policy%20-%20Canadian%20Cancer%20Statistics%20-%20English/Canadian%20Cancer%20Statistics%202011%20-%20English.ashx. Accessed June 26, 2011.
3. Statistics Canada. Available at: http://www.statcan.gc.ca. Accessed June 26, 2011.
4. Stern RS. Dermatologists and office-based care of dermatologic disease in the 21st century. J Investig Dermatol Symp Proc 2004;9(2):126–30.

5. Thorpe KE, Florence CS, Joski P. Which medical conditions account for the rise in health spending? Health Aff (Millwood) 2004;22. W4-437–45.

6. Lopez AD, Murray CC. The global burden of disease, 1990-2020. Nat Med 1998;4(11):1241–3.

7. The Lewin Group, Inc. The burden of skin diseases 2005. The Society for Investigative Dermatology and The American Academy of Dermatology Association. Available at: http://www.lewin.com/content/publications/april2005skindisease.pdf. Accessed June 21, 2011.

8. Schofield J, Grindlay D, Williams H. Skin conditions in the UK: a Health Care Needs Assessment. Watford (UK): Centre of Evidence Based Dermatology, University of Nottingham; 2009.

9. Leider M, Rosenblum M. A dictionary of dermatological words, terms and phrases. New York: Blakiston; 1968. p. 440.

10. Papier A, Chalmers RJ, Byrnes JA, et al. Framework for improved communication: the Dermatology Lexicon Project. J Am Acad Dermatol 2004;50(4):630–4.

11. Ackerman AB. Need for a complete dictionary of dermatology early in the 21st century. Arch Dermatol 2000;136:23.

12. Practice of dermatology. American Academy of Dermatology. Available at: http://www.aad.org/. Accessed June 29, 2011.

13. Cutaneous science. National Institute of Arthritis and Nusculoskeletal and Skin Diseases. Available at: http://www.niams.nih.gov/. Accessed June 29, 2011.

14. Skin Cochrane Reviews. The Cochrane Collaboration. Available at: www.skin.cochrane.org. Accessed June 29, 2011.

15. VanBeek M, Beach S, Braslow L, et al. Highlights from the report of the working group on "Core measures of the burden of skin diseases". J Invest Dermatol 2007;127(12):2701–6.

16. Who ICD Revision Project and ICD-11. Available at: http://web.ilds.org/cms/index.php?page=Introduction. Accessed June 21, 2011.

17. Johnson MT, Roberts J. Skin conditions and related need for medical care among persons 1-74 years. United States, 1971-1974. Vital Health Stat 11 1978;(212):i–v, 1–72.

18. Johnson MT. Defining the burden of skin disease in the United States—a historical perspective. J Investig Dermatol Symp Proc 2004;9(2):108–10.

19. Papp K, Valenzuela F, Poulin Y, et al. Epidemiology of moderate-to-severe plaque psoriasis in a Canadian surveyed population. J Cutan Med Surg 2010; 14(4):167–74.

20. Barbeau M, Bpharm HL. Burden of atopic dermatitis in Canada. Int J Dermatol 2006;45(1):31–6.

21. Kliewer EV, Demers AA, Elliott L, et al. Twenty-year trends in the incidence and prevalence of diagnosed anogenital warts in Canada. Sex Transm Dis 2009;36(6):380–6.

22. Marra F, Ogilvie G, Colley L, et al. Epidemiology and costs associated with genital warts in Canada. Sex Transm Infect 2009;85(2):111–5.

23. Pope E. Epidermolysis bullosa care in Canada. Dermatol Clin 2010;28(2):391–2, xiii.

24. Smith JA. The impact of skin disease on the quality of life of adolescents. Adolesc Med 2001;12(2):vii, 343–53.

25. Barankin B, DeKoven J. Psychosocial effect of common skin diseases. Can Fam Physician 2002; 48:712–6.

26. The Skin Cancer Foundation. Skin Cancer Facts. Available at: http://www.skincancer.org/Skin-Cancer-Facts/. Accessed June 26, 2011.

27. Cancer Facts & Figures 2011. Available at: http://www.cancer.org/acs/groups/content/@epidemiologysurveilance/documents/document/acspc-029771.pdf. Accessed June 26, 2011.

28. Edwards BK, Ward E, Kohler BA, et al. Annual report to the nation on the status of cancer, 1975-2006, featuring colorectal cancer trends and impact of interventions (risk factors, screening, and treatment) to reduce future rates. Cancer 2010;116(3):544–73.

29. Cancer Trends Progress Report - 2009/2010 Update. Available at: http://progressreport.cancer.gov/doc_detail.asp?pid=1&did=2009&chid=93&coid=920&mid=#trends. Accessed June 26, 2011.

30. Rogers HW, Weinstock MA, Harris AR, et al. Incidence estimate of nonmelanoma skin cancer in the United States, 2006. Arch Dermatol 2010;146(3):283–7.

31. Donaldson MR, Coldiron BM. No end in sight: the skin cancer epidemic continues. Semin Cutan Med Surg 2011;30(1):3–5.

32. Government of Canada SC. CANSIM—Results. Available at: http://www5.statcan.gc.ca/cansim/a16?id=1020532&lang=eng&pattern=&stByVal=3&requestID=2011070323523337105&MBR%5B%27AGE%27%5D=1&MBR%5B%27GEO%27%5D=1&MBR%5B%27SEX%27%5D=1&MBR%5B%27CAUSEOFDEATH%27%5D=4616&retrLang=eng&syear=2000&eyear=2007&exporterId=TABLE_HTML_TIME_AS_COLUMN&__checkbox_accessible=true&action%3Aa23=Retrieve+now. Accessed July 4, 2011.

33. Skin cancer prevention. SunSmart Saskatchewan. Available at: http://www.saskcancer.ca/Background%20Document. Accessed June 26, 2011.

34. Public Health Agency of Canada. Cancer surveillance on-line. Available at: http://dsol-smed.phac-aspc.gc.ca/dsol-smed/cancer/index_e.html. Accessed June 26, 2011.

35. Murray CJ, Lopez AD. Global mortality, disability, and the contribution of risk factors: global burden of disease study. Lancet 1997;349(9063):1436–42.

36. Halioua B, Beumont MG, Lunel F. Quality of life in dermatology. Int J Dermatol 2000;39:801–6.

37. Golics C, Basra M, Finlay A, et al. Adolescents with skin disease have specific quality of life issues. Dermatology 2009;218(4):357–66.

38. Qureshi AA, Freedberg I, Goldsmith L, et al. Report on "Burden of Skin Disease" Workshop NIAMS, September 2002. J Investig Dermatol Symp Proc 2004;9(2):111–9.

39. Evers AW, Lu Y, Duller P, et al. Common burden of chronic skin diseases? Contributors to psychological distress in adults with psoriasis and atopic dermatitis. Br J Dermatol 2005;152(6):1275–81.

40. Hong J, Koo B, Koo J. The psychosocial and occupational impact of chronic skin disease. Dermatol Ther 2008;21(1):54–9.

41. Both H, Essink-Bot M, Busschbach J, et al. Critical review of generic and dermatology-specific health-related quality of life instruments. J Invest Dermatol 2007;127(12):2726–39.

42. Chen SC, Bayoumi AM, Soon SL, et al. A catalog of dermatology utilities: a measure of the burden of skin diseases. J Investig Dermatol Symp Proc 2004;9(2):160–8.

43. Ware JE Jr, Sherbourne CD. The MOS 36-item short-form health survey (SF-36). I. Conceptual framework and item selection. Med Care 1992;30(6):473–83.

44. Goldberg DP. The detection of psychiatric illness by questionnaire: a technique for the identification and assessment of non-psychotic psychiatric illness. Oxford (England): Oxford U. Press; 1972. p. xii, 156.

45. Finlay A, Khan G. Dermatology Life Quality Index (DLQI)—a simple practical measure for routine clinical use. Clin Exp Dermatol 1994;19(3):210–6.

46. Basra M, Fenech R, Gatt R, et al. The Dermatology Life Quality Index 1994-2007: a comprehensive review of validation data and clinical results. Br J Dermatol 2008. Available at: http://onlinelibrary.wiley.com.proxy.lib.sfu.ca/doi/10.1111/j.1365-2133.2008.08832.x/full. Accessed June 29, 2011.

47. Lewis V, Finlay AY. 10 Years experience of the Dermatology Life Quality Index (DLQI). J Investig Dermatol Symp Proc 2004;9(2):169–80.

48. Badia X, Mascaro JM, Lozano R. Measuring health-related quality of life in patients with mild to moderate eczema and psoriasis: clinical validity, reliability and sensitivity to change of the DLQI. The Cavide Research Group. Br J Dermatol 1999;141:698–702.

49. de Korte J, Mombers FM, Sprangers MA, et al. The suitability of quality-of-life questionnaires for psoriasis research: a systematic literature review. Arch Dermatol 2002;138:1221–7.

50. Chren M, Lasek RJ, Quinn LM, et al. Skindex, a quality-of-life measure for patients with skin disease: reliability, validity, and responsiveness. J Invest Dermatol 1996;107(5):707–13.

51. Gupta MA, Gupta AK. The Psoriasis Life Stress Inventory: a preliminary index of psoriasis-related stress. Acta Derm Venereol 1995;75(3):240–3.

52. Martin AR, Lookingbill DP, Botek A, et al. Health-related quality of life among patients with facial acne - assessment of a new acne-specific questionnaire. Clin Exp Dermatol 2001;26(5):380–5.

53. Wiebe S, Guyatt G, Weaver B, et al. Comparative responsiveness of generic and specific quality-of-life instruments. J Clin Epidemiol 2003;56(1):52–60.

54. Brunner HI, Klein-Gitelman MS, Miller MJ, et al. Minimal clinically important differences of the child-hood health assessment questionnaire. J Rheumatol 2005;32(1):150–61.

55. Lam C, Young N, Marwaha J, et al. Revised versions of the Childhood Health Assessment Questionnaire (CHAQ) are more sensitive and suffer less from a ceiling effect. Arthritis Rheum 2004;51(6):881–9.

56. Huber AM, Hicks JE, Lachenbruch PA, et al. Validation of the Childhood Health Assessment Questionnaire in the juvenile idiopathic myopathies. Juvenile Dermatomyositis Disease Activity Collaborative Study Group. J Rheumatol 2001;28(5):1106–11.

57. Barnard D, Woloski M, Feeny D, et al. Development of disease-specific health-related quality-of-life instruments for children with immune thrombocyto-penic purpura and their parents. J Pediatr Hematol Oncol 2003;25(1):56–62.

58. Gold MR, Siegel RG, Weinstein MC, editors. Cost-Effectiveness in health and medicine. New York: Oxford University Press; 1996.

59. Drummond M, O'Brien B, Stoddart GL, et al. Methods for the economic evaluation of health care pro-grammes. Toronto: Oxford Medical Publishers; 1998.

60. Tan JKL. Psychosocial impact of acne vulgaris: evaluating the evidence. Skin Therapy Lett 2004;9(7):1–3, 9.

61. Chren M, Weinstock MA. Conceptual issues in measuring the burden of skin diseases. J Investig Dermatol Symp Proc 2004;9(2):97–100.

62. Parks L, Balkrishnan R, Hamel–Gariépy L. the importance of skin disease as assessed by "willingness-to-pay". J Cutan Med Surg 2003;7(5):369–71.

63. Lundberg L, Johannesson M, Silverdahl M, et al. Quality of life, health-state utilities and willingness to pay in patients with psoriasis and atopic eczema. Br J Dermatol 1999;141:1067–75.

64. Delfino M Jr, Holt EW, Taylor CR, et al. Willingness-to-pay stated preferences for 8 health-related quality-of-life domains in psoriasis: a pilot study. J Am Acad Dermatol 2008;59(3):439–47.

65. Radtke M, Schäfer I, Gajur A, et al. Willingness-to-pay and quality of life in patients with vitiligo. Br J Dermatol 2009;161(1):134–9.

66. Cham PM, Chen SC, Grill JP, et al. Reliability of self-reported willingness-to-pay and annual income in patients treated for toenail onychomycosis. Br J Dermatol 2007;156:922–8.

67. Schmitt J, Meurer M, Klon M, et al. Assessment of health state utilities of controlled and uncontrolled

psoriasis and atopic eczema: a population-based study. Br J Dermatol 2008;158:351–9.

68. Coons SJ, Rao S, Keininger DL, et al. A comparative review of generic quality-of-life instruments. Pharmacoeconomics 2000;17:13–35.

69. Cohen JW, Krauss NA. Spending and service use among people with the fifteen most costly medical conditions, 1997. Health Aff (Millwood) 2003;22(2): 129–38.

70. Dehkharghani S, Bible J, Chen JG, et al. The economic burden of skin disease in the United States. J Am Acad Dermatol 2003;48(4):592–9.

71. Bernatsky S, Hudson M, Panopalis P, et al. The cost of systemic sclerosis. Arthritis Rheum 2009;61(1): 119–23.

72. Wasel N, Poulin Y, Andrew R, et al. A Canadian self-administered online survey to evaluate the impact of moderate-to-severe psoriasis among patients. J Cutan Med Surg 2009;13(6): 294–302.

73. Mahler R, Jackson C, Ijacu H. The burden of psoriasis and barriers to satisfactory care: results from a Canadian patient survey. J Cutan Med Surg 2009;13(6):283–93.

74. Lynde CW, Poulin Y, Guenther L, et al. The burden of psoriasis in Canada: insights from the pSoriasis Knowledge IN Canada (SKIN) survey. J Cutan Med Surg 2009;13(5):235–52.

75. Workplace injury and illness summary. Available at: http://www.bls.gov/news.release/osh.nr0.htm. Accessed June 27, 2011.

76. Occupational skin exposures and diseases take toll on the workplace. 2010. Available at: http://www.infectioncontroltoday.com/topics/national-institute-for-occupational-safety-and-health-niosh.aspx. Accessed June 27, 2011.

77. Lushniak BD. Occupational contact dermatitis. Dermatol Ther 2004;17(3):272–7.

78. Lushniak BD. The importance of occupational skin diseases in the United States. Int Arch Occup Environ Health 2003;76(5):325–30.

79. Health and Safety Report. 2010. Available at: http://www.ccohs.ca/newsletters/hsreport/issues/2010/10/ezine.html?id=29032&link=1#ontopic. Accessed June 27, 2011.

80. Schalock PC, Zug KA. Protection from occupational allergens. Curr Probl Dermatol 2007;34:58–75.

81. Government of Canada PHAOC. Melanoma Skin Cancer Facts and Figures—Public Health Agency Canada. Available at: http://www.phac-aspc.gc.ca/cd-mc/cancer/melanoma_skin_cancer_figures-cancer_peau_melanome_figures-eng.php. Accessed June 26, 2011.

82. SEER Cancer Statistics Review 1975-2008. Available at: http://seer.cancer.gov/csr/1975_2008/index.html. Accessed June 21, 2011.

83. Bann CM, Fehnel SE, Gagnon DD. Development and validation of the Diabetic Foot Ulcer Scale-short form (DFS-SF). Pharmacoeconomics 2003; 21(17):1277–90.

84. Bergner M, Bobbitt RA, Carter WB, et al. The Sickness Impact Profile: development and final revision of a health status measure. Med Care 1981;19(8): 787–805.

85. Chren M, Lasek RJ, Flocke SA, et al. Improved discriminative and evaluative capability of a refined version of skindex, a quality-of-life instrument for patients with skin diseases. Arch Dermatol 1997; 133(11):1433–40.

86. Rhee JS, Matthews BA, Neuburg M, et al. Creation of a quality of life instrument for nonmelanoma skin cancer patients. Laryngoscope 2005;115(7):1178–85.

87. Goldberg D. The detection of psychiatric illness by questionnaire a technique for the identification and assessment of non-psychotic psychiatric illness. London; New York: Oxford University Press; 1972.

88. Chren M, Lasek RJ, Sahay AP, et al. Measurement properties of skindex-16: A brief quality-of-life measure for patients with skin diseases. J Cutan Med Surg 2001;5(2):105–10.

89. Doward LC, McKenna SP, Kohlmann T, et al. The international development of the RGHQoL: a quality of life measure for recurrent genital herpes. Qual Life Res 1998;7(2):143–53.

90. Landgraf JM, Abetz L, Ware JE Jr. Child health questionnaire (CHQ): a user's manual. 1st edition. Boston: The Health Institute, New England Medical Center; 1996.

91. Anderson RT, Rajagopalan R. Development and validation of a quality of life instrument for cutaneous diseases. J Am Acad Dermatol 1997;37(1):41–50.

92. Whalley D, McKenna SP, Dewar AL, et al. A new instrument for assessing quality of life in atopic dermatitis: international development of the Quality of Life Index for Atopic Dermatitis (QoLIAD). Br J Dermatol 2004;150(2):274–83.

93. Aftergut K, Carmody T, Cruz PD. Use of the HIV-DERMDEX quality-of-life instrument in HIV-infected patients with skin disease. Int J Dermatol 2001; 40(7):478–81.

94. Chen SC, Yeung J, Chren M. Scalpdex: a quality-of-life instrument for scalp dermatitis. Arch Dermatol 2002;138(6):803–7.

95. McKenna SP, Whalley D, Dewar AL, et al. International development of the Parents' Index of Quality of Life in Atopic Dermatitis (PIQoL-AD). Qual Life Res 2005;14(1):231–41.

96. Balkrishnan R, McMichael AJ, Camacho FT, et al. Development and validation of a health-related quality of life instrument for women with melasma. Br J Dermatol 2003;149(3):572–7.

Services Available and Their Effectiveness

Christine Ahn, BA[a], Scott A. Davis, MA[a],*,
Tushar S. Dabade, MD[a], Alan B. Fleischer Jr, MD[a],
Steven R. Feldman, MD, PhD[a,b,c]

KEYWORDS

- Dermatology • Skin care • Self-care • Generalist care
- Specialist care • Subspecialist care

The impact of skin disease in the United States is significant and growing. In 2004, skin diseases were 1 of the top 15 groups of medical conditions that experienced the greatest increase in both prevalence and health care spending from 1987 to 2000. Approximately 1 of 3 people in the United States have 1 or more of the 3000 identified skin diseases at any given time. In a joint project by the American Academy of Dermatology (AAD) and the Society for Investigative Dermatology,

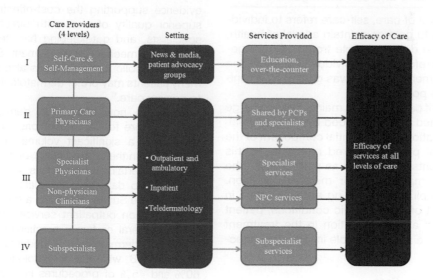

Funding/Conflicts of Interest: The Center for Dermatology Research is supported by an educational grant from Galderma Laboratories, L.P. Dr Feldman has received research, speaking and/or consulting support from Galderma, Abbott Labs, Warner Chilcott, Leo, Amgen, Astellas, Centocor, National Biologic Corporation, and Stiefel/GSK. Dr Fleischer has received research, speaking and/or consulting support from Astellas, Centocor, Amgen, Abbott, Galderma, Stiefel, Medicis, and Intendis. Dr Dabade, Mr Davis and Ms Ahn have no conflicts to disclose.

[a] Department of Dermatology, Center for Dermatology Research, Wake Forest School of Medicine, Medical Center Boulevard, Winston-Salem, NC 27157-1071, USA
[b] Department of Pathology, Center for Dermatology Research, Wake Forest School of Medicine, Medical Center Boulevard, Winston-Salem, NC 27157-1071, USA
[c] Department of Public Health Sciences, Center for Dermatology Research, Wake Forest School of Medicine, Medical Center Boulevard, Winston-Salem, NC 27157-1071, USA
* Corresponding author.
E-mail address: scdavis@wakehealth.edu

the total economic burden of skin disease in 2004 was estimated at $96 billion, taking into account the annual cost of skin disease of $39.3 billion (direct medical costs and lost productivity costs) and the additional economic burden of skin disease on quality of life estimated at $56.2 billion.[1]

This article describes the range of services available for patients with skin disease in the United States. Within the structure of health care systems, 4 levels of care are characterized and discussed: self-care and management, generalist care, specialist care, and subspecialist care. Within each level, this article discusses the profiles of individuals involved in delivering medical care, the location or setting in which these services are provided, the capacity and specific activities of care providers, and current literature on the efficacy of these different levels of care.

FOUR LEVELS OF HEALTH CARE PROVIDERS
Level 1: Self-care and Self-management

In the first level of care, self-care refers to individuals' actions to gain or maintain a level of health, which may be distinguishable from self-management, which refers to an individual's modification of a management plan that was guided by a clinician at some point.

This level of care is guided mainly by knowledge that is obtained and understood by the individual. Patient education is an essential component of the framework of patient-centered medicine. In this setting, patients are enlisted as partners with the physician in managing their medical condition. With noncompliance becoming a central issue in the treatment of dermatologic conditions, patient knowledge of and participation in the treatment of their disease play a vital role in providing effective care.

Level 2: Primary Care

Primary care refers to care provided by physicians who have received postgraduate training in pediatrics, family or general practice, and internal medicine. Primary care physicians (PCPs) are trained to have fundamental knowledge of common diseases of all organ systems, thus they serve the role to make basic diagnoses and provide nonsurgical treatment of common medical conditions. They often provide the first contact for an undiagnosed health concern, as well as continuing care for most patients.

PCPs provide substantial medical care to patients with dermatologic conditions. From 1990 to 1994, 5% of all outpatient visits to internists and 7% of all visits to family physicians

were for dermatologic diseases.[2] In 1998, nondermatologists were estimated to provide care for 56% of visits for common skin complaints, whereas dermatologists managed approximately 40% of outpatient visits for dermatologic problems.[3] Under managed care, which was the dominant mechanism of payment for the treatment of skin disease for many patient groups in the 1990s, primary care providers acted as the gatekeepers, serving as the first point of access to health care for the primary purpose of reducing health care cost and resource use. In 1996, Ramsay and Weary[4] suggested that public opinion still favored the idea of the Marcus Welby physician, a primary care provider capable of providing quality care in all aspects of medicine. However, treatment of skin conditions by dermatologists has been shown to be more cost-effective, because of the superior diagnostic skills of dermatologists in managing skin diseases and the ability of dermatologists to treat skin problems using less physician time.[5] Studies have provided consistent evidence supporting the cost-effectiveness and superior quality of care with direct access to specialists, and gatekeeping has ceased to be the primary mechanism of payment. Studies suggest that public perception has also shifted, and many patients may prefer dermatologic specialists to primary care.[6]

PCPs are now second to dermatologists in providing care for skin conditions. They continue to perform a significant volume of skin-related procedures in the United States, and almost exclusively treat certain skin conditions, such as impetigo. According to data from the National Ambulatory Medical Care Survey (NAMCS), a survey collecting information on outpatient services in the United States, general or family practitioners performed 12% of all dermatologic procedures in 2007 and 11% in 2008, whereas dermatologists performed 60% and 45% of procedures in 2007 and 2008, respectively.

Level 3: Specialists

Specialist care for skin disease is provided by the dermatology workforce in the United States, which includes dermatologists (physicians who have undergone at least 4 years of postgraduate training in the treatment of skin disease) as well as other health care practitioners supervised by dermatologists: nurse practitioners (NPs), physician assistants (PAs), and clinical triage assistants (CTAs). A smaller volume of dermatologic procedures are performed by plastic surgeons, who are specialists with some training in cutaneous surgery.

A shortage of physicians in the US dermatology workforce has been documented since 1999, because of a combination of increased demand for services, limited training positions for new physicians, and changes in the demographics and distribution of physicians. In more recent years, with an aging population and increasing prevalence of certain skin diseases such as melanoma and nonmelanoma skin cancer, and with greater access to specialists, the demand for dermatologic services has been increasing. Because of limited training positions for dermatologists in the United States, there has been limited increase of dermatologists compared with other specialties such as internal medicine and neurology (**Fig. 1**), and the overall size of the dermatology workforce continues to be smaller than other specialties such as orthopedic surgery, ophthalmology, and neurology (**Fig. 2**). Instead, data indicate a rapid influx of nonphysician clinicians (NPCs) or physician extender clinicians to the dermatology workforce to meet the increasing needs. These NPCs include NPs, physicians' assistants, and CTAs, who work with dermatologists to provide care.[7–10]

NPs are registered nurses, and most obtain master's degrees and sit for national certifying examinations. In many states, they are permitted to practice without physician supervision and are given prescriptive authority. PAs differ from NPs in that they are licensed health practitioners but cannot work autonomously. PAs are considered dependent health practitioners and are required to work with physicians. PA training is in the context of collaborative care, and in contrast to NPs, a PA is primarily trained by physicians, completing a 2-year to 2.5-year program consisting of primary care medical curricula and a year of internships mentored by physicians. Similar to NPs, PAs are required to sit for a general national certifying examination. Although the situation varies from state to state, physicians delegate certain responsibilities to PAs, some of which include prescriptive authority within their practice arrangements.

In 2010, Straka and colleagues[9] described a new member of the dermatology health care team: the CTA. CTAs are also described as phone nurses or call-back nurses, and do not have the certification of NPs or PAs, but have emerged in dermatology clinics to share some of the physicians' workload, increasing efficiency and enhancing the quality of care.

In a practice profile survey of randomly selected members of the AAD, the percentage of respondents who reported the use of PAs, NPs, or both in their dermatology practices increased 43% between 2002 (21%) and 2007 (30%). Thirty-six percent of respondents planned to hire NPCs by 2010. PAs were more prevalent than NPs in 2002, 2005, and 2007, with 23% of respondents

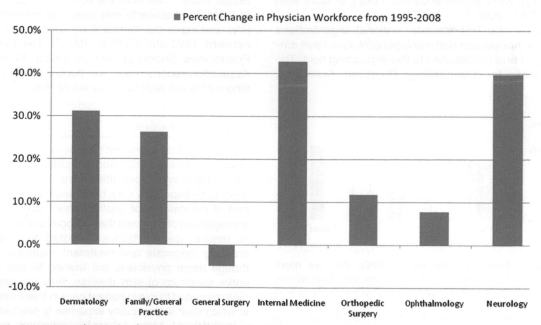

Fig. 1. Percentage change in physician workforce in the United States, NAMCS, 1995 to 2008. Between 1995 and 2008, the greatest percentage changes were in the internal medicine and neurology workforces, followed by dermatology. Orthopedic surgery and ophthalmology had smaller increases in physician workforce, whereas general surgery decreased.

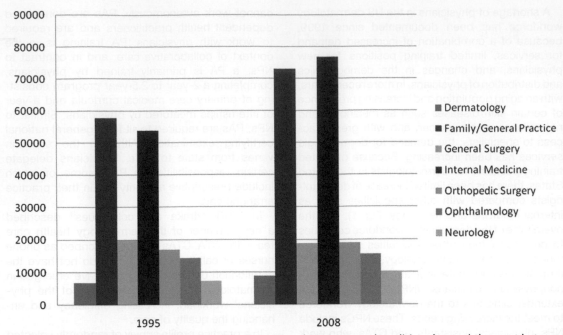

Fig. 2. Size of physician workforce by specialty in 1995 and 2008. Internal medicine changed the most between 1995 and 2008, exceeding the family and general practice physician workforce in 2008. Of the specialties studied, dermatology was the specialty with the smallest physician workforce in 2008.

reporting the use of PAs and 10% using NPs (**Fig. 3**). Younger cohorts of dermatologists and practices that spent 50% or more patient care time performing surgical and cosmetic dermatology were significantly more likely to work with NPCs in 2007.[8]

Over the last decade, national organizations for nonphysician dermatologic clinicians have emerged and contributed to this expanding field. The Society for Dermatology Physician Assistants,

which reported membership of 15 when it was founded in 1994, reported 1200 members in 2006, and estimates that there are more than 2200 dermatology PAs practicing in the United States today. Data from the American Academy of Physician Assistants estimated the number of PAs working in the dermatology specialty to be between 1800 and 2000 in 2007.[11] The Nurse Practitioners' Society of the Dermatology Nurses' Association reports more than 3000 members, of whom 71% are registered nurses or NPs.[12]

Level 4: Subspecialists

Subspecialist dermatologic care comes from physicians who have completed an additional 1 to 2 years of training in specialties within dermatology (**Box 1**). Subspecialty care becomes an important part of the delivery of quality patient care in the management of diseases that are complex enough to require specific training devoted to understanding diagnosis and treatment methods. Although these physicians are trained to see the entire spectrum of skin disease, they are especially recruited to join in patient care in these cases in which their subspecialty expertise is needed.

In 2010, 41 Mohs fellowship programs were approved under the American College of Mohs Surgery (ACMS), and more than 900 members of the ACMS.[13] These 1-year to 2-year fellowships

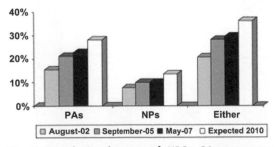

Fig. 3. Trends in the use of NPCs. PAs are more common than NPs as nonphysician members of the dermatology health care team. There was an overall increase in the use of NPCs from 2002 to 2007. (*Reprinted from* Resneck JS Jr, Kimball AB. Who else is providing care in dermatology practices? Trends in the use of nonphysician clinicians. J Am Acad Dermatol 2008;58:213; with permission from Elsevier. Copyright 2011.)

require trainees to participate in at least 500 Mohs micrographic surgery (MMS) cases under the supervision of an ACMS-approved Mohs surgeon.[14]

WHERE SERVICES ARE PROVIDED
Introduction

This section describes the setting in which skin diseases are seen and treated in the United States. Treatment and care for skin conditions are largely provided in the outpatient setting; however, inpatient dermatologic care makes up a significant component of dermatology, and is primarily provided in a consultative setting. A persistent undersupply of dermatologists, especially in specific geographic locations, has led to the emergence of other settings for the delivery of care, such as teledermatology. For rural patients with limited access to specialist care, teledermatology is used as a method of consultation between primary care providers and specialists.

Outpatient Dermatology

At all levels of care, most dermatologic services are provided in the outpatient setting. Approximately 10% of all outpatient visits are for skin-related conditions. As much as 25% of visits to PCPs are related to a skin-related complaint, with visits for a dermatologic condition as a chief complaint accounting for 6%. In 1999 and 2000, there were 35 million annual visits to dermatologists[3]; however, mean wait times for new patient appointments with dermatologists indicate unmet demands, reported as low as 31.1 days in solo

dermatologic practices to as high as 55.9 days in academic practices.[15]

The provision of this care has been studied using data from the NAMCS and the National Hospital Ambulatory Medical Care Survey (NHAMCS). These surveys are conducted by the National Center for Health Statistics to collect descriptive data based on samples of visits to office-based physician practices (NAMCS) and hospital emergency departments (EDs) and outpatient departments (OPDs).

Inpatient Dermatology

Management of skin diseases is often provided in the outpatient setting; however, certain subsets of skin diseases require hospital inpatient care. Since the adoption of the diagnosis-related group (DRG) system by Medicare in 1983, there have been significant changes in the management of hospitalized patients with skin diseases, and a shift in the dermatologists' role from a primary provider of care to a consultant. In a study by Kirsner and colleagues,[16] data from 2 databases, the Healthcare Cost and Utilization Project-3 Nationwide Inpatient Sample (HCUP-3 NIS) from 1992 to 1994 and the Medicare Provider Analysis and Review (MEDPAR) from 1990 to 1996, were used to identify dermatology-specific and dermatology-related DRGs to estimate the number of patients hospitalized for skin disease annually in the United States. In 1994, 468,014 discharges were classified under dermatology DRGs according to HCUP-3 NIS data, and 183,310 discharges were classified as such according to MEDPAR data. From 1992 to 1994, total discharges under dermatology-specific DRGs decreased, whereas total discharges of dermatology-related DRGs increased.

In 1997, 101 dermatology residency programs in the United States in the AAD were surveyed to determine inpatient dermatologic activity, and to compare this activity with 1982 levels before the introduction of DRGs. The chairpersons of 97 programs were surveyed and 71 responded (response rate 73%). Of the survey respondents, 24 (34%) institutions had dedicated dermatology beds, compared with 41 (58%) in 1982. Whereas most programs still relied on a rotating attending dermatologist as the person responsible for care of hospitalized patients with skin disease, the number of programs that relied on nondermatologist physicians to care for inpatients increased from 11 (15.5%) to 23 (32.4%), suggesting a shift of care. Furthermore, although the skin conditions for which patients were hospitalized did not change significantly, the frequency of hospitalization for these conditions has changed from an average of 119 patients admitted annually for dermatologic conditions in 1982 to 36.5 in 1997. Across all academic dermatology programs, 3687 patients were admitted annually.[17] This finding suggests that most hospital admissions with dermatology-specific or dermatology-related diagnoses have been admitted by physicians other than dermatologists at academic medical centers.

Despite the shift of primary responsibility of inpatient care away from specialists, dermatologists still play an essential role in providing care in the inpatient setting, working in consult with nondermatologist physicians. In a prospective study of dermatologic consultations at a major teaching hospital, the frequency, reasons for, and impact of inpatient dermatologic consultation were recorded for 8 months. During this period, consultations were requested for 591 patients who were either hospitalized or being evaluated in the ED or urgent care settings. In more than 60% of consults, the assessment of cutaneous condition and treatment was changed by dermatologic consultation, and 50% of consults resulted in substantial changes in treatment, requiring switching to or changing a systemic therapeutic agent. The diagnoses that were frequently missed by the referring service were drug eruption, papulosquamous eruptions, and skin infections, which are common conditions with established treatment. The most common outcome of dermatologic consultation was recommendation for topical steroids, systemic antibiotics, or antihistamines.[18]

Teledermatology

Teledermatology is a mode of delivery of dermatologic care using telecommunication technology to transfer medical information, usually in the form of store and forward (SAF) asynchronous still digital image technology (similar to e-mail) or real-time or live interactive (LI) videoconferencing. The substitution of digital images for dermatology physical examination has become a topic of discussion in recent years, because of the increasing popularity of telemedicine in the delivery of care to populations such as rural underserved, prisoners, military, or international patients.[19] The use of telecommunication technology in the treatment of skin conditions is advantageous because the manifestations of diseases are normally outwardly apparent. In addition, with a persistently high demand for the assessment and treatment of skin disorders, especially diseases like skin cancer that are increasing in prevalence and often require the intervention of a specialist, teledermatology

provides a setting where timely consultation among all levels of care providers is possible.

WHAT SERVICES ARE PROVIDED
Introduction

This section describes the range of services and the activities of different providers within different settings of dermatologic care. In self-care and self-management, care is delivered through patient initiative and education, through the use of over-the-counter (OTC) products, and the use of public resources such as support groups and advocacy groups. Physicians and NPCs provide a wide range of services for dermatologic conditions that may overlap but also vary based on the provider and the setting in which they are delivered.

Self-care/Management

Major sources of information for the patient include newspapers, magazines, personal accounts, Internet sources, and patient pamphlets through which national organizations such as the AAD provide information designed for public education.[20] In the AAD's Web-based resource, 60 common skin conditions are described with sections that provide several images and discuss the signs and symptoms, the common populations affected and causes, the diagnosis and treatment, and tips for patients with the condition. Other widely used sources of patient education material on the Internet include disease-specific national organizations such as the National Psoriasis Foundation (NPF), as well as more general Web sites such as http://WebMD.com, http://Wikipedia.org, and http://MedicineOnline.com.

Patient advocacy groups are also an important component of patient education and self-care. These groups provide an arena in which patients' views and needs can be represented and taken into consideration in health policy, patient education, and scientific research[21] The wide range of skin disorders has led to the development of many dermatologic patient groups. These groups range from national organizations for common skin diseases such as psoriasis and eczema to international organizations bringing together individuals and advocacy groups from different countries. The Coalition of Skin Diseases is a combined effort of 16 advocacy organizations in the United States that aims to generate awareness of skin disease, coordinate patient care issues, and, working in concert with the National Institute of Arthritis and Musculoskeletal and Skin Diseases, expand scientific research of skin disease.[22]

Patients provide self-care and management through the use of OTC products. In a report by the National Council on Patient Information and Education, 10% of adults reported using nonprescription, OTC medications to treat skin problems over a 6-month survey period.[23] OTC products are used to treat a wide variety of skin problems, ranging from general skin conditions such as dry or itchy skin, to more specific dermatologic conditions such as dermatitis, eczema, and psoriasis. Common OTC products available to treat such skin conditions include emollients, tars, shampoos, keratolytic products with salicylic acid, and topical corticosteroids, with the 2 most common products being hydrocortisone (HC) and benzoyl peroxide.

Services Provided by Physicians

PCPs, specialists, and subspecialists are involved (often in consultation with each other) in the evaluation, diagnosis, and treatment of dermatologic conditions.

OTC or prescription topical agents are commonly recommended by physicians in the treatment of common skin conditions, such as pruritis, eczema, acne, and psoriasis. Based on NAMCS data on dermatologic treatment in the outpatient setting and NHAMCS data on hospital OPD and ED dermatologic treatment from 1995 to 2007, the most common topical medications prescribed in outpatient visits with primary dermatologic diagnoses were Keflex (2.9%), liquid nitrogen (2.2%), and prednisone (1.6%). The most common topical medications prescribed in visits with primary dermatologic diagnoses in the inpatient setting were Keflex, Benadryl, and prednisone. In both the ED and OPD, Keflex was the most common (8.3%) and (4.0%), respectively, followed by Benadryl and prednisone.

In approximately 353 million visits to office-based US physicians from 1989 to 2008, topical OTC products were recommended, and were associated largely with dermatologists (33.5% of total OTC use), general/family practitioners (19.7%), and pediatricians (18.9%). The most commonly used therapeutics were anti-infectives (19.4%), followed by HC products (16.9%), acne products (14.5%), and moisturizers (12.2%) (**Table 1**). Comparison of dermatologist and nondermatologist use of these products revealed that nondermatologists used HC products nearly twice as often as dermatologists, whereas dermatologists used moisturizers more frequently than nondermatologists (**Table 2**). In an analysis of recommendation patterns of US physicians of OTC topical antipruritics, dermatologists accounted for 41% of

Table 1
Estimated frequency and percentage of topical OTC products recommended by dermatologists by therapeutic category, NAMCS, 1989 to 2008

Therapeutic Category	Frequency of Recommendation (Millions of Visits)	% of Total OTC Use
Anti-infective	31.1	19.6
HC	21.3	16.9
Acne	18.3	14.5
Moisturizer	15.3	12.2
Miscellaneous	15.3	12.1
Cleansers	14.5	10.0
Sunscreen	10.0	7.9
Keratolytic	9.2	7.3
Shampoo	5.1	4.1
Antipruritics	3.7	2.9
Antiseptics	1.6	1.3

Anti-infectives, HC, acne products, and moisturizers were the most frequent topical OTC products recommended by dermatologists, comprising more than half of total OTC use.

recommendations of OTC products, followed by family physicians (26%) and pediatricians (21%). The most common medications recommended were HC (72%) and diphenhydramine (15%), and OTC products were recommended more often for the pediatric age group.[24]

Linear regression analysis revealed that physician-recommended topical OTC use has decreased significantly over time among dermatologists and nondermatologists (P<.0001) Overall, physicians have been recommending HC, anti-infectives, keratolytics, and acne products at a decreasing rate, whereas dermatologists have been recommending moisturizers and sunscreens at an increasing rate.

Physicians also perform a wide range of procedures for dermatologic conditions, with most procedures provided by dermatologists (55%) and general and family physicians (19%), based on NAMCS data on outpatient dermatologic procedures between 1995 and 2008. Of the top 2 dermatologic procedures, dermatologists performed 66% of local excision/destruction and 79% of biopsies, and general and family practitioners performed the second largest proportion (29% of local excisions and destructions and 14% of biopsies). General and family physicians performed a larger proportion of some procedures than dermatologists, including incision with drainage of skin and subcutaneous tissue, closure

Table 2
Most commonly used OTC products and associated percentages of total OTC use by dermatologists and nondermatologists: NAMCS, 1989 to 2008

Rank	Dermatologists		Nondermatologists	
1	Hydrocortisone	(16.9)	Hydrocortisone	(32.6)
2	Benzoyl peroxide	(13.3)	Clotrimazole	(9.3)
3	Sunscreen	(7.4)	Bacitracin, neomycin, and polymyxin B (neosporin)	(7.2)
4	Bacitracin and polymyxin (polysporin)	(7.1)	Bacitracin	(5.4)
5	Salicylic acid	(5.8)	Medication(s) prescribed/provided OTC	(3.4)
6	Bacitracin	(3.9)	Benzoyl peroxide	(3.1)
7	Sulfacetamide	(3.4)	Povidone/Iodine	(3.0)
8	Cetaphil	(3.2)	Bacitracin and polymyxin (Polysporin)	(2.3)
9	Hydroquinone	(2.9)	Salicylic acid	(2.2)
10	Tar	(2.8)	Miconazole	(2.1)
11	Emollient/lotion/cream/moisturizer	(2.2)	Permethrin	(2.1)
12	Minoxidil	(1.8)	Eucerin	(1.8)
13	Aquaphor	(1.6)	Phenol	(1.7)
14	Selenium sulfide	(1.4)	Selenium sulfide	(1.6)

Hydrocortisone is the most common OTC topical product recommended by both dermatologists and nondermatologists, whereas dermatologists more often recommend sunscreen and moisturizers than other physicians.

of skin and subcutaneous tissue, nonexcisional debridement of wound, infection, or burn, and removal of nail, nail bed, or nail fold (**Table 3**). However, per physician, dermatologists perform more of skin-related procedures than any other specialty. Between 1995 and 2008, dermatologists annually performed within a range of 1111 to 2937 procedures per physician, and general and family practitioners performed 52 to 93 procedures per physician (**Table 4**).

In the inpatient setting, 2,221,960 procedures were performed in the ED and 13,762,165 procedures were performed in the OPD. The most common procedures performed in the ED were other local excision or destruction of lesion or tissue of skin and subcutaneous tissue (24%), other incision with drainage of skin and subcutaneous tissue (22%), removal of nail, nail bed, or nail fold (11%). The most common procedures performed in the OPD were other local excision or destruction of lesion or tissue of skin and subcutaneous tissue (36%), closure of skin and subcutaneous tissue of other sites (13%), and nonexcisional debridement of wound, infection, or burn (10%) (**Table 5**).

In the treatment of dermatologic conditions in the inpatient setting, advanced therapeutic regimens are used. Despite a decrease in dermatology inpatient activity, advanced therapeutic regimens such as Goeckerman therapy, extracorporeal photochemotherapy, skin grafts, pulse steroids or pulse immunosuppressants, and intravenous immunoglobulin treatments are available. Some of the skin conditions for which patients are hospitalized include psoriasis, dermatitis, bullous disease, drug reactions, icer/grafting, malignancy, and lupus.[16,17]

Unique Services Provided by Specialists

With their training and background, dermatologists provide more expertise in the treatment of skin disease. Nondermatologists refer patients with skin complaints to dermatologists at rates between 33% and 72%. During a 2-year study period at a general medicine clinic, 37.5% of patients presenting to their PCP were referred to a dermatologist, 68% of whom were referred on the initial evaluation. The most common reason for referral to a dermatologist was for a biopsy or excision of a suspicious lesion (26.1% of referrals), followed by referrals for evaluation of a lesion or eruption of uncertain origin (20.7%). A failure of response to treatment was the reason for 13.5% of referrals.[25] In a study on the basis for referrals to dermatologists, the most frequent reason for referral was for therapy, followed by diagnosis or a combination of diagnosis and therapy.[26]

Dermatologists are primary providers of cutaneous surgery procedures (skin excisions, intermediate repairs, complex repairs, skin flaps, and skin grafts), performing more skin surgery than

Table 3
Estimated frequency of top 10 common dermatologic procedures performed by physicians in the outpatient setting: NAMCS, 1995 to 2008[a]

Procedure (ICD-9 Code)	Estimated Frequency (Thousands)					Total (% of All Dermatologic Procedures)
	Dermatology	General and Family Practice	General Surgery	Plastic Surgery	All Other	
Local excision or destruction of lesion or tissue of skin and subcutaneous tissue (86.3)	100,180	30,185	7831	4344	9180	151,720 (50.9)
Closed biopsy of skin and subcutaneous tissue (86.11)	34,847	6167	957	354	1644	43,969 (14.7)
Incision with drainage of skin and subcutaneous tissue (86.04)	2460	3453	1104	176	1709	8902 (3.0)
Closure of skin and subcutaneous tissue of other sites (86.69)	652	3453	282	127	1961	6475 (2.2)
Injection of sclerosing agent into vein (39.92)	1097	52	509	406	3188	5252 (1.8)
Botulinum toxin injection[b]	1569	81	0	972	2468	5090 (1.7)
Nonexcisional debridement of wound, infection, or burn (86.28)	358	1533	1199	63	1687	4840 (1.6)
Chemosurgery of skin (86.24)	3987	106	0	83	638	4814 (1.6)
Removal of nail, nail bed, or nail fold (86.23)	116	2847	225	0	455	3643 (1.2)
Injection or tattooing of skin lesion or defect (86.02)	2915	35	0	40	202	3192 (1.1)
All other dermatologic procedures	14,618	7631	4043	8962	25,077	60,331
Total (% of all dermatologic procedures)	162,799 (55)	55,543 (19)	16,150 (5)	15,527 (5)	48,209 (16)	298,228 (100)

Dermatologists perform 55% of all dermatologic procedures, followed by general/family physicians. Local excisions are the most commonly performed dermatologic procedure, with dermatologists performing the largest proportion.

[a] NAMCS data from 2005 and 2006 were not included, because of inconsistencies in data collection.

[b] Identified by medication or reason-for-visit code for botulinum toxin.

any other specialist.[27,28] According to an analysis of data from 1998 to 1999 from the Center for Medicare and Medicaid Services (CMS), dermatologists performed 54% of all cutaneous surgery procedures identified during this 2-year span, compared with plastic surgeons (15%) and general surgeons (8%). Dermatologists performed most surgical excision of benign and malignant skin lesions (58%), immediate repairs (62%), and complex repairs (50%). They performed the most flaps of any other specialty (40%), and 20% of all grafts. Emergency room physicians performed

Table 4
Estimated number of annual skin-related procedures performed per physician: NAMCS, 1995 to 2008[a]

Year	Dermatologists	General Practice/Family Physicians	General Surgeons
1995	1111	68	42
1996	1145	69	51
1997	1572	89	60
1998	1590	67	37
1999	1626	61	60
2000	1327	58	37
2001	1653	63	67
2002	1828	75	86
2003	1624	75	81
2004	1996	93	96
2007	2937	71	130
2008	1795	52	67

Dermatologists perform more skin-related procedures annually, compared with all other specialties. The number of procedures performed per dermatologist has also increased since 1995, whereas the number of procedures per physician has remained relatively consistent for nondermatologists.
[a] NAMCS data from 2005 and 2006 were not included, because of inconsistencies in data collection.

more simple and intermediate closures, often associated with trauma, such as laceration repair. On a per physician basis, dermatologists performed the largest volume of complex repairs, intermediate repairs, and excisions. Dermatologists and plastic surgeons performed a similar volume of skin flaps and full-thickness skin grafts, whereas plastic surgeons performed more split-thickness skin graft procedures, often associated with their work with patients with burns.[28]

Dermatologists also perform the most outpatient cosmetic procedures in the United States, which continues to be a growing part of modern dermatology.[29] Based on NAMCS data from 1995 to 2008, the most common procedures performed in the office-based setting were sclerotherapy (20%), botulinum toxin injections (19%), chemical peels (18%), soft tissue fillers (12%), and liposuction (10%) (**Table 6**). The American Academy of Cosmetic Surgery (AACS) conducts a yearly procedural census to gather information about the number of cosmetic procedures performed by AACS members in the United States, who are mostly dermatologic surgeons, plastic surgeons, head and neck surgeons, oral and maxillofacial surgeons, general surgeons, plastic surgeons, or ocular plastic surgeons. In 2009, the AACS reported results from 254 completed

surveys (response rate 16%), and found that more than 17.5 million cosmetic procedures were performed in the United States by all cosmetic surgeons, and the total number of procedures performed by AACS members has increased by 8% since 2008.[30] Less-invasive procedures that have increased the most since 2005 are laser resurfacing, botulinum toxin injections, chemical peels, and soft tissue fillers, and the most commonly offered less-invasive cosmetic surgery procedures in 2009 were botulinum toxin injections, soft tissue fillers, and chemical peels. Based on NAMCS data on dermatologic procedures from 1995 to 2008, dermatologists performed 31% of all botulinum toxin procedures identified.

As specialists, dermatologists are also trained to interpret cutaneous pathology specimens. Up to 25% of dermatology residency curricula are devoted to dermatopathology, and there is similar representation of pathology presented in the dermatology board-certifying examination. In a study by Feldman and colleagues, pathology claims submitted to Medicare between 1999 and 2000 were analyzed to quantify the relative experience of dermatologists and pathologists in the interpretation of skin pathology specimens. Within all claims for skin-related diagnoses, dermatologists performed 9.7 million (31.2%), whereas pathologists performed 10.7 million (34.5%) and independent laboratories and group practices performed 10.2 million (32.8%). On a per physician basis, dermatologists read 1047 skin-related pathology cases per physician, which was similar to pathologists, who read 1155 cases per physician.[31] Dermatopathology is not only a component of the medical training of dermatologists, but it is also an integral part of the services that dermatologists provide.

Specialist NPCs

According to a survey of practice profiles, the level of supervision of PAs and NPs did not vary significantly among respondent dermatology practices.[8] Most dermatologists allowed NPCs to see new patients (77%) and established patients with new problems (85%), worsening existing problems (73%), and stable existing problems (99%). Respondents reported that NPCs spent more time seeing medical dermatology patients (79%) than working in cosmetic (9%) or noncosmetic surgery (12%).

PAs have had an emerging role in delivering dermatologic care. They are generally involved in handling routine patient care and education, which includes taking patient histories and performing physical examinations, ordering and interpreting

Table 5
Top 10 common dermatologic procedures and associated percentages performed in the hospital setting: NAMCS, 1995 to 2007

	ED Procedure (ICD-9 code)	(%)	OPD Procedure (ICD-9 code)	(%)
1.	Local excision or destruction of lesion or tissue of skin and subcutaneous tissue (86.3)	(24.4)	Local excision or destruction of lesion or tissue of skin and subcutaneous tissue (86.3)	(36.4)
2.	Incision with drainage of skin and subcutaneous tissue (86.04)	(22.5)	Closure of skin and subcutaneous tissue of other sites (86.59)	(13.0)
3.	Removal of nail, nail bed, or nail fold (86.23)	(11.4)	Nonexcisional debridement of wound, infection, or burn (86.28)	(9.9)
4.	Nonexcisional debridement of wound, infection, or burn (86.28)	(6.7)	Closed biopsy of skin and subcutaneous tissue (86.11)	(8.0)
5.	Closed biopsy of skin and subcutaneous tissue (86.11)	(5.3)	Incision with drainage of skin and subcutaneous tissue (86.04)	(5.1)
6.	Closure of skin and subcutaneous tissue of other sites (86.59)	(4.6)	Removal of nail, nail bed, or nail fold (86.23)	(3.1)
7.	Ultraviolet light therapy (99.82)	(3.2)	Chemosurgery of skin (86.24)	(2.4)
8.	Debridement of nail, nail bed, or nail fold (86.27)	(2.5)	Botulinum toxin injection[a]	(2.2)
9.	Injection of sclerosing agent into vein (39.93)	(2.3)	Debridement of nail, nail bed, or nail fold (86.27)	(1.8)
10.	Botulinum toxin injection[a]	(2.2)	Ultraviolet light therapy (99.82)	(1.3)

The most common procedure in the ED and OPD is local excision or destruction of lesions or tissue of skin and subcutaneous tissue. Ultraviolet light therapy is provided in these settings, and botulinum toxin injections comprise an equal proportion of procedures in both settings.
[a] Identified by medication or reason-for-visit code for botulinum toxin.

laboratory tests, and diagnosing and implementing treatment plans. Most PAs receive surgical training as part of PA school curricula, and are often involved in performing more common dermatologic minor procedures such as biopsies, liquid nitrogen destruction, surgical excisions and minor repairs (such as skin grafts and Mohs surgery closings), lasers, cryotherapy, phototherapy, chemical peels, collagen, botulinum toxin injections, hair transplants, and liposuction.[7,11] In a study of NAMCS data on the use of PAs in all practices including dermatology, dermatologic symptoms were evaluated frequently by PAs, accounting for 14% of all PA visits.[32]

The role of CTAs in delivering dermatologic health care has been described more recently. In a prospective observational study examining the range of duties and responsibilities of CTAs, standardized observers with clinical backgrounds monitored the work of CTAs for 2 consecutive days at 10 office sites. CTAs performed an average of 90 activities/interventions per day per office, with 35% of these functions being direct patient-related activities. In direct activities with patients, CTAs typically handle telephone calls with patients, triage patients with urgent clinical

problems, report laboratory results, and answer clinical questions about physician-developed treatment protocols.[9]

Subspecialist Care

Subspecialist care is provided by dermatology subspecialties, including cosmetic dermatology, dermatopathology, Mohs surgery, and pediatric dermatology, among others (see **Table 1**). These subspecialties meet specific needs of patients with skin conditions. Cosmetic dermatology may include dermatologists who have completed fellowships in surgical dermatology, specializing in performing cosmetic procedures that range from minimally invasive procedures such as botulinum toxin, fillers, photo rejuvenation, and laser surgery, to surgical procedures including liposuction, blepharoplasty, and rhinoplasty. Although dermatologists completing standard residencies show competency in dermatopathology, dermatopathologists specialize in looking at the pathology of cutaneous specimens at the cellular level. Although many skin diseases may be identified by clinical appearance, dermatopathologists specialize in examining skin biopsies that may

Table 6
Frequency and associated percentage of cosmetic procedure visits: NAMCS, 1995 to 2008[a]

	Cosmetic Procedure	Frequency (Thousands)	(%)
1.	Sclerotherapy	5252	(19.7)
2.	Botulinum toxin injection	5089	(19.1)
3.	Chemical peel	4813	(18.0)
4.	Soft tissue fillers	3193	(12.0)
5.	Liposuction	2587	(9.7)
6.	Dermabrasion	2251	(8.4)
7.	Mammoplasty	1780	(6.7)
8.	Facial rhytidectomy	535	(2.0)
9.	Epilation of skin	491	(1.8)
10.	Hair transplantation	405	(1.5)
11.	Rhinoplasty	230	(0.9)
12.	Collagen	39	(0.1)
	Total	13,945,401	(100)

Sclerotherapy, botulinum toxin injections, and chemical peels were the most commonly performed cosmetic procedures from 1995 to 2008.

[a] NAMCS data from 2005 and 2006 were not included, because of inconsistencies in data collection.

provide more information. One subspecialty that has experienced growth more recently is Mohs surgery within surgical dermatology. MMS is the surgical removal of skin cancer and other malignancies, followed by microscopic examination of histologic sections of the entire surgical margin of excised tissue. This method was developed to ensure complete removal of malignancies and spare surrounding tissue, especially in areas where this is important, such as the face, nose, and eyes.[33,34] With the increase in the prevalence of melanoma and nonmelanoma cancer, this subspecialty field has been growing. Retrospective studies have reported referral rates for MMS for nonmelanoma skin cancer of 30.7%,[35] 32.7%,[36] and 30.8%.[37] Pediatric dermatology is a subspecialty that deals with the complex diseases of neonates, hereditary skin diseases, and skin disorders of the pediatric population. Conditions that are commonly treated are acne, atopic dermatitis, hair and nail disorders, pigmentation disorders, and psoriasis.

EFFICACY OF TREATMENT OR CARE

This section discusses the efficacy of the services and treatment provided on all levels of dermatologic care. It is important to consider the efficacy on each level, because both nonprescription and prescription treatments are used in the management of common skin disease. Efficacy is measured in literature on many different levels: management of outcomes, patient satisfaction, adherence to treatments, diagnostic accuracy, cost-effectiveness.

Self-care and Self-management

Although public resources such as newspapers, magazines, and the Internet can provide patient education for many dermatologic conditions, the readability of these materials is an important consideration in the effectiveness of these resources. General guidelines state that public education materials should be written at the sixth-grade to eighth-grade level. In a study of patient-oriented online resources for dermatologic conditions, 3 commonly accessed Internet sources (http://WebMD.com, http://Wikipedia.org, and http://MedicineOnline.com) were compared with electronic pamphlets provided on the Web site of the AAD for readability. Using the Flesch readability ease score and Flesch-Kincaid grade level as measures of readability, http://Wikipedia.org was the most difficult to comprehend, followed by the AAD electronic pamphlets. These pamphlets and http://MedicineOnline.com materials were the most concise, averaging 1200 words or less.[38]

In a study comparing patient education material on psoriasis from the AAD, the NPF, material from textbooks, and health-related articles from *Time*, *Newsweek*, and the *New York Times*, material from AAD and NPF scored the highest Flesch-Kincaid grade levels, ranging from grade 11 to 12, and material from the Arthritis Foundation brochures on methotrexate and psoriatic arthritis was scored at the eighth-grade level and had the highest Flesch reading ease score. Among the news publications, *Newsweek* had the highest Flesch reading ease score, followed by *Time* and the *New York Times*, which both were written at grade level 11 (**Table 7**).[39]

Patient advocacy groups can also contribute significantly to patient perspectives and knowledge of disease through psychological and moral support provided through these services. Nijsten and Bergstresser[21] propose a possible way of increasing the coherence and impact of all involved in dermatologic care by creating an alliance between governmental health authorities, health insurance, media, and the population that will serve as a link between patients and health care providers (**Fig. 4**). The effectiveness of those

Table 7
Readability of education materials for patients with psoriasis

Document	Flesch-Kincaid Grade Level	Flesch Reading Ease Score[a]
AF: methotrexate	8	62
AF: psoriatic arthritis	8	60
NPF: tar	9	60
Newsweek: medicine	9	60
Epstein: psoriasis	9	53
AF: Reiter syndrome	10	53
Lowe: psoriasis	10	51
Time: health	11	52
Lowe: PUVA	11	51
New York Times: skin troubles	11	51
AAD: Psoriasis	11	44
NPF: UVB	12	48
NPF: PUVA	12	48
NPF: Methotrexate	12	39

AF patient materials have the highest readability, with the highest Flesch reading ease score, and are written at a Flesh-Kincaid grade level of 8. Material from the NPF is among the lowest readability.

Abbreviations: AF, Arthritis Foundation; PUVA, psoralen plus ultraviolet A.

[a] Flesch reading ease score is between 0 and 100, with higher scores indicating material that is easier to read.

Data from Feldman SR, Vanarthos J, Fleischer AB Jr. The readability of patient education materials designed for patients with psoriasis. J Am Acad Dermatol 1994; 30(2 Pt 1):284–6.

educational efforts has been shown in patients with psoriasis and members of the NPF. Members of the NPF were more often affected by more extensive psoriasis; however, they were more likely to have knowledge of the available therapies for this condition, reported that psoriasis had less impact on their daily lives than patients from the general US population, and reported higher satisfaction with their current therapies.[40] Thus, patients with more knowledge of their disease may have more realistic expectations of their outcomes of therapies, leading them to be more satisfied with their treatment, and also may be more informed about coping strategies that help them to decrease the impact of the disease on their quality of life.[21]

In a study of patient perspectives on self-care, most adults indicated an increasing preference of self-treating conditions over seeing a doctor.[41] Federal law mandates that medication should be available in an OTC form unless there is specific reason to restrict access through prescriptions; however, dermatologists have had mixed feelings toward changes of prescription medications to OTC status, such as the change in topical HC in 1979. The medical concern behind the OTC availability of HC was that inappropriate use or application of an OTC product may not only be ineffective or result in adverse side effects that are concomitant with the medication, but misuse of OTC products may also mask the development and delay accurate diagnoses of skin cancers or other skin conditions. Thus, assessing the efficacy of self-care in the treatment of skin diseases requires consideration of safety and efficacy, as well as the ability of patients to use the medication appropriately.

Despite the controversy surrounding HC, self-management with OTC products such as HC has been shown to be safe and effective, depending on patterns of use and self-treatment. One study sought to determine compliance with label directions of OTC HCs by examining self-reported patterns of use in adults and children.[42] In this study, 2000 adults in the United States were identified as users of OTC HC in the last 6 months through a telephone survey, and respondents were asked about the conditions they were treating with OTC HC and the frequency and duration of their use of the product. Eighty-three percent of adults used OTC HC for conditions that were consistent with the label. In 98% of cases, HC was applied less than or equal to 4 times daily, and in 92% of cases, it was applied for less than or equal to 7 days, which are consistent with the label. In an overall calculation of compliance, which accounted for the condition treated, and the frequency and duration of use, 73% of adult respondents were deemed compliant with the OTC label, and 27% were deemed noncompliant for 1 or more reasons. However, studies using objective electronic monitors have shown that self-reports typically overestimate compliance; therefore it is possible that compliance was lower.[43]

In a study of self-application of topical creams, 20 healthy volunteers were recruited to assess the technique and precision of test subjects' application of a test cream. Volunteers were instructed to apply a fluorescent test cream to the entire surface of their body except the head and neck and skin covered by underwear. When application sites were measured under Wood's ultraviolet radiation, as much as 31% of the skin surface targeted for application did not show fluorescence and was thus considered untreated. The most commonly neglected site was the back, followed by the feet (in particular the sole), breast, legs,

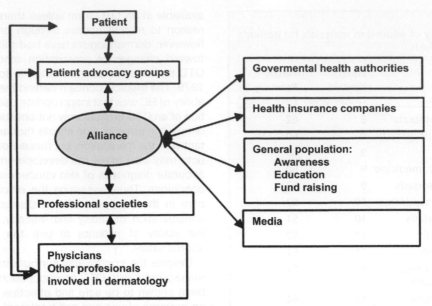

Fig. 4. Proposed method of increasing coherence and impact of all involved in dermatologic care. The proposed mechanism of increasing coherence and the impact of dermatologic care is creating an alliance that will serve as a link between professional societies, physicians, and other health care professions and patients and patient advocacy groups. (*Reprinted from* Nijsten T, Bergstresser PR. Patient advocacy groups: let's stick together. J Invest Dermatol 2010;130(7):1758; with permission from Macmillan Publishers Ltd. Copyright 2010.)

arms, and hands (in order of decreasing rates of neglected areas).[44] In a series of studies on sunscreen users on a sunny day at the beach, despite the fact that 65% of sunbathers used 1 or more sunscreens, the median sun protection factor used was estimated to be 5 to 6. Study subjects tended to apply the sunscreen in smaller amounts than directed, and many did not reapply it as necessary.[45]

The result may be a false sense of security when patients do not realize how they are supposed to take an OTC medication like sunscreen. When deciding what products to bring to market, manufacturers typically err on the safe side and strive to minimize the risk of adverse effects from overdosing. Although the safety concerns are understandable, the emphasis on safety often results in products the efficacy of which is easily impaired by underdosing or failure to use the product regularly.[46] Patients' frequent inability to understand or follow label directions thus becomes a major limitation to the efficacy of self-care.

Effectiveness of PCP and Specialist Care

In response to the introduction of managed care, the experience of PCPs and dermatologists in treating skin conditions has been well defined in previous literature. For optimal patient safety and outcomes of care, it is important to consider the

effectiveness of the different services of various dermatologic health care providers.

Despite direct access to specialists, the imbalance of supply and demand for dermatologic services because of the shortage of dermatologists has been only moderately corrected by the influx of NPC specialists.[47] According to NAMCS data up to 2008, PCPs continue to perform a significant proportion of skin-related procedures.

Based on NAMCS data from 1990 to 1994, 39% of all visits for a single dermatologic diagnosis were to PCPs. Referrals for these dermatology-related visits was more common (5.8%) than referrals for all office visits to PCPs (4.5%, $P<.001$). The referral rate for dermatology-related conditions by internists ranged from 16.6% to 46.5%, 6.8% to 18.% for pediatricians, and 8.2% to 23% for family/general practitioners. The number of visits per dermatologic episode was estimated at 5.8 for family/general practitioners, 5.9 for internists, and 9.3 for pediatricians. The most frequent diagnoses associated with referral were common dermatologic problems, which suggests that managing skin problems may be difficult for primary care providers, because of the greater likelihood of referral for skin disorders than other medical conditions, and the frequent need to refer patients with common skin problems.[5]

Based on data from the CMS Web site, dermatologists perform more surgical procedures on the skin than other specialty.[27] Skin diseases are not a large part of the workload for primary care providers, and the relative amount of continuing exposure to dermatologic problems varies widely. A calculation of the percent of outpatient care time per physician shows that dermatologists spent 86.9% of outpatient time on dermatologic conditions, compared with 4.1% for internists, 6.2% for family physicians, 8.1% for pediatricians, and 2.9% for all other physicians.[48] Dermatologists also have special expertise in the management of skin conditions. They identify and provide higher diagnostic accuracy, and provide more cost-effective treatment of patients with skin disease by requiring less physician time and lower referral rates.[49] In US medical schools surveyed in 1986, the mean requirement of medical education in dermatology was 21 hours, most often within the first 2 preclinical years. Only about 1 of 3 medical students had an opportunity to participate in a clerkship in dermatology, and several schools did not provide any students with clerkships.[50] However, Wagner and colleagues show that even a 4-week clerkship in dermatology is not sufficient for nondermatologists to provide quality care. When 37 medical student and resident groups were asked to name malignant and benign skin diseases and indicate the advisability of a biopsy, dermatology residents' performance was significantly better than other resident groups, and there was no difference in performance among internal medicine residents who had 4 weeks of previous training in dermatology and those who had none. Similarly, there was no difference in the pretest and posttest scores of senior medical students after a 4-week clerkship in dermatology.[51] In addition, there is evidence that PCPs may not always use the most recent treatment consensus guidelines for common skin diseases. For example, evidence-based guidelines dictate that topical retinoids should be preferred over older alternatives such as antibiotics and benzoyl peroxide for first-line treatment of acne.[52] However, in a study comparing pediatricians' and dermatologists' patterns of treatment of acne vulgaris, dermatologists prescribed topical retinoids at 46.1% of acne visits by patients ages 10 to 18 years, whereas pediatricians prescribed retinoids at 12.1% of visits by the same age group.[53]

Patient satisfaction is also an important component of efficacy to consider. In a prospective survey study, 150 consecutive patients seen in an outpatient dermatology clinic were surveyed to complete a survey on their opinions on the efficacy, costs, and desirability of direct access to dermatologic specialty care. Of 115 respondents, 39% of respondents were on an initial visit, 50% of respondents had previously seen another physician, and 30% had been referred by another physician. Of the 50% who had previously seen another physician, two-thirds had received therapy, and only one-third of these individuals believed that the therapy had any benefit. Twenty-three percent of respondents reported having more than 5 visits to a different physician before seeing a dermatologist, and only 6% of respondents believed a generalist could adequately treat their skin disease. Overall, 87% of respondents described direct access to dermatology as being "very important" to their health care.[6] In a study comparing patients' confidence in skin care by primary care providers and dermatologists, patients had overall high rates of satisfaction with the treatment rendered by both physicians, but satisfaction was significantly higher for dermatologists delivering treatment of skin disease, and most patients preferred access to dermatologists for skin problems.[54]

Teledermatology

Previous studies have reported mixed results regarding the effectiveness of teledermatology. In a systematic review of literature addressing the diagnostic accuracy and concordance of teledermatology, approximately two-thirds of studies that compared diagnoses made through clinic dermatology and teledermatology found that diagnoses made face-to-face were more accurate.[55] In a prospective observational study of 116 adults, office-based and remote clinicians made concordant diagnoses based on physical examination and digital images, respectively, in 61% to 64% of all cases. This rate of agreement was reported to be even greater (>75%) when photographic quality was high and office-based clinician certainty was high.[56] Diagnostic concordance between teledermatology and clinic dermatology were comparable, with LI teledermatology being better than SAF teledermatology. When comparing management of disease, the accuracy of teledermatology and clinic dermatology was equivalent for clinical management of skin conditions, although teledermatology had lower rates of management accuracy in specific notable conditions such as malignant lesions. Some of the practical advantages of teledermatology were the levels of patient satisfaction, which were comparable in both teledermatology and clinic settings, and the reduction in the number of clinic visits and the time to treatment.[55]

Subspecialist Care

The efficacy of subspecialist over specialist care has been a topic of debate for certain areas in procedural dermatology, such as MMS. The controversy stems from critics questioning the need to remove all cancerous cells to achieve a cure, a lack of prospective randomized trials, a documented overestimation of cure rates, and the fact that current treatment options for skin cancer are already considered extremely effective. In addition, certain patient groups, such as patients with history of dementia, spinal chronic arthritis, or poor sphincter control, pose special challenges. In the literature, MMS has low documented overall complication rates (1.6%), and a high clearance rate for most cancers of the skin.[57–59] In recent years, several medical specialties have shifted toward providing increasing procedural care in the outpatient setting. In response, the Joint Commission Accreditation of Health Care Organizations proposed a safety standard that would require physicians to retain hospital privileges and credentials by performing a minimum number of annual procedures in the hospital setting. The safety of MMS, which is almost always performed in the physician office, has been supported by low adverse event rates (1.64%), and low rates of infection (1%–3%), more consistent with clean procedures than clean contaminated procedures.[60]

There are growing concerns that an increasing number of physicians and nonphysicians are providing cosmetic procedures such as botulinum injections and laser therapy, with limited regulation on cosmetic training. In Minneapolis, dentists have begun marketing cosmetic treatments such as botulinum toxin and dermal filler treatments.[61] Dermatologists are trained through cosmetic dermatology fellowships, or cosmetic training within procedural dermatology fellowships. In a study of public perception of dermatologists as surgeons, respondents reported greater confidence in the surgical skills of plastic surgeons, except for the treatment of skin cancer. Although the public often views plastic surgeons as perhaps the original source of cosmetic or aesthetic surgery, participants rated the cosmetic appearance of surgical scars from dermatologists and plastic surgeons as equivalent.[62]

Complications to Assessing Efficacy

The effectiveness of dermatologic treatments provided by physicians is complicated by low patient adherence, which has been documented as a common problem in dermatology.[63] Although higher levels of adherence have been shown to improve outcomes for patients with common dermatologic conditions such as atopic dermatitis and psoriasis, an estimated 33% to 50% of

patients are nonadherent to dermatologic treatment.[64,65] In a prospective study, 17 first-time patients receiving prescription for previously untried topically administered drug were surveyed for adherence and dosing (mostly for topical corticosteroids), and patient drug containers were

List of Acronyms	
AACS	American Academy of Cosmetic Surgery
AAD	American Academy of Dermatology
ACMS	American College of Mohs Surgery
CMS	Center for Medicare and Medicaid services
CTA	Clinical triage assistant
DRG	Diagnosis-related group
ED	Emergency Department
HC	Hydrocortisone
HCUP-3 NIS	Healthcare Cost and Utilization Project-3 Nationwide Inpatient Sample
JCAHO	Joint Commission Accreditation of Health Care Organizations
LI	Live Interactive
MEDPAR	Medicare Provider Analysis and Review
MMS	Mohs micrographic surgery
NAMCS	National Ambulatory Medical Care Survey
NCHS	National Center for Health Statistics
NHAMCS	National Hospital Ambulatory Medical Care Survey
NIAMS	National Institute of Arthritis and Musculoskeletal and Skin Diseases
NP	Nurse practitioner
NPC	Non-physician clinician
NPF	National Psoriasis Foundation
OPD	Outpatient Department
OTC	Over-the-counter
PA	Physician assistant
PCP	Primary care physician
PUVA	Psoralen plus ultraviolet A
SAF	Store and forward
SID	Society for Investigative Dermatology
SPF	Sun protection factor
US	United States

weighed. Two patients did not fill prescriptions at all, only 1 patient used the recommended dosage, and other patients underdosed the new topical treatments, with a general median of 35% of the expected individual dosages used.[66]

As a general consideration, caution must be applied when assessing the efficacy of treatment methods because physicians are often limited to seeing patients with skin diseases for whom self-care or management or other previously physician-directed therapy has failed. Assessing efficacy at this level imparts selection bias because it does not accurately represent the unknown population for which self-care or management was successful.

REFERENCES

1. Bickers DR, Lim HW, Margolis D, et al. The burdens of skin diseases: 2004 a joint project of the American Academy of Dermatology Association and the Society for Investigative Dermatology. J Am Acad Dermatol 2006;55(3):490–500.

2. Feldman SR, Fleischer AB Jr, Williford PM, et al. Increasing utilization of dermatologists by managed care: an analysis of the National Ambulatory Medical Care Survey, 1990-1994. J Am Acad Dermatol 1997; 37(5 Pt 1):784–8.

3. Stern RS. Dermatologists and office-based care of dermatologic disease in the 21st century. J Investig Dermatol Symp Proc 2004;9(2):126–30.

4. Ramsay DL, Weary PE. Primary care in dermatology: whose role should it be? J Am Acad Dermatol 1996; 35(6):1005–8.

5. Feldman SR, Fleischer AB Jr, Chen JG. The gatekeeper model is inefficient for the delivery of dermatologic services. J Am Acad Dermatol 1999;40(3): 426-32.

6. Owen SA, Maeyens E Jr, Weary PE. Patients' opinions regarding direct access to dermatologic specialty care. J Am Acad Dermatol 1997;36(2 Pt 1):250–6.

7. Baker KE. Will a physician assistant improve your dermatology practice? Semin Cutan Med Surg 2000;19(3):201–3.

8. Resneck JS Jr, Kimball AB. Who else is providing care in dermatology practices? Trends in the use of nonphysician clinicians. J Am Acad Dermatol 2008;58(2):211–6.

9. Straka BT, Wiser TH, Feldman SR, et al. The clinical triage assistant: a new member of the dermatology health care team. J Am Acad Dermatol 2010;63(6): 1103–5.

10. White SM, Geronemus R. Should non-physicians perform cosmetic procedures? Dermatol Surg 2002;28(9):856–9.

11. Arnold T. Physician assistants in dermatology. J Clin Aesthet Dermatol 2008;1(2):28–31.

12. About DNA. 2011. Available at: http://www.dnanurse.org/utilities/about_dna. Accessed April 28, 2011.

13. Jesitus J. Mohs surgeons wrestle with increasing skin cancer rates, scrutiny by insurers. 2010. Available at: http://www.modernmedicine.com/modernmedicine/Modern+Medicine+Now/Mohs-surgeons-wrestle-with-increasing-skin-cancer-/ArticleStandard/Article/detail/692414. Accessed May 2, 2011.

14. Mohs micrographic surgery training. American College of Mohs Surgery; 2011. Available at: http://www.mohscollege.org/acms/training.php. Accessed April 28, 2011.

15. Resneck JS Jr, Tierney EP, Kimball AB. Challenges facing academic dermatology: survey data on the faculty workforce. J Am Acad Dermatol 2006;54(2): 211–6.

16. Kirsner RS, Yang DG, Kerdel FA. Inpatient dermatology. The difficulties, the reality, and the future. Dermatol Clin 2000;18(3):383–90, vii.

17. Kirsner RS, Yang DG, Kerdel FA. Dermatologic disease accounts for a large number of hospital admissions annually. J Am Acad Dermatol 1999; 41(6):970–3.

18. Falanga V, Schachner LA, Rae V, et al. Dermatologic consultations in the hospital setting. Arch Dermatol 1994;130(8):1022–5.

19. Vallejos QM, Quandt SA, Feldman SR, et al. Teledermatology consultations provide specialty care for farmworkers in rural clinics. J Rural Health 2009; 25(2):198–202.

20. For the public. American Academy of Dermatology; 2011. Available at: http://www.aad.org/for-the-public/home. Accessed May 10, 2011.

21. Nijsten T, Bergstresser PR. Patient advocacy groups: let's stick together. J Invest Dermatol 2010;130(7): 1757–9.

22. Coalition of Skin Diseases. Coalition of Skin Diseases. 2011. Available at: http://www.coalitionofskindiseases.org. Accessed April 7, 2011.

23. Americans take healthcare into their own hands: consumers increasingly comfortable with self-medication. Consumer Healthcare Products Association; 2011. Available at: http://www.chpa-info.org/Consumer_Survey_SM.aspx. Accessed May 9, 2011.

24. Duque MI, Vogel CA, Fleischer AB Jr, et al. Over-the-counter topical antipruritic agents are commonly recommended by office-based physicians: an analysis of US practice patterns. J Dermatolog Treat 2004;15(3):185–8.

25. Lowell BA, Froelich CW, Federman DG, et al. Dermatology in primary care: prevalence and patient disposition. J Am Acad Dermatol 2001;45(2):250–5.

26. Eaglstein WH, Laszlo KS. Patient referrals to a dermatologist. The referring physician's perspective. Arch Dermatol 1996;132(3):292–4.

27. Roenigk RK. Dermatologists perform more skin surgery than any other specialist: implications for

health care policy, graduate and continuing medical education. Dermatol Surg 2008;34(3): 293–300.

28. Shaffer CL, Feldman SR, Fleischer AB Jr, et al. The cutaneous surgery experience of multiple specialties in the Medicare population. J Am Acad Dermatol 2005;52(6):1045–8.

29. Housman TS, Hancox JG, Mir MR, et al. What specialties perform the most common outpatient cosmetic procedures in the United States? Dermatol Surg 2008;34(1):1–7.

30. American Academy of Cosmetic Surgery Procedural Census Trends, 2005-2009. American Academy of Cosmetic Surgery; 2011. Available at: http://www.cosmeticsurgery.org/media/2009_fact_sheet_trends.pdf. Accessed March 15, 2011.

31. Hancox JG, Neville JA, Chen J, et al. Interpretation of dermatopathology specimens is within the standard of care of dermatology practice. Dermatol Surg 2005;31(3):306–9.

32. Clark AR, Monroe JR, Feldman SR, et al. The emerging role of physician assistants in the delivery of dermatologic health care. Dermatol Clin 2000; 18(2):297–302.

33. Mohs micrographic surgery overview. American College of Mohs Surgery; 2011. Available at: http://www.mohscollege.org/about/overview.php. Accessed May 2, 2011.

34. When does my skin cancer need Mohs surgery? American College of Mohs Surgery; 2011. Available at: http://www.mohscollege.org/about/indicators.php. Accessed May 10, 2011.

35. Miller PK, Roenigk RK, Brodland DG, et al. Cutaneous micrographic surgery: Mohs procedure. Mayo Clin Proc 1992;67(10):971–80.

36. Welch ML, Anderson LL, Grabski WJ. How many nonmelanoma skin cancers require Mohs micrographic surgery? Dermatol Surg 1996;22(8):711–3.

37. Gaston DA, Naugle C, Clark DP. Mohs micrographic surgery referral patterns: the University of Missouri experience. Dermatol Surg 1999;25(11):862–6.

38. Tulbert BH, Snyder CW, Brodell RT. Readability of patient-oriented online dermatology resources. J Clin Aesthet Dermatol 2011;4(3):27–33.

39. Feldman SR, Vanarthos J, Fleischer AB Jr. The readability of patient education materials designed for patients with psoriasis. J Am Acad Dermatol 1994; 30(2 Pt 1):284–6.

40. Nijsten T, Rolstad T, Feldman SR, et al. Members of the National Psoriasis Foundation: more extensive disease and better informed about treatment options. Arch Dermatol 2005;141(1):19–26.

41. Consumer Healthcare Products Association. Americans take healthcare into their own hands: consumers increasingly comfortable with self-medication. 2011. Available at: http://www.chpa-info.org/Consumer_Survey_SM.aspx. Accessed May 9, 2011.

42. Ellis CN, Pillitteri JL, Kyle TK, et al. Consumers appropriately self-treat based on labeling for over-the-counter hydrocortisone. J Am Acad Dermatol 2005;53(1):41–51.

43. Balkrishnan R, Carroll CL, Camacho FT, et al. Electronic monitoring of medication adherence in skin disease: results of a pilot study. J Am Acad Dermatol 2003;49(4):651–4.

44. Ulff E, Maroti M, Kettis-Lindblad A, et al. Single application of a fluorescent test cream by healthy volunteers: assessment of treated and neglected body sites. Br J Dermatol 2007;156(5):974–8.

45. Wulf HC, Stender IM, Lock-Andersen J. Sunscreens used at the beach do not protect against erythema: a new definition of SPF is proposed. Photodermatol Photoimmunol Photomed 1997;13(4):129–32.

46. Cramer JA. Microelectronic systems for monitoring and enhancing patient compliance with medication regimens. Drugs 1995;49(3):321–7.

47. Kimball AB, Resneck JS Jr. The US dermatology workforce: a specialty remains in shortage. J Am Acad Dermatol 2008;59(5):741–5.

48. Fleischer AB Jr, Herbert CR, Feldman SR, et al. Diagnosis of skin disease by nondermatologists. Am J Manag Care 2000;6(10):1149–56.

49. Feldman SR, Li J. Special expertise of dermatologists in the delivery of skin care. In: Barker J, Burgdorf W, editors. The challenge of skin diseases in Europe. 3rd edition. Berlin: ABW Wissenschaftsverlag; 2010. p. 19–22.

50. Federman DD. Medical student education in dermatology. Arch Dermatol 1985;121(12):1503.

51. Wagner RF Jr, Wagner D, Tomich JM, et al. Diagnoses of skin disease: dermatologists vs. nondermatologists. J Dermatol Surg Oncol 1985;11(5):476–9.

52. Zaenglein AL, Thiboutot DM. Expert committee recommendations for acne management. Pediatrics 2006;118(3):1188–99.

53. Yentzer BA, Irby CE, Fleischer AB Jr, et al. Differences in acne treatment prescribing patterns of pediatricians and dermatologists: an analysis of nationally representative data. Pediatr Dermatol 2008;25(6):635–9.

54. Federman DG, Reid M, Feldman SR, et al. The primary care provider and the care of skin disease: the patient's perspective. Arch Dermatol 2001; 137(1):25–9.

55. Warshaw EM, Hillman YJ, Greer NL, et al. Teledermatology for diagnosis and management of skin conditions: a systematic review. J Am Acad Dermatol 2011;64(4):759–72.

56. Kvedar JC, Edwards RA, Menn ER, et al. The substitution of digital images for dermatologic physical examination. Arch Dermatol 1997;133(2): 161–7.

57. Bene NI, Healy C, Coldiron BM. Mohs micrographic surgery is accurate 95.1% of the time for melanoma

in situ: a prospective study of 167 cases. Dermatol Surg 2008;34(5):660–4.

58. Cook JL, Perone JB. A prospective evaluation of the incidence of complications associated with Mohs micrographic surgery. Arch Dermatol 2003;139(2): 143–52.

59. Garcia C, Holman J, Poletti E. Mohs surgery: commentaries and controversies. Int J Dermatol 2005;44(11):893–905.

60. Hancox JG, Venkat AP, Coldiron B, et al. The safety of office-based surgery: review of recent literature from several disciplines. Arch Dermatol 2004; 140(11):1379–82.

61. Rollins S. Botox treatments, coming to a dentist's office near you? Time; 2011. Available at: http://healthland.time.com/2011/03/03/botox-treatments-coming-to-a-dentists-office-near-you/. Accessed May 4, 2011.

62. Chung V, Alexander H, Pavlis M, et al. The public's perception of dermatologists as surgeons. Dermatol Surg 2011;37(3):295–300.

63. Greenlaw SM, Yentzer BA, O'Neill JL, et al. Assessing adherence to dermatology treatments: a review of self-report and electronic measures. Skin Res Technol 2010;16(2):253–8.

64. Carroll CL, Feldman SR, Camacho FT, et al. Better medication adherence results in greater improvement in severity of psoriasis. Br J Dermatol 2004; 151(4):895–7.

65. Serup J, Lindblad AK, Maroti M, et al. To follow or not to follow dermatological treatment–a review of the literature. Acta Derm Venereol 2006;86(3):193–7.

66. Storm A, Benfeldt E, Andersen SE, et al. A prospective study of patient adherence to topical treatments: 95% of patients underdose. J Am Acad Dermatol 2008;59(6):975–80.

Models of Care and Organization of Services

Alina Markova, BA[a],[*], Michael Xiong, BA[a],
Jenna Lester, BA[a], Nancy J. Burnside, MD[a],[b]

KEYWORDS

- Models of care • Dermatology • Physician extenders
- Teledermatology • VAMC • PPO • HMO • Fee-for-service

This article examines the overall organization of services and delivery of health care in the United States. Health maintenance organization (HMO), fee-for-service (FFS), preferred provider organizations (PPOs), and the Veterans Health Administration (VHA) are discussed, with a focus on structure, outcomes, and areas for improvement. An overview of wait times, malpractice, telemedicine, and the growing population of physician extenders in dermatology is also provided.

HMO

An HMO is a type of managed care plan in which a network of designated health care providers (eg, physicians, nurse practitioners [NPs], therapists) is available to enrollees. Under the HMO model, there is a gatekeeper (GA), usually a primary care physician (PCP), whom the patient must first see to obtain a referral to a specialist. By contracting with a specific network of health care providers, and by emphasizing preventive care, HMOs are able to keep costs low. However, this cost cutting may also lead to certain disadvantages, including restricted access to specialists within the HMO network, and lack of coverage for procedures that the HMO may deem unnecessary. Under the Medicare HMO plan (also known as Medicare Advantage), patients are enrolled in traditional Medicare A and B, along with an HMO that offers extra services not covered by Medicare alone, such as prescription drugs, eyeglasses, and dental care.[1–3]

FFS

In an FFS system, health care services are unbundled and paid for separately. The advantage of an FFS model is that patients have the freedom and flexibility to choose any physician and hospital, not just those restricted to a certain network. The trade-off for this autonomy is that patients often have to pay higher copayments and deductibles. A copayment is a set fee, usually in the range of $20 to $40, which patients pay per visit to the physician. The amount of the copayment may differ between physicians in primary care and specialty settings. A deductible differs in that the amount paid is usually a percentage of the total costs for a service. The insurance then covers the remainder of the costs. Depending on variations in insurance policies and treatment plans, patients may be required to pay copayments, deductibles, or both. Physicians under the FFS system receive payment for each type of service rendered, such as an office visit, test, procedure, or other health care services. Because a GA is not required under FFS, patients typically have direct access to specialists. Medicare FFS is also known as traditional Medicare, in which

Funding: None.

Financial disclosures: The authors have nothing to disclose.

[a] Alpert Medical School of Brown University, 222 Richmond Street, Box G-9286, Providence, RI 02912, USA

[b] Department of Dermatology, Providence Veterans Affairs Medical Center, 830 Chalkstone Avenue, Providence, RI 02908, USA

* Corresponding author.

E-mail address: alina_markova@brown.edu

Dermatol Clin 30 (2012) 39–51

doi:10.1016/j.det.2011.09.005

patients are enrolled in Medicare A and B, and pay higher deductibles and premiums to gain access to a wider network of physicians compared with Medicare HMO (**Fig. 1**).[1–3]

PPOs are health care providers that assemble in a network to provide cost-sharing benefits to their subscribers. The network of physicians affiliated with a particular PPO provides care on an FFS basis usually to a group of patients belonging to the same employer group. As a result of this arrangement, the patient receives care from a network of providers at a discounted rate, and the providers have access to an increased pool of patients.[4] PPOs have become increasingly popular as a result of the aversion many people have to the rigidity inherent in an HMO. Compared with HMOs, PPOs have more care options for the subscriber, fewer care restrictions, and less overhead cost for the provider, and more reasonable administrative costs for purchasers.[5] This situation has caused an increase in the number of people who want to be enrolled in a PPO and in turn may create added demand for physicians to affiliate themselves with a PPO.

The Patient Protection and Affordable Care Act has called for significant health insurance reform in the United States. Of relevance to dermatology, the zoster vaccine was included in the first round of preventative services guidelines.[6] This act also included a 10% excise tax on indoor ultraviolet tanning, which took effect on July 1, 2010. This bill restructured payments to Medicare Advantage insurance companies to begin in 2012. These changes will adjust local Medicare spending levels, with bonuses for plans achieving high-quality scores. Such modifications may decrease the availability of Medicare Advantage plans, causing patients to revert to the traditional Medicare plan. Physician payments will be affected variably, depending on the contracted rates of the geographic area compared with those of Medicare.

Although there is a clear trend of improved skin cancer outcomes when diagnosed by dermatologists, and with increasing numbers of dermatologists, the health care outcomes of skin diseases when treated by nondermatologists are not so tangible. In addition to increasing and standardizing the education of skin diseases among nondermatologists, there should be a concurrent movement to educate the public about skin cancer, as well as to increase the number of

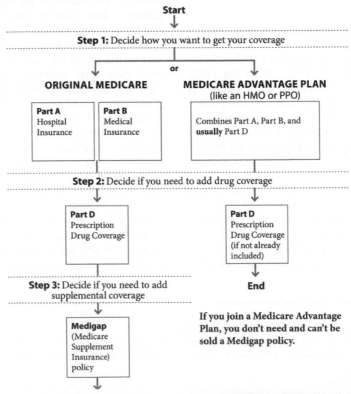

Fig. 1. Medicare coverage choices (*Official Medicare Handbook 2009*). (*From* Centers for Medicare and Medicaid Services. Medicare & You. U.S. Department of Health and Human Services, 2009.)

medical students admitted to dermatology residency programs. Through this 3-pronged approach, there is promise that dermatologic health outcomes will improve.

The increase to popularity of PPOs can be attributed in part to their ability to keep costs low for providers, purchasers, and subscribers. Subscribers are given the option to visit in-network providers, allowing the subscriber to benefit from the lower cost-sharing benefits of the networked providers.[4] Although there are financial benefits to remaining in the network, the subscriber is not restricted from seeing physicians outside the approved group of providers.

PPOs have gained favorability among providers for several reasons. Many providers believe that their relationship with the PPO network is more collegial than that with an HMO. Physicians may believe PPOs are less intrusive in their health care practices, are more accommodating to providers' preferred methods of reimbursement, and are more inclusive in their network composition.[5]

However, many argue that the unrestrictive nature of PPOs would benefit from moderation. PPOs operate on an FFS basis, thus generating revenue from services or procedures. This system may allow for potential abuse, including excessive use of health care to generate a profit. PPO networks are generally laissez-faire when it comes to the health care decisions of the providers and may exacerbate the issue of cost and sustainability. Providers can freely make health care decisions that can lead to excessive use of health care resources.

PPOs AND DERMATOLOGY

As of 1995, patients enrolled in a PPO accounted for 60% of the care provided by dermatologists to managed care patients.[7] This number has likely increased considering the greater prevalence of PPOs covering US employees since 1995 (**Fig. 2**). **Table 1** reveals that for HMO subscribers, 14% of common skin complaints are seen by a dermatologist, whereas 31% of these complaints are seen by a nondermatologist. In contrast, PPO subscribers comprise 22% of such visits to dermatologists, and only 8% to non-dermatologists. The difference in accessing dermatologic care between HMO patients and PPO patients could be attributed to the inclusive and easy-to-access PPO physician networks or the restrictive nature of HMOs in their referrals to specialty care.[7]

Despite the number of dermatologists seeing PPO patients, there still seems to be some friction between dermatologists and managed care organizations. The problems causing this friction may not be entirely relevant to PPOs, which are less restrictive by nature; however, the problems are prevalent when comparing a dermatologist in a PPO network with a dermatologist in private practice. Dermatologists have reported problems when trying to seek separate reimbursement for certain surgical procedures that are performed as part of a regular office visit.[8] Reimbursement issues surrounding bundled payments may present a fundamental flaw with respect to the successful integration of dermatology into a managed care situation. If there are reimbursement difficulties for in-office procedures, many

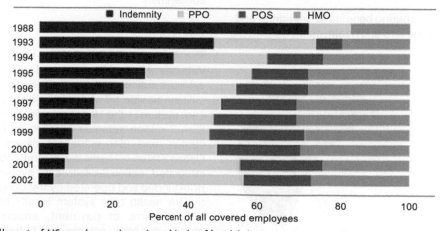

Fig. 2. Enrollment of US employees in various kinds of health benefit arrangements, selected years 1988 to 2002. (*From* Hurley RE, Strunk BC, White JS. The puzzling popularity of the PPO. Health Aff (Millwood) 2004;23(2): 56–68; with permission.)

Table 1
Number of visits (millions) and percentage distribution for common skin complaints to dermatologists and nondermatologists compared

Type of Payment	Dermatologists (n [millions] [%])	Nondermatologists (n [millions] [%])
PPO	3.4 (22)	1.6 (8)
HMO	2.2 (14)	6.1 (31)
Medicare	2.7 (17)	2.8 (14)
Medicaid	0.3 (2)	1.5 (8)
Commercial insurance	3.3 (21)	4.6 (24)
Other	3.7 (24)	2.9 (15)
Total	15.6	19.6

Data from Stern RS. Managed care and the treatment of skin disease, 1995. Continued growth and emerging dominance. Arch Dermatol 1998;134(9):1089–91.

dermatologists may not choose to be a part of a PPO network.

However, in examining this same predicament from a different vantage point, one notices a different problem. If dermatologists are allowed full reimbursement for office surgical procedures with minimal restriction, as is characteristic of a PPO, this could cause the health care system to incur unnecessary costs. With certain restriction, physicians may be more likely to use these procedures more discriminately, thereby preventing unnecessary use of services.

In addition, **Fig. 3** displays the frequency with which dermatologists deviate from the managed care prescription drug formulary. Their deviation is a reflection of the restrictive nature of the formulary. There is clearly dissatisfaction with the managed care system. It is not universally well received by dermatologists.[8]

AREAS FOR IMPROVEMENT: PPOs AND DERMATOLOGY

PPOs offer cost-sharing benefits to providers, and, as a result, purchasers and health care subscribers can enjoy health care at a more affordable cost. Given that 60% of managed care patients seen by dermatologists in 1995 were enrolled in a PPO, it seems that PPO patients have not needed additional incentive to access dermatologic care. Furthermore, a larger percentage of US employees were covered under a PPO in 2002 than 1995 (exhibit 1) thus it can be reasonably hypothesized that the number of PPO patients accessing dermatologic care has also increased. Regulating the amount and type of care that is given may control 1 unflattering aspect of PPOs: their inability to successfully contain costs.[5] These increased measures to manage care not only help control costs, but may also give preferred provider networks more influence in quality improvement. Networks can make demands of providers that result in better outcomes for patients. This method of action may cause PPO networks to resemble HMOs in many ways, but ideally PPOs will continue to provide choice and flexibility and become more efficient and focused on quality and cost containment.

THE VHA

The VHA was established by the US Department of Veterans Affairs (VA) to provide health care for veterans suffering from conditions related to their military service.[9] The VHA is the largest health care system in the United States, caring for more than 8 million veterans enrolled in 138 medical centers and 909 outpatient clinics within the United States.[10,11] This is a centrally administered, integrated, national health care system. Although both funded and operated by the US government, the VA health care system mostly refrains from FFS systems of payment, endorsing better care over high volume of better-reimbursed services.[9,12] The main aim of the VHA is to provide health care to eligible veterans to improve their

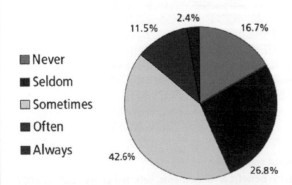

■ Never
■ Seldom
□ Sometimes
■ Often
■ Always

2.4%
11.5%
16.7%
42.6%
26.8%

Fig. 3. Frequency of deviation by dermatologists from prescription formulary.

health and functional status, with a focus on service-connected conditions (those related to their military service). Because of the influx of veterans and growing cost of the VA health care system, the US Congress limited VA medical care to veterans with low socioeconomic status or those with a service-connected condition. These prerequisites to care account for the higher level of comorbidities and lower socioeconomic status in the VA population.[9] In the United States, the VA health system provides medical care to more than 65,000 homeless persons each year, making the VA the largest provider of care to this population.[9] Whereas Medicare and Medicaid must be funded in accordance with the number of beneficiaries, the VA system may be funded at a level chosen by Congress.[9] In an effort to improve overall health care value, the VA has been divided into 21 veterans integrated service networks (VISNs), each made up of 7 to 10 VA hospitals, 25 to 30 ambulatory care clinics, several nursing homes, and counseling centers.[9] VISNs allow this federally run health care system to have a decentralized structure by promoting accountability and effectiveness at the most appropriate management level. Community-based outpatient clinics were created to provide better continuity of care with more convenient points of access for veterans. In addition, the National Formulary was instituted for prescription, nonprescription medicines, and medical supplies. Veterans rated their satisfaction with their health care services a score of 79 on the American Customer Satisfaction Index versus a score of 70 for private-sector hospitals.[9] Patients from the VA scored higher compared with their community colleague care systems in adjusted overall quality (67% vs 51%), chronic disease care (72% vs 59%), and preventive care (64% vs 44%), but not for acute care (53% vs 55%).[13,14] Health care policy should acknowledge the improved ability of the VA health system to provide quality care at lower costs and should focus efforts on incentivizing other providers in all health care systems to adopt these practices (**Fig. 4**).[10]

The VA dermatology specialty care clinics encompass clinics in general dermatology, dermatologic surgery, melanoma screening, chronic skin disease, and phototherapy.

The nationwide centralization of the VA health care system allows for comprehensive comparative effectiveness research, a tool to providing

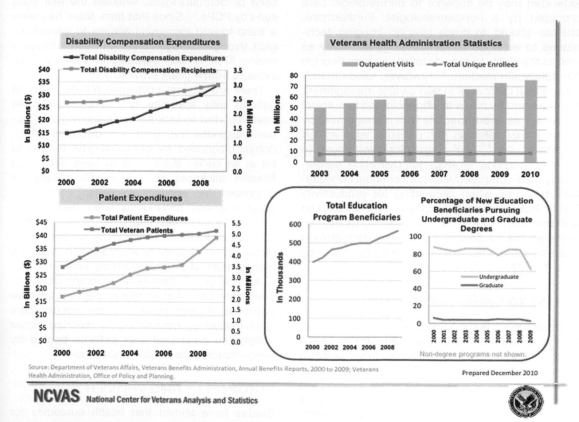

Fig. 4. Trends in the use of VA programs and services. (*From* United States Office of Veterans Affairs. National Center for Veterans Analysis and Statistics. Available at: http://www.va.gov/vetdata/Quick_Facts.asp.)

a high value of patient-centered medical care.[12] This large network's research products have the benefit of generalizability to other health care systems.[12,14] The VHA has undertaken the mission to evaluate teledermatology as a method of providing broader and faster access to a dermatologist for enrolled veterans. Results of this primary effort have revealed that the diagnostic accuracy of an in-person dermatology visit (usual care) is 5% to 19% better than teledermatology.[15] When teledermatologists with dermatoscopy training are included, the diagnostic accuracy improves for circumscribed skin lesions, although it still does not exceed usual care. Whereas store-and-forward (SAF) teledermatology is currently more widely used in the VA, live interactive teledermatology may have better diagnostic and management concordance with usual care.[15] Although overall management accuracy was equivalent for both SAF teledermatology and usual care, the former showed significantly lower accuracy for malignant skin lesions (eg, squamous cell carcinoma, basal cell carcinoma, and melanoma). Although this study has suggested gaps between teledermatology and in-person care, teledermatology (by a dermatologist or dermatology physician extender) may be superior to dermatologic care provided by a nondermatologist. Furthermore, studies should examine specific imaging techniques to enhance teledermatology accuracy as well as the ability to provide follow-up care through this telehealth medium.[15] However; teledermatology clinical outcomes in skin cancer management as measured by times to diagnosis and to surgical treatment were comparable with management by conventional referrals for patients with limited access to care.[16] SAF dermatology was found to be a cost-saving strategy for delivering dermatology care compared with conventional consultation methods, when accounting for productivity loss.[16] Patients reported relatively high satisfaction with teledermatology.[15] Further research is needed to determine the best way to provide dermatology in areas without access to in-person dermatology care (**Fig. 5**).

ACCESS TO DERMATOLOGY CARE

Dermatologists responding to a survey conducted by the American Academy of Dermatology (AAD) in 2009 reported that 35% of their practice revenue is from private FFS, 31% from Medicare FFS (traditional Medicare), 12% from Medicare HMO, 7% from self-pay medical and surgical patients, 7% from self-pay cosmetic patients, 4% from Tricare, and 3% from Medicaid.[17] In 1990, about one-third of skin disease visits were

Flow of clinical care

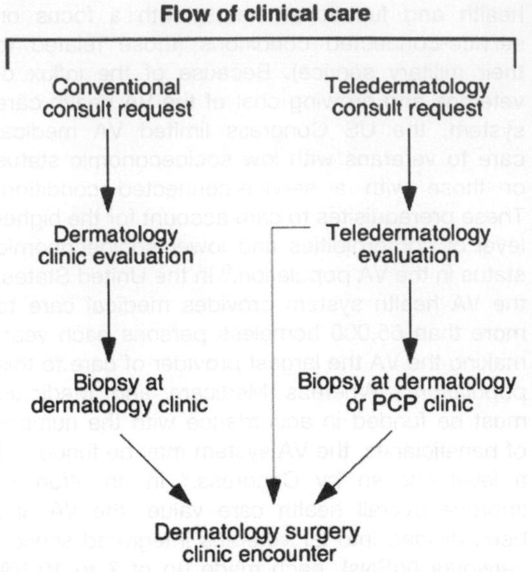

Fig. 5. Flow of clinical care. (*Data from* Solberg L. Lessons for non-VA care delivery systems from the U.S. Department of Veterans Affairs Quality Enhancement Research Initiative: QUERI Series. Implement Sci 2009;4:9.)

seen by dermatologists, whereas the rest were seen by PCPs.[18] Since that time, there has been a trend toward increasing access to dermatologists through managed care, with dermatologists seeing 37% of skin diseases in 1994, a slight increase from 4 years previously.[19]

There are several postulates for the influx of patients into specialty practices. PCPs have been reported to lack sufficient training to effectively diagnose and treat skin disorders. Melanomas diagnosed by dermatologists tended to be at an earlier stage, and to have decreased Breslow thickness compared with melanomas diagnosed by nondermatologists.[20] Moreover, patients whose melanomas were detected by dermatologists had improved survival rates compared with their peers seen by nondermatologists. Other studies have reaffirmed that the management of skin diseases by nondermatologists is not so effective as by dermatologists.[21–24] There may also be an increased desire to improve patient satisfaction. Patients whose skin disorders were treated by dermatologists reported higher satisfaction compared with patients treated by nondermatologists for skin disorders.[25]

OUTCOMES OF HMO VERSUS FFS

Studies have shown that health outcomes for patients with HMO coverage may be better than for those with FFS coverage, especially with regard to melanoma outcomes. Certain cancers, including melanoma, female breast, cervix, and prostate, were diagnosed at an earlier stage for enrollees of Medicare HMO compared with Medicare FFS.[26] Another study similarly showed that patients in Medicare HMO plans had their melanomas diagnosed at an earlier stage compared with patients enrolled in Medicare FFS.[27] Specifically, 32.1% of melanoma cases were diagnosed at the in situ stage for Medicare HMO patients, compared with 23.5% among Medicare FFS patients. Moreover, patients in Medicare HMOs had increased survival compared with the Medicare FFS cohort; median survival was an extra 26 months. This improvement in survival disappeared when controlling for stage at diagnosis, suggesting that the extended survival was a result of diagnosis at an earlier stage rather than an inherent advantage of Medicare HMO treatment methods.

Earlier diagnosis and increased survival in HMO patients may be a result of the HMO effect, in which patients in HMOs are more likely to visit their PCPs on a regular basis, thus allowing for increased screening opportunities.[22] The improved survival of HMO patients compared with FFS patients was seen only when melanoma was the patient's first diagnosed cancer. For patients who had a previous history of cancer, there were no differences in stage at diagnosis or survival between HMO and FFS patients. One explanation for this phenomenon is that patients who have a previous history of cancer may be more vigilant in screening for melanoma regardless of whether they are in an HMO or FFS system, thus negating any early diagnosis advantages that an HMO system had. That no improvement in survival was seen once the likelihood of early diagnosis was equalized may further imply that HMOs do not have inherently superior treatment modalities compared with FFS.

However, a different study showed that non-Hispanic whites with melanomas as a second or later cancer diagnosis still had their melanomas diagnosed at an earlier stage in HMO plans compared with FFS.[28] This finding suggests that HMOs have superior detection methods compared with FFS that cannot be fully compensated for by increased patient vigilance. Although Hispanic patients were more likely to have their melanomas diagnosed at an earlier stage with an HMO versus FFS, the earlier diagnosis was not associated with increased survival.

IMPROVING DERMATOLOGY CARE

With conflicting data regarding patient outcomes in HMO and FFS systems, it is difficult to construct definitive guidelines for improving dermatologic care. Nonetheless, there are broad trends that may elucidate methods to improve patient outcomes. Physician supply has been shown to positively correlate with improved skin disease outcomes. A retrospective study of more than 1500 cases of melanoma diagnosed in 1994 showed that each additional dermatologist per 10,000 population was associated with a 39% increased odds of early diagnosis.[29] The same investigators also showed that each additional dermatologist per 100,000 population was associated with a reduction in melanoma mortality by 0.19 cases per 100,000.[30] A similar trend for diagnosis and mortality existed for family physicians, although to a lesser degree. However, an increase in the number of general internists was associated with a later stage of melanoma diagnosis, and worse survival. The difference in outcomes between family physicians and general internists may be a result of family physicians' more extensive training in dermatology and dermatologic procedures compared with general internists.[31,32] Although there is debate regarding the ability of PCPs to significantly improve dermatologic outcomes, it is clear that increasing the number of dermatologists leads to better outcomes for patients with skin diseases.[20,21,23,24,33–35]

SUPPLY AND DEMAND

Demand for dermatologists has remained high and unmet, whereas supply has not changed.[36] The demand can be accounted for via several factors, including the growing and aging population,[37] the increasing incidence of various skin diseases, such as atopic dermatitis, melanoma, and nonmelanoma cutaneous malignancies,[38–40] and the easing of access to dermatologists by managed care programs.[41] The supply of dermatologists has consistently remained less than demand.[42,43] A lack of significant expansion of dermatology training programs for the past 3 decades has caused the number of dermatologists to remain stagnant at about 10,600, or 3.6 per 100,000 population.[44] Although some dermatology residency programs have increased the number of admittances, others have closed completely, such that there was a net decline of residency spots from 2007 to 2008.[45]

In 2007, 33% of dermatology practices were actively seeking to hire a new associate, and 30% of practices employed physician assistants (PAs) or NPs.[36] Moreover, there has been a broadening scope toward cosmetic and surgical dermatology, which further decreases the availability of noncosmetic and nonsurgical dermatologic care.[46] Given the undersupply of dermatologists in the United States, and a positive correlation between the number of dermatologists and patient outcomes, efforts should be made to expand the quantity of annual dermatology trainees.

Although there is a clear trend of improved skin cancer outcomes when diagnosed by dermatologists, and with increasing numbers of dermatologists, the health care outcomes of skin diseases when treated by nondermatologists are not so tangible. In addition to increasing and standardizing the education of skin diseases among nondermatologists, there should be a concurrent movement to educate the public about skin cancer, as well as increasing the number of medical students admitted to dermatology residency programs. Through this 3-pronged approach, there is promise that dermatologic health outcomes will improve.

INCREASING PATIENT AWARENESS

Lack of patient awareness of skin cancer risks, especially among minority populations, has been associated with later-stage diagnosis and worse prognosis of skin cancers.[47] Moreover, a recent survey showed that a significantly smaller percentage of minorities have had a full-body skin examination performed by a physician, perform self-skin examinations, or apply sunscreen, compared with whites.[48] Among all races, most adults in the United States do not practice adequate sun protection,[49] yet ultraviolet radiation exposure is the most important modifiable risk factor for all skin cancers.[50] Moreover, patients who are more knowledgeable and aware of melanoma tend to seek out medical treatment sooner, and to have thinner lesions at diagnosis.[36,51–53] Patient delay in seeking out treatment has been proposed as the most important factor in preventing early diagnosis of melanoma.[54,55] Other studies have shown that workers at risk for noncancerous occupational skin disorders, such as contact dermatitis and eczema, lack knowledge of the risks and preventive measures of these skin disorders.[56–58] Given the public's insufficient awareness of the risks and preventive measures of a wide spectrum of skin diseases, including melanoma, nonmelanoma cutaneous cancers, and noncancerous skin disorders, it is recommended that public health efforts increase to educate communities about skin safety practices. Increasing patient education of chronic skin diseases (eg, psoriasis and actinic dermatitis) through helping the patient understand the specific disease, ways for self-management, and techniques of coping have been shown to increase the quality of life of the patient, as well as reduce the severity of the skin condition.[59] Public health efforts should also be tailored toward specific populations. In the state of California, the disease burden of melanoma among Hispanics is higher compared with non-Hispanic whites, a result of linguistic barriers, less awareness of risks and symptoms, and differing melanoma patterns.[60] Patient education may thus be an additional component toward improving overall health outcomes.

INCREASING TRAINING OF NONDERMATOLOGISTS

Most physicians have limited exposure to dermatology during medical school and residency.[61–63] With numerous studies showing that nondermatologists lack sufficient training and knowledge in diagnosing and managing skin disease,[21,23,33,34,64,65] it is important to improve dermatology education among PCPs. A recent survey has shown that PCPs are increasingly interested in medical education with regard to skin cancer.[66] The use of dermoscopy as part of PCP residency training has recently been implemented, and studies have shown that PCPs have increased diagnostic accuracy with the use of dermoscopy in triaging suspicious lesions.[67,68] There has also been a rapid increase in the availability of online continuing medical education (CME) programs, although the lack of standardization has made the effectiveness of such programs difficult to evaluate.[69–71] An evaluation of 20 different educational training programs designed for PCPs showed that most were able to significantly improve knowledge, competence, confidence, diagnostic performance, or systems outcomes.[72] Although numerous programs have suggested improved effectiveness of PCPs in diagnosing skin diseases after undergoing educational programs, many of the programs are highly diverse in their teaching techniques, and results have varied. There may be a role for implementation of a standardized, robust training program across primary care residencies.[16]

PHYSICIAN EXTENDERS

The increasing wait times and shortage in the dermatology workforce have created the need for physician extenders in dermatology practices.[43,73] Physician extenders are nonphysician clinicians such as NPs, PAs, and aestheticians.[74] NPs are registered nurses often with a master's degree, who may practice without physician supervision and with prescriptive authority. PAs generally complete a 2-year training program, require physician supervision, and may have limited prescriptive authority. Nursing and medical state boards regulate NPs and PAs, respectively. Aestheticians are not considered an extension of medical practice, and are regulated by state boards of cosmetology.[74] Nearly all physician extenders (99%) see established patients with stable conditions, but 77% reported also seeing new patients (**Table 2**).[74] Only 10% of dermatologists reported that their physician extenders received formal dermatology training, but more than one-half reported that they had some dermatology rotation in their respective training schools. Most physician extenders were specialty-trained in the office or at external lectures.[74] The AAD recommends that dermatologists provide on-site supervision to physician extenders and personally see new patients as well as any established patients with significant new problems.[74] The Florida House Bill 699 requires that only a board-certified dermatologist or plastic surgeon can

supervise off-site PAs and NPs engaged in dermatology or skin care services. From July 1, 2011 such supervision was limited to 1 office within 25 miles of the physician's primary place of practice or in a contiguous county.

Although certain gaps in the dermatology workforce are being addressed by the growing population of physician extenders, the number of dermatologists has not experienced a similar boom (**Fig. 6**). The supply of dermatologists is limited by the availability of dermatology residency training positions, particularly by Medicare's freezing of funds to create more residency spots, emphasis on expanding the primary care trainee programs, and the decreased focus of hospitals to support trainees in an almost entirely outpatient specialty.[73]

WAIT TIMES

Secondary to the dermatology workforce shortage, dermatologic care delivery has been significantly

Table 2
The role of physician extenders

Patient types seen by physician extenders and frequency of formal presentation of patient to physician during extender visit

	Respondents Whose Extenders See This Patient Type (%)	Mean Percentage of Patient Type Formally Presented to Physician During Extender Visit (%)[a]
New patients	77	46
Established patients with new problems	85	36
Established patients with worsening existing problems	73	53
Established patients with stable existing problems	99	25

Physician extender practice characteristics among general dermatologists vs surgically or cosmetically focused dermatologists

	Mean Reported Extender Percentage Time Spent with:		
	Medical Dermatology Patients (%)	Surgical Dermatology Patients (%)	Cosmetic Dermatology Patients (%)
General dermatologists with extenders[b]	83	9	8
Surgically or cosmetically focused dermatologists with extenders[c]	72	18	10

Respondents who did not report both data on their own patient care hours and those of their extenders were excluded from this analysis.
[a] Among respondents whose extenders see this patient type.
[b] General dermatologists were defined as those with greater than 50% of their patient care hours in medical dermatology.
[c] Surgically or cosmetically focused dermatologists were defined as those with 50% or more of their patient care hours in cosmetic and surgical dermatology combined.

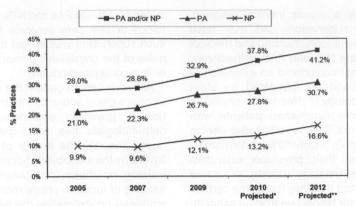

Fig. 6. Projected trends in employment of physician extenders by type of extender. (*Data from* Kostecki J. American Academy of Dermatology Association's dermatology practice profile survey 2009 report. Schaumburg (IL): 2009.)

affected, as reflected in growing wait times for patient appointments.[73] When benchmarks wait times were set at 3 weeks for a new patient appointment and 2 weeks for an established patient appointment, 1 study demonstrated that more than 60% of dermatologists exceeded these criteria. Responding dermatologists reported median wait times of 35 days for a new patient appointment and 25 days for a return patient.[73] Dermatologists also reported seeing an average of 160 patients and spending 35 hours seeing patients each week. Both new patient and established patient wait times were significantly lower in areas with "just enough" or "too many" dermatologists versus those areas with "too few dermatologists".[73]

MALPRACTICE

Although professional liability premiums for dermatologists are lower than those of high-risk specialties, these payments have mimicked the increase in medicine as a whole. Median premiums were highest for practices with more than 10% cosmetics ($10,200 vs $8,215 for noncosmetics) and for those with more than 30% in noncosmetic surgery ($9,584 vs $8,233 for <30%).[73] Premiums were also higher in American Medical Association-defined "crisis states," and in those with state liability caps more than $250,000 in place.

ROLE OF PHARMACEUTICALS

Dermatologic drug development has fallen behind those for other fields such as oncology, cardiology, and neurology. Although cutting-edge research using combinatorial chemistry, ultrahigh-throughout screening, genomics, proteomics, and recombinant DNA technologies is being used to develop drugs in various specialties, large pharmaceuticals have for

the most part ignored dermatology. The goal of multinational pharmaceutical corporations is to produce blockbuster drugs, those that may attain peak annual sales of $1 billion or more. In dermatology, it is more difficult to find blockbusters. Large companies with proper resources to develop advanced drugs may choose to ignore dermatology, whereas smaller companies who may have the

List of Acronyms	
AAD	American Academy of Dermatology
AMA	American Medical Association
CBOC	Community-based outpatient clinic
CME	Continuing Medical Education
DA	Direct access
FFS	Fee-for-service
GA	Gatekeeper
HMO	Health Maintenance Organization
LI	Live interactive [teledermatology]
NP	Nurse practitioner
OSD	Occupational skin disorder
PA	Physician assistant
PCP	Primary care physician
PPACA	Patient Protection and Affordable Care Act
PPO	Preferred Provider Organization
SAF	Store-and-forward [teledermatology]
SES	Socioeconomic status
UV	Ultraviolet
VA	Veterans Affairs [health system]
VAMC	Veterans Affairs Medical Center
VHA	Veterans Health Administration
VISN	Veterans Integrated Service Network

desire do not have the resources. Dermatologic drug innovation has thus stagnated, and the current lines of therapy often use the same targets or general mechanisms of action as previous drugs.[75]

SUMMARY

The United States has a dynamic health care system with a variety of approaches to dermatologic care. Outcomes among PPOs, HMOs, FFS, and VAMC are comparable and are improved with increasing supply of dermatologists. Our diversity in care also provides us with the unique opportunity to work to incorporate successful strategies from each system to best manage skin disease.

REFERENCES

1. Official Medicare Website. May 13, 2011. Available at: http://www.medicare.gov. Accessed June 15, 2011.
2. Medicare and You handbook 2012. Centers for Medicare & Medicaid Services. Available at: http://www.medicare.gov/Publications/Pubs/pdf/10050.pdf. Accessed September 7, 2011.
3. AARP Medicare Website. May 13, 2011. Available at: http://aarp.org/health/medicare-insurance/. Accessed June 15, 2011.
4. Gabel J, Ermann D. Preferred provider organizations: performance, problems, and promise. Health Aff (Millwood) 1985;4(1):24–40.
5. Hurley RE, Strunk BC, White JS. The puzzling popularity of the PPO. Health Aff (Millwood) 2004;23(2):56–68.
6. Resneck JS Jr. An analysis of health system reform for dermatologists: elements and implications of the Patient Protection and Affordable Care Act. J Am Acad Dermatol 2010;63(4).706–15.
7. Stern RS. Managed care and the treatment of skin disease, 1995. Continued growth and emerging dominance. Arch Dermatol 1998;134(9):1089–91.
8. Scheinfeld N, Jesitus J, Sonnenreich P. At a glance: dermatology trends in managed care. P T 2008;33(6):365–7.
9. Kizer KW, Dudley RA. Extreme makeover: transformation of the veterans health care system. Annu Rev Public Health 2009;30:313–39.
10. Gao J, Moran E, Almenoff P, et al. Variations in efficiency and the relationship to quality of care in the veterans health system. Health Aff (Millwood) 2011;30(4):655–63.
11. 2010. Available at: http://www.va.gov. Accessed June 15, 2011.
12. Atkins D, Kupersmith J, Eisen S. The Veterans Affairs experience: comparative effectiveness research in a large health system. Health Aff (Millwood) 2010;29(10):1906–12.
13. Asch SM, McGlynn E, Hogan M, et al. Comparison of quality of care for patients in the Veterans Health Administration and patients in a national sample. Ann Intern Med 2004;141(12):938–45.
14. Solberg L. Lessons for non-VA care delivery systems from the U.S. Department of Veterans Affairs Quality Enhancement Research Initiative: QUERI Series. Implement Sci 2009;4:9.
15. Warshaw EM, Greer N, Hillman Y, et al. Teledermatology for diagnosis and management of skin conditions: a systematic review. J Am Acad Dermatol 2011;64(4):759–72.
16. Pak HS, Datta S, Triplett C, et al. Cost minimization analysis of a store-and-forward teledermatology consult system. Telemed J E Health 2009;15(2):160–5.
17. Kostecki J. American Academy of Dermatology Association's dermatology practice profile survey 2009 report. Schaumburg (IL): 2009.
18. Thompson TT, Feldman SR, Fleischer AB Jr. Only 33% of visits for skin disease in the US in 1995 were to dermatologists: is decreasing the number of dermatologists the appropriate response? Dermatol Online J 1998;4(1):3.
19. Feldman SR, Fleischer AB Jr, Williford PM, et al. Increasing utilization of dermatologists by managed care: an analysis of the National Ambulatory Medical Care Survey, 1990-1994. J Am Acad Dermatol 1997;37(5 Pt 1):784–8.
20. Pennie ML, Soon SL, Risser JB, et al. Melanoma outcomes for Medicare patients: association of stage and survival with detection by a dermatologist vs a nondermatologist. Arch Dermatol 2007;143(4):488–94.
21. Chen SC, Pennie ML, Kolm P, et al. Diagnosing and managing cutaneous pigmented lesions: primary care physicians versus dermatologists. J Gen Intern Med 2006;21(7):678–82.
22. Morrison A, O'Loughlin S, Powell FC. Suspected skin malignancy: a comparison of diagnoses of family practitioners and dermatologists in 493 patients. Int J Dermatol 2001;40(2):104–7.
23. Chen SC, Bravata DM, Weil E, et al. A comparison of dermatologists' and primary care physicians' accuracy in diagnosing melanoma: a systematic review. Arch Dermatol 2001;137(12):1627–34.
24. Carli P, De Giorgi V, Palli D, et al. Dermatologist detection and skin self-examination are associated with thinner melanomas: results from a survey of the Italian Multidisciplinary Group on Melanoma. Arch Dermatol 2003;139(5):607–12.
25. Owen SA, Maeyens E, Weary PE. Patients' opinions regarding direct access to dermatologic specialty care. J Am Acad Dermatol 1997;36(2):250–6.
26. Riley GF, Potosky AL, Lubitz JD, et al. Stage of cancer at diagnosis for Medicare HMO and fee-for-service enrollees. Am J Public Health 1994;84(10):1598–604.

27. Kirsner RS, Wilkinson JD, Ma F, et al. The association of Medicare health care delivery systems with stage at diagnosis and survival for patients with melanoma. Arch Dermatol 2005;141(6):753–7.

28. Rouhani P, Arheart KL, Kirsner RS. Differences in melanoma outcomes among Hispanic Medicare enrollees. J Am Acad Dermatol 2010;62(5):768–76.

29. Roetzheim RG, Pal N, van Durme DJ, et al. Increasing supplies of dermatologists and family physicians are associated with earlier stage of melanoma detection. J Am Acad Dermatol 2000;43(2): 211–8.

30. van Durme DJ, Ullman R, Campbell RJ, et al. Effects of physician supply on melanoma incidence and mortality in Florida. Southern Medical Journal 2003; 96(7):656–60.

31. Jones TP, Boiko PE, Piepkorn MW. Skin biopsy indications in primary care practice: a population-based study. J Am Board Fam Pract 1996;9(6): 397–404.

32. Boiko PE, Koepsell TD, Larson EB, et al. Skin cancer diagnosis in a primary care setting. J Am Acad Dermatol 1996;34(4):608–11.

33. Ramsay DL, Fox AB. The ability of primary care physicians to recognize the common dermatoses. Arch Dermatol 1981;117(10):620–2.

34. Mccarthy GM, Lamb GC, Russell TH, et al. Primary care based dermatology practice–internists need more training. J Gen Intern Med 1991;6(1):52–6.

35. Cassileth BR, Clark WH Jr, Lusk EJ, et al. How well do physicians recognize melanoma and other problem lesions? J Am Acad Dermatol 1986;14(4): 555–60.

36. Kimball AB, Resneck JS. The US dermatology workforce: a specialty remains in shortage. J Am Acad Dermatol 2008;59(5):741–5.

37. Kosmadaki MG, Gilchrest BA. The demographics of aging in the United States–implications for dermatology. Arch Dermatol 2002;138(11):1427–8.

38. Thestrup-Pedersen K. Atopic eczema: what has caused the epidemic in industrialized countries and can early intervention modify the natural history of atopic eczema? J Cosmet Dermatol 2003;2:9.

39. Jemal A, Saraiya M, Patel P, et al. Recent trends in cutaneous melanoma incidence among whites in the United States. J Natl Cancer Inst 2001;93(9):678–83.

40. Rogers HW, Weinstock MA, Harris AR, et al. Incidence estimate of nonmelanoma skin cancer in the United States, 2006. Arch Dermatol 2010;146(3): 283–7.

41. Ferris TG, Chang Y, Blumenthal D, et al. Leaving gatekeeping behind–effects of opening access to specialists for adults in a health maintenance organization. N Engl J Med 2001;345(18):1312–7.

42. Resneck J Jr. Too few or too many dermatologists? Difficulties in assessing optimal workforce size. Arch Dermatol 2001;137(10):1295–301.

43. Resneck J Jr, Kimball AB. The dermatology workforce shortage. J Am Acad Dermatol 2004;50(1):50–4.

44. Smart D. Physician characteristics and distribution in the US. USA: AMA Press; 2007.

45. Education ACfGM. Accredited Program List. May 13, 2011. Available at: http://www.acgme.org/adspublic/reports/accredited_programs.asp?accredited=1. Accessed June 15, 2011.

46. Kimball AB. Dermatology: a unique case of specialty workforce economics. J Am Acad Dermatol 2003; 48(2):265–70.

47. Pipitone M, Robinson JK, Camara C, et al. Skin cancer awareness in suburban employees: a Hispanic perspective. J Am Acad Dermatol 2002;47(1):118–23.

48. Imahiyerobo-Ip J, Ip I, Jamal S, et al. Skin cancer awareness in communities of color. J Am Acad Dermatol 2011;64(1):198–200.

49. Santmyire BR, Feldman SR, Fleischer AB Jr. Lifestyle high-risk behaviors and demographics may predict the level of participation in sun-protection behaviors and skin cancer primary prevention in the United States: results of the 1998 National Health Interview Survey. Cancer 2001;92(5):1315–24.

50. Armstrong B. How sun exposure causes skin cancer: an epidemiological perspective. In: Prevention of Skin Cancer. Boston: Kluwer Academic Publishers; 2004. p. 89–116.

51. Richard MA, Grob JJ, Avril MF, et al. Delays in diagnosis and melanoma prognosis (I): the role of patients. Int J Cancer 2000;89(3):271–9.

52. Schmid-Wendtner MH, Baumert J, Stange J, et al. Delay in the diagnosis of cutaneous melanoma: an analysis of 233 patients. Melanoma Res 2002; 12(4):389–94.

53. Rampen FH, Rumke P, Hart AA. Patients' and doctors' delay in the diagnosis and treatment of cutaneous melanoma. Eur J Surg Oncol 1989; 15(2):143–8.

54. Temoshok L, DiClemente RJ, Sweet DM, et al. Factors related to patient delay in seeking medical attention for cutaneous malignant melanoma. Cancer 1984;54(12):3048–53.

55. Krige JE, Isaacs S, Hudson DA, et al. Delay in the diagnosis of cutaneous malignant melanoma. A prospective study in 250 patients. Cancer 1991; 68(9):2064–8.

56. Schwanitz HJ, Riehl U, Schlesinger T, et al. Skin care management: educational aspects. Int Arch Occup Environ Health 2003;76(5):374–81.

57. Berndt U, Wigger-Alberti W. Efficacy of a barrier cream and its vehicle as protective measures against occupational irritant contact dermatitis. Contact Dermatitis 2000;42(2):77–80.

58. Itschner L, Hinnen U, Elsner P. Prevention of hand eczema in the metal-working industry: risk awareness and behaviour of metal worker apprentices. Dermatology 1996;193(3):226–9.

59. de Bes J, Legierse CM, Prinsen CA, et al. Patient education in chronic skin diseases: a systematic review. Acta Derm Venereol 2011;91(1):12–7.

60. Pollitt RA, Clarke CA, Swetter SM, et al. The expanding melanoma burden in California hispanics: importance of socioeconomic distribution, histologic subtype, and anatomic location. Cancer 2011;117(1):152–61.

61. Wise E, Singh D, Moore M, et al. Rates of skin cancer screening and prevention counseling by US medical residents. Arch Dermatol 2009;145(10):1131–6.

62. Moore MM, Geller AC, Zhang Z, et al. Skin cancer examination teaching in US medical education. Arch Dermatol 2006;142(4):439–44.

63. Little JM Jr, Hall MN, Pettice YJ. Teaching dermatology: too dependent on dermatologists? Fam Med 1993;25(2):92–4.

64. Gerbert B, Maurer T, Berger T. Primary care physicians as gatekeepers in managed care. Primary care physicians' and dermatologists' skills at secondary prevention of skin cancer. Arch Dermatol 1996;132:1030–8.

65. Feldman SR, Fleischer AB Jr. Skin examinations and skin cancer prevention counseling by US physicians: a long way to go. J Am Acad Dermatol 2000;43(2 Pt 1):234–7.

66. Anderson RT, Dziak K, McBride J, et al. Demand for continuing medical education programs on cancer care among primary care physicians in North Carolina. N C Med J 2004;65(3):130–5.

67. Argenziano G, Puig S, Zalaudek I, et al. Dermoscopy improves accuracy of primary care physicians to triage lesions suggestive of skin cancer. J Clin Oncol 2006;24(12):1877–82.

68. Dolianitis C, Kelly J, Wolfe R, et al. Comparative performance of 4 dermoscopic algorithms by nonexperts for the diagnosis of melanocytic lesions. Arch Dermatol 2005;141(8):1008–14.

69. Casebeer L, Kristofco R, Strasser S. Standardizing evaluation of online continuing medical education: physician knowledge, attitudes, and reflection on practice. J Contin Educ Health Prof 2004;24:68–75.

70. Curran VR, Fleet L. A review of evaluation outcomes of web-based continuing medical education. Med Educ 2005;39(6):561–7.

71. Durbec F, Vitry F, Granel-Brocard F, et al. The role of circumstances of diagnosis and access to dermatological care in early diagnosis of cutaneous melanoma: a population-based study in France. Arch Dermatol 2010;146(3):240–6.

72. Goulart JM, Quigley EA, Dusza S, et al. Skin cancer education for primary care physicians: a systematic review of published evaluated interventions. J Gen Intern Med 2011;26(9):1027–35.

73. Suneja T, Smith ED, Chen GJ, et al. Waiting times to see a dermatologist are perceived as too long by dermatologists: implications for the dermatology workforce. Arch Dermatol 2001;137(10):1303–7.

74. Resneck JS Jr, Kimball AB. Who else is providing care in dermatology practices? Trends in the use of nonphysician clinicians. J Am Acad Dermatol 2008;58(2):211–6.

75. Altman DJ. The roles of the pharmaceutical industry and drug development in dermatology and dermatologic health care. Dermatol Clin 2000;18(2):287–96.

Dermatologic Health Disparities

Kesha J. Buster, MD[a],*, Erica I. Stevens, BS[b],
Craig A. Elmets, MD[a]

KEYWORDS

- Health disparities • Dermatology • Education • Workforce
- Atopic dermatitis • Skin cancer • Research

Health disparity refers to "a chain of events signified by a difference in: (1) environment, (2) access
to, use of, and quality of care, (3) health status, or
(4) a particular health outcome that deserves scrutiny."[1] Disparities can be broad and across
a variety of demographic variables including, but
not limited to, race, age, sex, education, and
health insurance status. The 2010 US Department
of Health and Human Services National Healthcare
Disparities Report confirms substantial health
care–related barriers. The report identified access
to and quality of care as inadequate, particularly
for ethnic minorities and persons with low
income.[2] Over the 8 years that the Agency for
Healthcare Research and Quality (AHRQ) has reported on the status of health care quality and
disparities, they have observed that although
quality of care is improving, access to care and
the state of health disparities are not.[2] In collaboration with the AHRQ, the Institute of Medicine
Committee on Future Directions for the National
Healthcare Quality and Disparities Reports identified 8 national priority areas to be addressed,
including population health, safety, and access.
Evidence of health disparities across race,
ethnicity, and socioeconomic status was demonstrated for all 8 priority areas.

The paucity of and great need for data on epidemiology, natural history, clinical presentation,
complications, and treatment of specific skin
diseases in people of color has also been
highlighted recently in the dermatologic literature.[3]
According to a recent report, "empiric evidence
regarding access to and use of dermatologic
care services [in minority populations] is scant."[4]

RACE AND ETHNICITY

Race is a poorly defined term that, at times, is used
interchangeably with the term ethnicity. In practical
terms, race is a political and social construct more
than a biological phenomenon.[5] By contrast,
ethnicity refers to "...large groups of people
classed according to common racial, national,
tribal, religious, linguistic, or cultural origin or background."[6] Despite the complexities of defining race
and ethnicity, health disparities between those
who define themselves as white compared with
others clearly exist. Since 1974 the number of
office visits to dermatologists nearly doubled
(from 18 million to 36 million by 2000), and the
majority of patients seen by dermatologists are
white (92%)—whereas this number for nondermatologists is 84%.[7] The reasons for lower use of
dermatologic care by racial minorities are unclear.

For this appraisal of dermatologic health disparities, skin cancer and atopic dermatitis were
selected for review because each is relatively
common, and the association with health disparities has been examined for both diagnoses. Clearly
there are numerous other skin diseases seen
by both dermatologists and nondermatologists

Funding: Dr Buster was supported by an NIH T32 grant.
Disclosures: The authors have nothing to disclose.
[a] Department of Dermatology, University of Alabama at Birmingham, 1530 3rd Avenue, South EFH 414,
Birmingham, AL 35294, USA
[b] University of Alabama at Birmingham School of Medicine, 1530 3rd Avenue, South FOT 1203, Birmingham,
AL 35294, USA
* Corresponding author.
E-mail address: kbuster07@yahoo.com

including acne, rosacea, psoriasis, and many others, but there are few to no data on dermatologic health disparities related to those conditions. Other topics addressed in this review include health reform and the dermatologic workforce, dermatologic education, and research.

SKIN CANCER

Skin cancer morbidity and mortality are disproportionally higher in blacks, Hispanics, and people of low socioeconomic status (SES).[8–12] Melanoma is more common in non-Hispanic whites and people of high SES,[13] yet blacks, Hispanics, people of low SES,[13,14] and older-age persons often present with more advanced disease or have increased mortality.[8–10,15,16] The 5-year melanoma survival is 74.1% for blacks compared with 92.9% for whites.[16] Nonmelanoma skin cancer (NMSC) in blacks is uncommon, with an incidence of 3.4 per 100,000.[17] Despite the lower incidence of NMSC in ethnic minorities, blacks as a whole present with later stage or more aggressive squamous cell carcinomas.[9] The less educated tend to have lower skin cancer screening rates and more often have poor or inaccurate perceptions of their skin cancer risk.[18,19] Like the less educated, ethnic minorities, the elderly, and people with lower income may be more likely to have inaccurate skin cancer risk perceptions.[19] Lack of insurance and increased age also negatively affect skin cancer outcomes.[14,20]

ATOPIC DERMATITIS

The incidence of childhood eczema in the United States is approximately 10.7%.[21] Large-scale reports estimate the prevalence to be between 8.3% and 18.1%,[21–23] and it may be increasing.[24,25] Black race or multiracial background significantly correlates with eczema prevalence.[21] Similarly, black and Asian children are more often seen for the diagnosis of AD than are white children,[25,26] suggesting increased prevalence or severity of this disorder among these racial minorities. Just as increased SES is associated with higher rates of melanoma,[13,14] education beyond high school by a household member is significantly associated with the increased prevalence of eczema.[21] It is unclear whether, like skin cancer, the morbidity of atopic dermatitis is increased with decreased SES. Beyond race, urban setting, health insurance status, single-mother household, and smaller family size are also associated with increased risk of childhood eczema.[21] Presence of eczema appears to be significantly greater in the insured than in the uninsured[21]; however, one consideration is that those without insurance are often without health care access as well and thus are not diagnosed, leading to prevalence data that in all probability are an underestimate.

Multiple studies have shown that breastfeeding is associated with a reduced risk of atopic dermatitis, as well as a variety of other ailments (eg, asthma, obesity, childhood leukemia, and diabetes).[27,28] As a result, the American Academy of Pediatrics[29] and the US Surgeon General[30] have established recommendations to increase breastfeeding initiation and duration. The current level of breastfeeding costs the United States an estimated excess of $13 billion annually[28] in preventable health care costs and death. These costs hold particularly true for populations in which disparities in health care are most prevalent, including blacks, younger women, the less educated, and lower income women.[31,32] Such disparities may help to explain the increased risk of AD among some racial minorities, but conflicts with the increased rate of AD in high SES children.

HEALTH CARE REFORM AND THE DERMATOLOGY WORKFORCE

The Patient Protection and Affordability of Care Act and the Reconciliation Act was passed and signed into law in March 2010 (**Fig. 1**). Despite the varied and polarized opinions on the legislation, it is clear that some of the measures would improve health disparities. Recent figures indicate that there are more than 50 million (16.7%) uninsured persons in the United States, and this number has been increasing since 2000.[33] Ten percent of those uninsured are children (7.5 million).[33] Of the insured, 30.6% are covered by government programs such as Medicare (43.4 million) and Medicaid (47.8 million).[33] The United States economy loses $207 billion each year as a result of the poorer health and decreased lifespan of uninsured persons, and in 2008 $43 billion was spent on the uncompensated health care of the uninsured.[34] A major goal of the health care reform act is to increase insurance coverage to nearly all Americans, thereby providing cost sharing and leading to lower overall premiums. By 2014, the individual mandate for health insurance purchase by most Americans will be enforced and at that time health insurance exchanges will open. It is estimated that the number of uninsured nonelderly people will decline to 21 million within 2 years of this mandate.[35] The majority of nonelderly persons remaining uninsured will be unauthorized immigrants (approximately 30%) and those eligible for, but not

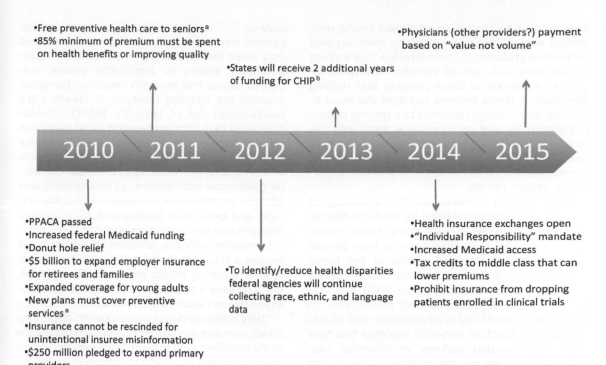

•Free preventive health care to seniors[a]
•85% minimum of premium must be spent
 on health benefits or improving quality

•States will receive 2 additional years
 of funding for CHIP[b]

•Physicians (other providers?) payment
 based on "value not volume"

2010   2011   2012   2013   2014   2015

•PPACA passed
•Increased federal Medicaid funding
•Donut hole relief
•$5 billion to expand employer insurance
 for retirees and families
•Expanded coverage for young adults
•New plans must cover preventive
 services[a]
•Insurance cannot be rescinded for
 unintentional insuree misinformation
•$250 million pledged to expand primary
 providers

•To identify/reduce health disparities
 federal agencies will continue
 collecting race, ethnic, and language
 data

•Health insurance exchanges open
•"Individual Responsibility" mandate
•Increased Medicaid access
•Tax credits to middle class that can
 lower premiums
•Prohibit insurance from dropping
 patients enrolled in clinical trials

Fig. 1. Major provisions of the Patient Protection and Affordability Care Act (PPACA). [a] This does not include skin cancer examinations. [b] CHIP, Child Health Insurance Program. (*Data from* Healthcare.gov. Understand the law. Available at: http://www.healthcare.gov. Accessed April 12, 2011.)

enrolled in Medicaid (approximately 25%).[36] The specific effects of this legislation on dermatologic health disparities are not known. The dramatic increase in insured patients would likely lead to a shift in care of previously uninsured patients from emergency rooms and urgent care centers to primary and specialty care offices. To address the increased need, the legislation dedicated $250 million to expand the primary care workforce.[37] This funding will help to some extent; however, some specialties—including dermatology—already have a shortage of providers. According to the 2009 American Academy of Dermatology (AAD) practice profile survey,[38] 38% of dermatologists report that there is a shortage of dermatologists in their community. This shortage was greatest in rural settings. Nearly one-third of survey respondents indicated that they were actively looking for another dermatologist to join their practice.[38] The average wait time for new patients was 33.9 days, and for established patients was 17.9 days.[38] These results are similar to the previous surveys done in 2007, 2005, and 2002. These shortages exist despite the fact that a majority of dermatologists' patient care time is dedicated to medical dermatology (67.1%), with only 25.1% on noncosmetic surgical dermatology and 7.8% on cosmetics.[38] The

anticipated increase in insured patients coupled with a lack of funding to expand the dermatology workforce may only worsen the current shortage. In order for dermatologists to provide a sufficient amount of dermatologic care, innovative methods to prevent excessive patient wait times and lack of access to dermatologic care are needed.

DERMATOLOGY EDUCATION AND HEALTH DISPARITIES

A variety of studies have found that medical students in the United States are exposed to very little dermatology in comparison with other clinical specialties. United States medical students receive an average of between 16 and 22 hours of dermatologic training—less than 1% of their undergraduate medical education.[39–41] Consequently, fewer than 40% of primary care residents indicate that their medical school curriculum has adequately prepared them to manage common skin conditions.[42] Similarly, a recent survey of United Kingdom students found that the majority (55.7%) believed that their undergraduate medical education did not provide adequate education in dermatology.[43]

In a recent United States survey, 47% of dermatologists and dermatology residents reported that their medical training (medical school and/or residency) was inadequate in training them on skin conditions in blacks.[44] Those who felt their training in this area was lacking identified the need for greater exposure to black patients and training materials.[44] These findings highlight the need to expose dermatology residents to a diverse patient population as well as to provide them with the didactics, textbooks, and peer-reviewed literature necessary to prepare them to address special considerations in skin of color, to prevent disparities in quality of care.

There is little research on the adequacy of current dermatologic training to produce dermatologists with cross-cultural competence, confidence, and skill in treating patients from diverse backgrounds. A PubMed search of the terms dermatology, residency, and education reveals just one published paper since 2000 that addresses residency training and ethnic skin. In that study,[45] 52.4% of chief residents and 65.9% of program directors surveyed reported that their residency provided lectures or didactics integrating ethnic skin into the curriculum. This finding and the knowledge of the growing proportion of ethnic minorities in the United States population (**Fig. 2**) underscore the need for a vigorous assessment of medical education to ensure dermatologists are adequately prepared to provide quality care to patients of diverse racial and ethnic backgrounds.

DISPARITIES IN RESEARCH

It is well known that racial and ethnic minorities have been historically underrepresented in medical research.[46–48] This situation may be a reflection of study recruitment,[49] minorities' disinterest or distrust,[48,50] lack of access,[48] or other factors. Limited minority participation in research studies may affect the applicability of clinical trial results, potentially leading to detrimental patient outcomes. Given this research disparity, Congress enacted the National Institutes of Health (NIH) Revitalization Act of 1993, PL 103-43,[51] which mandated that both women and racial minorities be represented in clinical research. The NIH defines clinical research as: (1) patient-oriented research, which includes (a) mechanisms of human disease, (b) therapeutic interventions, (c) clinical trials, and (d) development of new technologies; (2) epidemiologic and behavioral studies; and (3) outcomes research and health services research.[51]

Consistent with this, a review of the literature reveals a steady increase in dermatologic clinical studies involving ethnic minorities. By contrast, there remains a scarcity of robust basic dermatologic research examining skin of color.[3]

There is little evidence on how health disparities affect dermatologic research. A systematic review of the literature failed to identify any research citing specific barriers to subject participation in dermatologic research.[48] A study analyzing survey responses of black and white parents of pediatric dermatology patients found that black parents had significantly less trust in the medical research community ($P = .03$), were 3 times more likely to believe their child would be "treated like a guinea pig" if they participated in research ($P = .03$), and were significantly less likely to enroll their children in a clinical study in the setting of being cared for by an established provider ($P = .0001$).[52] The investigators also found that black parents had less exposure to research advertisements.[52] Despite these findings, their study found that black parents were as likely as white parents to enroll their children in low-risk research studies. This finding is consistent with data on pediatric cancer clinical trials, in which minority children are proportionately represented.[53] With such limited data, however, it is clear that additional studies are needed to determine what and how health disparities challenge dermatologic research so that barriers to minority participation may be targeted and overcome.

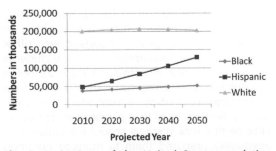

Fig. 2. Projections of the United States population by race with the resident population numbers represented in thousands. Thus the projected white population in 2050 is approximately 200 million citizens. (*Data from* U.S. Census Bureau. U.S. Population Projections. Available at: http://www.census.gov/population/www/projections/downloadablefiles. html. Accessed April 21, 2011.)

SUMMARY

As a dermatologic community, our work is cut out for us. Health care disparities in dermatology clearly exist, but need better definition to be properly addressed. There is inadequate epidemiologic data on dermatologic health disparities, and the current data are effectively limited to the diagnoses of skin cancer and atopic dermatitis or eczema

List of Acronyms	
AAD	American Academy of Dermatology
AD	Atopic dermatitis
AHRQ	Agency for Healthcare Research and Quality
AMA	American Medical Association
ATDCTF	Access to Dermatologic Care Task Force
NMSC	Nonmelanoma skin cancer
SES	Socioeconomic status

Ample room exists to further explore the extent and nature of these and other inequities across a spectrum of dermatologic diseases. In addition, a variety of health disparities exist beyond those detailed in this article, including those secondary to culture or language barriers, additional socioeconomic barriers (transportation, education, and literacy), age, disability, differential treatment, and outcomes. Potential solutions that merit further exploration include patient navigators, patient-centered medical homes, professional translators, child care, and literacy assistance, among others.[54]

Addressing the need for further health disparities research is an identified priority of the National Institute of Arthritis and Musculoskeletal and Skin Disease,[3] but this has not yet been fully recognized by the dermatologic research community. Institutions in the United States are increasingly establishing minority health research centers with goals focused on reducing health disparities. These goals range from enhancing minority health research infrastructure and training skilled minority health researchers to providing patient-focused and community-focused programs to directly eliminate inequities.[55,56] Such efforts present an opportunity for dermatologic researchers and providers to fill in the major gaps in current knowledge and literature by establishing health disparity–focused careers within supportive academic environments.

Increased research as well as collaboration between dermatologic organizations that aim to eliminate health care disparities will help dermatologists to develop united and clear set goals. Recently the AAD created the Access to Dermatologic Care Task Force (ATDCTF) with the goal "to raise awareness among dermatologists of health disparities affecting populations identified by but not exclusive to race/ethnicity, SES, geography, gender, age, and disability status and to develop policies that increase access for these groups to dermatologic services."[57] The ATDCTF also serves as the link between the AAD and other physician organizations focused on reducing health care inequities, such as the American Medical Association (AMA). The AMA Commission to End Health Disparities focuses on collaboration to "increase awareness among physicians and health professionals; use evidence-based and other strategies; and advocate for action, including governmental, to eliminate disparities in health care and strengthen the health care system."[58] Through increased research, awareness, education, outreach, and public policy, dermatologic and general health disparities can be decreased resulting in improved health for all Americans.

REFERENCES

1. Carter-Pokras O, Baquet C. What is a "health disparity"? Public Health Rep 2002;117(5):426–34.
2. Agency for Healthcare Research and Quality. 2010 national healthcare disparities report. Available at: http://www.ahrq.gov/qual/nhdr10/nhdr10.pdf. Accessed May 1, 2011.
3. Taylor SC, Kelly AP, Dupree NE, et al. Health disparities in arthritis and musculoskeletal and skin diseases-the dermatology session: National Institute of Arthritis and Musculoskeletal and Skin Diseases, Bethesda, Maryland, December 15-16, 2000. J Am Acad Dermatol 2002;47(5):770–3.
4. McMichael AJ, Jackson S. Issues in dermatologic health care delivery in minority populations. Dermatol Clin 2000;18(2):229–33, viii.
5. Bigby M. Epidemiology of cutaneous disease. In: Kelly AP, Taylor SC, editors. Dermatology for skin of color. New York: McGraw Hill Medical; 2009. p. 16.
6. Rapp SR, Feldman SR, Graham G, et al. The Acne Quality of Life Index (Acne-QOLI): development and validation of a brief instrument. Am J Clin Dermatol 2006;7(3):185–92.
7. Stern RS. Dermatologists and office-based care of dermatologic disease in the 21st century. J Investig Dermatol Symp Proc 2004;9(2):126–30.
8. Wingo PA, Bolden S, Tong T, et al. Cancer statistics for African Americans, 1996. CA Cancer J Clin 1996;46(2):113–25.
9. Gloster HM Jr, Neal K. Skin cancer in skin of color. J Am Acad Dermatol 2006;55(5):741–60 [quiz: 761–4].
10. Weinstock MA. Nonmelanoma skin cancer mortality in the United States, 1969 through 1988. Arch Dermatol 1993;129(10):1286–90.
11. Geller AC, Miller DR, Lew RA, et al. Cutaneous melanoma mortality among the socioeconomically disadvantaged in Massachusetts. Am J Public Health 1996;86(4):538–43.

12. Reyes-Ortiz CA, Goodwin JS, Freeman JL, et al. Socioeconomic status and survival in older patients with melanoma. J Am Geriatr Soc 2006;54(11): 1758–64.

13. Linos E, Swetter SM, Cockburn MG, et al. Increasing burden of melanoma in the United States. J Invest Dermatol 2009;129(7):1666–74.

14. Roetzheim RG, Pal N, Tennant C, et al. Effects of health insurance and race on early detection of cancer. J Natl Cancer Inst 1999;91(16):1409–15.

15. Byrd KM, Wilson DC, Hoyler SS, et al. Advanced presentation of melanoma in African Americans. J Am Acad Dermatol 2004;50(1):21–4 [discussion: 142–3].

16. Altekruse SF, Kosary CL, Krapcho M, et al, editors. SEER cancer statistics review, 1975-2007. Bethesda (MD): NCI; 2010.

17. Scotto J, Fears TR, Fraumeni JF. Incidence of non-melanoma skin cancer in the United States. NIH Pub. no. 83–2433. Bethesda (MD): U.S. Dept. of Health and Human Services, National Institutes of Health; 1983.

18. Coups EJ, Geller AC, Weinstock MA, et al. Prevalence and correlates of skin cancer screening among middle-aged and older white adults in the United States. Am J Med 2010;123(5):439–45.

19. Buster KJ, You Z, Fouad M, et al. Skin cancer risk perceptions: a comparison across ethnicity, age, education, gender, and income. J Am Acad Dermatol August 27, 2011. [Epub ahead of print].

20. Bilimoria KY, Balch CM, Wayne JD, et al. Health care system and socioeconomic factors associated with variance in use of sentinel lymph node biopsy for melanoma in the United States. J Clin Oncol 2009; 27(11):1857–63.

21. Shaw TE, Currie GP, Koudelka CW, et al. Eczema prevalence in the United States: data from the 2003 National Survey of Children's Health. J Invest Dermatol 2011;131(1):67–73.

22. Asher MI, Montefort S, Bjorksten B, et al. Worldwide time trends in the prevalence of symptoms of asthma, allergic rhinoconjunctivitis, and eczema in childhood: ISAAC Phases One and Three repeat multicountry cross-sectional surveys. Lancet 2006; 368(9537):733–43.

23. Worldwide variation in prevalence of symptoms of asthma, allergic rhinoconjunctivitis, and atopic eczema: ISAAC. The International Study of Asthma and Allergies in Childhood (ISAAC) Steering Committee. Lancet 1998;351(9111):1225–32.

24. Laughter D, Istvan JA, Tofte SJ, et al. The prevalence of atopic dermatitis in Oregon schoolchildren. J Am Acad Dermatol 2000;43(4):649–55.

25. Horii KA, Simon SD, Liu DY, et al. Atopic dermatitis in children in the United States, 1997-2004: visit trends, patient and provider characteristics, and prescribing patterns. Pediatrics 2007;120(3):e527–34.

26. Janumpally SR, Feldman SR, Gupta AK, et al. In the United States, blacks and Asian/Pacific Islanders are more likely than whites to seek medical care for atopic dermatitis. Arch Dermatol 2002;138(5): 634–7.

27. Ip S, Chung M, Raman G, et al. Breastfeeding and maternal and infant health outcomes in developed countries. Evid Rep Technol Assess (Full Rep) 2007;(153):1–186.

28. Bartick M, Reinhold A. The burden of suboptimal breastfeeding in the United States: a pediatric cost analysis. Pediatrics 2010;125(5):e1048–56.

29. Gartner LM, Morton J, Lawrence RA, et al. Breast-feeding and the use of human milk. Pediatrics 2005;115(2):496–506.

30. Office of the Surgeon General. The Surgeon General's call to action to support breastfeeding 2011. Available at: http://www.surgeongeneral.gov/ topics/breastfeeding/factsheet.html. Accessed May 15, 2011.

31. Nommsen-Rivers LA, Chantry CJ, Cohen RJ, et al. Comfort with the idea of formula feeding helps explain ethnic disparity in breastfeeding intentions among expectant first-time mothers. Breastfeed Med 2010;5(1):25–33.

32. Ahluwalia IB, Morrow B, Hsia J, et al. Who is breastfeeding? Recent trends from the pregnancy risk assessment and monitoring system. J Pediatr 2003;142(5):486–91.

33. DeNavas-Walt C, Proctor BD, Smith JC. Income, poverty, and health insurance coverage in the United States: 2009. In: Bureau USC, editor. Washington, DC: U.S. Government Printing Office; 2010. p. 22–4.

34. Office of the Legislative Counsel. Compilation of patient protection and affordable care act. Available at: http:// docs.house.gov/energycommerce/ppacacon.pdf. Accessed May 2, 2011.

35. Congressional Budget Office. Estimate of the effects of the insurance coverage provisions contained in the Patient Protection and Affordable Care Act (Public Law 111-148) and the Health Care and Education Reconciliation Act of 2010 (P.L. 111-152). March 2011. Available at: http://www.cbo.gov/ budget/factsheets/2011b/HealthInsuranceProvisions. pdf. Accessed May 2, 2011.

36. Elmendorf D. CBO's analysis of the major health care legislation enacted in March 2010. March 30, 2011. Available at: http://www.cbo.gov/ftpdocs/ 121xx/doc12119/03-30-HealthCareLegislation.pdf. Accessed May 2, 2011.

37. Healthcare.gov. Understand the law. Available at: http://www.healthcare.gov. Accessed April 12, 2011.

38. Kostecki J. Dermatology practice profile survey 2009 report. Schaumburg (IL): American Academy of Dermatology Association; 2009 [Database provided to authors].

39. McCleskey PE, Gilson RT, DeVillez RL. Medical student core curriculum in dermatology survey. J Am Acad Dermatol 2009;61(1):30–35.e4.

40. Knable A, Hood AF, Pearson TG. Undergraduate medical education in dermatology: report from the AAD Interdisciplinary Education Committee, Subcommittee on Undergraduate Medical Education. J Am Acad Dermatol 1997;36(3 Pt 1):467–70.

41. Ramsay DL, Mayer F. National survey of undergraduate dermatologic medical education. Arch Dermatol 1985;121(12):1529–30.

42. Hansra NK, O'Sullivan P, Chen CL, et al. Medical school dermatology curriculum: are we adequately preparing primary care physicians? J Am Acad Dermatol 2009;61(1):23–29.e1.

43. Chiang YZ, Tan KT, Chiang YN, et al. Evaluation of educational methods in dermatology and confidence levels: a national survey of UK medical students. Int J Dermatol 2011;50(2):198–202.

44. Buster KJ, Yang L, Elmets CA. Are dermatologists confident in treating skin disease in African-Americans? [abstract 235]. J Invest Dermatol 2011. [Epub ahead of print].

45. Nijhawan RI, Jacob SE, Woolery-Lloyd H. Skin of color education in dermatology residency programs: does residency training reflect the changing demographics of the United States? J Am Acad Dermatol 2008;59(4):615–8.

46. Adams-Campbell LL, Ahaghotu C, Gaskins M, et al. Enrollment of African Americans onto clinical treatment trials: study design barriers. J Clin Oncol 2004;22(4):730–4.

47. Advani AS, Atkeson B, Brown CL, et al. Barriers to the participation of African-American patients with cancer in clinical trials: a pilot study. Cancer 2003; 97(6):1499–506.

48. Spears CR, Nolan BV, O'Neill JL, et al. Recruiting underserved populations to dermatologic research: a systematic review. Int J Dermatol 2011;50(4): 385–95.

49. Roberson NL. Clinical trial participation. Viewpoints from racial/ethnic groups. Cancer 1994;74(Suppl 9): 2687–91.

50. Corbie-Smith G, Thomas SB, Williams MV, et al. Attitudes and beliefs of African Americans toward participation in medical research. J Gen Intern Med 1999;14(9):537–46.

51. U.S. Department of Health and Human Services. NIH policy and guidelines on the inclusion of women and minorities as subjects in clinical research. Available at: http://grants.nih.gov/grants/funding/women_min/guidelines_amended_10_2001.htm. Accessed May 10, 2011.

52. Shaw MG, Morrell DS, Corbie-Smith GM, et al. Perceptions of pediatric clinical research among African American and Caucasian parents. J Natl Med Assoc 2009;101(9):900–7.

53. Bleyer WA, Tejeda HA, Murphy SB, et al. Equal participation of minority patients in U.S. national pediatric cancer clinical trials. J Pediatr Hematol Oncol 1997;19(5):423–7.

54. Sauaia A, Dellavalle RP. Health care inequities: an introduction for dermatology providers. Dermatol Clin 2009;27(2):103–7, v.

55. University of Alabama at Birmingham Minority Health and Health Disparities Research Center. Available at: http://mhrc.dopm.uab.edu/. Accessed on May 1, 2011.

56. Temple University School of Medicine Center for Minority Health and Health Disparities. Available at: http://www.temple.edu/medicine/departments_centers/research/minority_health.htm. Accessed on May 14, 2011.

57. American Academy of Dermatology Access to Dermatologic Care Task Force. Available at: http://www.aad.org/forms/cctf/default.aspx. Accessed May 14, 2011.

58. American Medical Association Commission to End Health Care Disparities. Available at: http://www.ama-assn.org/ama/pub/physician-resources/public-health/eliminating-health-disparities/commission-end-health-care-disparities.page. Accessed May 14, 2011.

A Review of Health Outcomes in Patients with Psoriasis

Kai Li, BS[a], April W. Armstrong, MD, MPH[b],*

KEYWORDS

• Psoriasis • Treatments • Health outcomes • Resources

Psoriasis is a chronic inflammatory skin disorder that affects 2% to 4% of the United States population.[1] Patients with psoriasis present with scaly and erythematous patches and plaques on the skin.[2] Psoriasis is associated with significant comorbidities and affects patients' quality of life. Successful management of psoriasis patients depends on clinicians' understanding of the various treatment options as well as their recognition of associated comorbidities.

PSORIASIS SUBTYPES

Psoriasis varies greatly in clinical presentation and ranges from mild disease with isolated patches to extensive disease with confluent plaques involving multiple areas of the body. Plaque psoriasis is the most common subtype, affecting 80% to 90% of those with psoriasis.[2] Plaque psoriasis is characterized by erythematous patches or plaques with silvery scales. Other subtypes of psoriasis include guttate, pustular, inverse, and erythrodermic forms. Guttate psoriasis appears as small, drop-shaped lesions on the trunk, limbs, and scalp, and it is sometimes associated with upper respiratory infections.[1] Pustular psoriasis is characterized by multiple pustules on the skin, whereas inverse psoriasis presents with erythematous patches in the intertriginous areas. Erythrodermic psoriasis is characterized by widespread erythema and scaling of the skin.[1]

Measurement of Disease Severity

In clinical practice, psoriasis disease severity is estimated primarily by using the total body surface area (TBSA) involved. Typically, TBSA involvement of less than 2% is considered mild disease, 2% to 10% is moderate disease, and greater than 10% is severe psoriasis. In clinical trials, researchers often use the Psoriasis Area and Severity Index (PASI) to assess disease severity. PASI is a validated disease-severity instrument that integrates area of involvement with erythema, scaling, and induration of psoriatic plaques. PASI ranges from 0 (no disease) to 72 (maximal disease). About 25% to 30% of patients with psoriasis are classified as having moderate-to-severe disease.[3]

Prevalence and Incidence

The National Institute of Arthritis and Musculoskeletal and Skin Diseases estimates that the prevalence of psoriasis in the United States is approximately 4%,[1] whereas psoriasis has a worldwide prevalence of approximately 2% to 3%.[3] Currently, more than 5 million adults have psoriasis, and 260,000 new cases are diagnosed annually in the United States.[4] Psoriasis appears to affect men and women equally. Although psoriasis can affect all age groups, the onset of psoriasis tends to peak between the ages of 20 and 30 and between ages 50 and 60.[1,3] Patients with

Funding sources: There were no sources of funding.
Dr Armstrong is an investigator and consultant for Abbott and Centocor.
[a] Department of Dermatology, University of California Davis Health System, University of California Davis, 3301 C Street, Suite 1400, Sacramento, CA 95816, USA
[b] Dermatology Clinical Research Unit, Teledermatology Program, Department of Dermatology, University of California Davis Health System, University of California Davis School of Medicine, 3301 C Street, Suite 1400, Sacramento, CA 95816, USA
* Corresponding author.
E-mail address: aprilarmstrong@post.harvard.edu

Dermatol Clin 30 (2012) 61–72
doi:10.1016/j.det.2011.08.012
0733-8635/12/$ – see front matter Published by Elsevier Inc.

derm.theclinics.com

early onset of psoriasis tend to have greater disease severity and a family history of psoriasis.[5]

BURDEN OF PSORIASIS
Impact of Psoriasis on Quality of Life

Psoriasis has a major impact on health-related quality of life that is comparable to other major medical diseases such as cancer, arthritis, hypertension, heart disease, diabetes, and depression.[1,6] In a review of quality-of-life studies from January 1966 to April 2000, investigators found that patients with psoriasis reported physical discomfort, impaired emotional functioning, and negative body image and self-image, as well as limitations in daily activities, social contacts, and work.[6] The severity of the psoriasis was directly correlated to lower levels of quality of life. A population-based survey looking at the association between quality of life and extent of disease showed that nearly 60% of patients with psoriasis report that the disease affects their everyday life and 26% report a change or discontinuation of daily activities.[7]

Economic Burden of Psoriasis

The estimated total direct and indirect health care cost of psoriasis in the United States is 11.25 billion dollars annually, with direct medical costs estimates ranging from 650 million to 4.3 billion dollars.[8,9] The cost of psoriasis in the United States is multidimensional. Total cost includes medical and prescription drug costs, patient expenditures, lost work time, reduced productivity, and diminished quality of life. In a case comparison of 56,528 patients with psoriasis versus the general population, patients with psoriasis had significantly greater health care resource use ($5529 vs $3509), higher total drug use ($1604 vs $822), and greater overall medical costs ($3925 vs $2687).[10]

Psychosocial Burden of Psoriasis

Epidemiologic studies show that the psychosocial burden of psoriasis is one of the most challenging aspects of disease management.[11] Psoriasis affects daily activities of living for nearly 60% of patients, especially in women, younger patients, and those afflicted with moderate-to-severe psoriasis.[7,12] Psychosocial consequences of having psoriasis include decreased self-esteem and stigmatization in social relations and employment. In a questionnaire given to 17,350 patients with psoriasis, as many as two-thirds of patients report that the disease has limited their daily activities in areas such as sleeping, sexual activity, use of

hands, walking, sitting for long periods of time, and performing job duties.[13,14]

Owing to visibility of psoriatic lesions, patients with severe psoriasis are especially vulnerable to social stigmatization. Patients have reported being asked to leave hair salons and barbershops, public pools, and health clubs. Compared with patients with psoriasis affecting regions of the body usually covered by clothing, patients with visible plaques that affect hands, arms, and head rate their psoriasis as more disabling.[13,15] Furthermore, the patients' disease severity is directly correlated with lower ratings of self-esteem and a fear of social isolation.[11,14]

This psychological stress from psoriasis can permeate employment and result in financial loss. A two-year study by the National Psoriasis Foundation (NPF) found that having psoriasis is associated with decreased household incomes and reduced employment opportunities, especially for patients with moderate-to-severe disease. Compared with those without psoriasis, psoriasis patients have lower income and are less likely to work full-time. Furthermore, psoriasis was reported as the primary reason for unemployment in 17% of patients with severe psoriasis.[16] An estimated 60% of patients missed an average of 26 days of work each year due to complications of psoriasis.[16]

Psoriasis is also related to decreased sexual intimacy and decreased libido in 30% to 70% of patients.[17,18] In a study conducted by Gupta and Gupta,[17] 40.8% of 120 patients surveyed reported that the disease impacted their sexual activity. The affected group also reported more joint pains, greater area of scaling, and greater pruritus severity. In addition, psoriasis patients had higher depression scores. A recent study has suggested that these comorbidities may contribute to decreased sexual functioning in psoriasis patients.

PSORIASIS COMORBIDITIES

Psoriasis is associated with comorbid conditions, including depression, arthritis, diabetes, hypertension, metabolic syndrome, and cardiovascular events. These comorbid conditions may occur concurrently or years after development of psoriasis.[19,20]

Shared Mechanisms Between Psoriasis and Comorbidities

The presence of rheumatologic and cardiovascular comorbidities among psoriasis patients suggests that a systemic inflammatory process may underlie these disease processes. For example, some studies suggest that increased amounts of pro-inflammatory cytokines, such as tumor necrosis factor-alpha and interleukin-1, may be linked to depression.[21] Furthermore, psoriasis may predispose patients to increased risk of atherosclerotic disease through a chronic, proinflammatory state that fosters the development of the metabolic syndrome.[22] One proposed mechanism for the association between the formation of atherosclerotic lesions and increased proinflammatory cytokines is that chronic inflammation may lead to increased oxidative modifications of lipoproteins, which are more atherogenic than native lipproteins.[19]

Psychiatric Comorbidity in Psoriasis

Multiple studies have documented higher rates of depression among psoriasis patients compared to control populations.[23–26] Recent studies have shown that psoriasis seems to be an independent risk factor for developing depressive symptoms.[27] Although chronic medical conditions have shown to be associated with depression, the prevalence of active suicidal ideation seemed to be higher in psoriasis patients.[23] Furthermore, a population-based cohort study in the United Kingdom found that psoriasis patients are more likely to be diagnosed with depression, anxiety, or suicidality compared with the general population. Specifically, compared with patients without psoriasis, patients with severe psoriasis have a 72% increased likelihood of having comorbid psychiatric conditions and those with mild psoriasis have a 38% increased likelihood.[26] In addition, young men appeared to be at the highest risk for displaying depression symptoms.

Rheumatologic, Cardiovascular, and Malignancy Comorbidities

Patients with psoriasis have an increased frequency of psoriatic arthritis, cardiovascular diseases, and certain types of malignancies compared with the general population. Psoriatic arthritis affects an estimated 25% to 34% of patients with psoriasis.[28] Although it can develop at any age, psoriatic arthritis most commonly appears approximately 10 years after the onset of psoriasis in most patients.[3] Psoriatic arthritis is characterized by tenderness and swelling of the affected joints. Early diagnosis and treatment are essential in the prevention of progressive joint damage. Although severity of psoriatic arthritis varies greatly, the most severe form of the disease can severely interfere with activities of daily living.[29]

Several epidemiologic studies have suggested an association between cardiovascular diseases and psoriasis.[30–33] In a large population study of patients from the United Kingdom, investigators found that psoriasis conferred an independent risk of myocardial infarctions after adjusting for traditional cardiovascular risk factors. Specifically, the relative risk was found to vary with age and severity of disease. For example, the relative risk of a 30-year-old person with severe psoriasis was 3.1, whereas that for a 60-year-old person with severe disease was 1.36.[34] Increasing epidemiologic evidence suggests that psoriasis may also be associated with diabetes and hypertension.[31,35]

Several studies suggest that psoriasis patients are more likely to have dyslipidemia compared with the general population.[36,37] In these studies, the levels of triglycerides, total cholesterol, low-density lipoprotein, and very-low-density lipoprotein were higher in psoriasis patients compared with the control groups.[36,37] Furthermore, compared with the general population, researchers have found that psoriasis patients are more likely to develop metabolic syndrome, which is characterized by abdominal obesity, elevated cholesterol and triglycerides, elevated blood pressure and insulin resistance, and elevated fasting blood glucose levels.[38] In a 2003 to 2006 cross-sectional health survey of 6546 participants, the prevalence of metabolic syndrome was found to be 40% in the United States among psoriasis patients compared with 23% among controls.[39] The most common presenting feature of metabolic syndrome seen in psoriasis patients was abdominal obesity. Metabolic syndrome confers a threefold to ninefold risk of developing type 2 diabetes and twofold to threefold risk of having an adverse cardiovascular event such as coronary heart disease, stroke, or myocardial infarctions.[40,41]

Studies examining malignancy risks in psoriasis patients are often complicated by the relatively rare occurrence of cancers in this population. Some studies suggest that psoriasis may be associated with increased risk of malignancies, including lymphomas, solid organ tumors, and nonmelanoma skin cancers.[42] In a prospective study of 6905 psoriasis patients that were followed for 9 years, these patients were 1.4 times more likely to develop malignancy compared with the general population.[43] Researchers have speculated that the apparent increased risk of malignancy might be related to psoriasis treatments, among other factors. Notably, the use of psoralen plus ultraviolet A (PUVA) and cyclosporine has been linked to the development of squamous cell carcinoma in psoriasis patients.[44] Previous treatment with retinoids or immunosuppressants also significantly increases the risk of malignancy.[45] In a 15-year prospective study of 1380 patients first treated with PUVA from 1975 to 1976, the relative risk of malignant melanoma was 1.1 after 15 years and 5.4 after 20 years.[46] The risk was greatest among patients who have had at least 250 PUVA treatments.[46]

Recommendations for Assessment of Comorbidities in Psoriasis

Comorbid conditions in psoriasis are becoming increasingly well recognized in the medical community. The NPF has proposed screening recommendations for dermatologists.[20] NPF recommends that psoriasis be approached as a multisystem disorder that may necessitate referrals to other specialists. Dermatologists are encouraged to inquire about the development of rheumatologic and cardiovascular diseases.[47] Specifically, it is recommended that physicians screen for cardiovascular risk factor according to the American Heart Association (AHA) recommendations. Beginning at age 20, physicians should inquire about risk factors such as family history of coronary heart disease, smoking, alcohol intake, physical activity, and diet. Screening should occur at least every 2 years with measurements of blood pressure, body mass index, waist circumference, and pulse. Measurements of fasting lipids and fasting glucose should be done at least every 5 years, or 2 years if risk factors are present. When patients reach age 40 years, the 10-year risk of developing coronary heart disease should be assessed with a multiple risk factor score every 5 years, or more often if risk factors change. Risk factors used in the global risk assessment includes age, sex, smoking status, systolic blood pressure, and lipid levels.[20]

Lifestyle Changes and Risk Modification

For some psoriasis patients, the large psychosocial burden of the disease may be associated with greater alcohol consumption, smoking, and increased food intake. Alcohol abuse has been linked to a higher incidence and severity of psoriasis, with some studies showing that abstinence from alcohol alone may be associated with psoriasis remission in some patients.[48–51] A recent cross-sectional study by Herron and colleagues[33] found that the prevalence of obesity in patients with psoriasis was higher than that of the general population (34% vs 18%). The prevalence of smoking was also greater (25% vs 9%). Smoking has also been linked with increased psoriasis severity. In a hospital-based cross-section study, smoking more than 20 cigarettes a day was associated with a more than twofold increase in severity of disease.[52,53]

The NPF recommends several lifestyle changes for psoriasis patients. Patients are encouraged to exercise at least three times a week for 20 minutes along with cessation of smoking and moderate alcohol intake.[20] Patients are also encouraged to modify eating habits. For patients already suffering from metabolic syndrome, the AHA guidelines recommend a target body mass index of less than 25, and physical activity for at least 30 minutes each day. Although not officially endorsed by the NPF, participation in psychotherapy or social support groups may help patients with learning disease coping mechanisms and reducing the psychosocial burden. Studies have also shown that, compared with pharmacotherapy alone, psychotherapy can lead to significant reduction in disease severity and psychosocial distress.[54]

TREATMENTS

Treatments for psoriasis need to be tailored to patients based on a variety of factors, including type of psoriasis, disease severity, medical coverage, and access to care. Treatments with topical agents, such as topical steroids and topical vitamin D agents, constitute the first line of therapy for mild-to-moderate disease. However, topical therapy alone is often inadequate for moderate-to-severe psoriasis. For patients with moderate-to-severe disease, phototherapy, systemic therapy, or biologics should be considered. Whereas large body surface area involvement will often necessitate systemic treatments, psoriasis involving critically functioning body regions, such as the hands and feet, sometimes warrant consideration for systemic therapy.[8,55–59]

Defining Treatment Goals

The primary goals in the treatment of psoriasis include reduction of disease severity and improvement of quality of life.[60] Before starting any treatment, dermatologists need to have a detailed discussion with patients regarding chronicity of the disease and help set realistic expectations based on disease severity and selected therapy. Clinicians and patients need to work together to achieve and maintain long-term control of psoriasis while monitoring for adverse effects. Specifically, clinicians need to document changes in psoriasis disease activity at each visit to evaluate effectiveness of treatment. Regular conversations on setting realistic therapeutic goals and encouraging patients to adhere to the treatment regimen are important steps to achieving disease control.

Topical Treatments

Topical treatments are usually considered the first-line therapy for patients with mild psoriasis because of their limited side-effect profiles.[61,62] However, because of the difficulties involved with application to large body surface areas, topical agents are generally used in patients with less than 10% TBSA involvement.[63] Patients with moderate-to-severe psoriasis will often have inadequate response to topical treatments alone, but topical therapy is a useful adjunct to systemic therapy in patients with moderate-to-severe disease.[64]

Corticosteroids are the most commonly prescribed topical agents for their antiinflammatory and antiproliferative properties. These properties are mediated through transcriptional regulation of genes encoding for inflammatory mediators, which leads to downstream inhibition of lymphocyte activation and a reduction in dermal edema and vascular permeability.[65] Topical steroid preparations are available in a variety of potencies; their selection should be based on disease severity, affected body location, and patient preference for vehicles.[66,67] Adverse effects of long-term use of topical corticosteroids include epidermal atrophy, acneiform eruptions, allergic contact dermatitis, and tachyphylaxis. In rare cases, long-term widespread use of high-potency topical steroids is associated with suppression of the hypothalamic-pituitary-adrenal axis.[68] Calcipotriene is a vitamin D3 analog that binds to the keratinocyte receptor and promotes terminal differentiation and inhibition of the proliferation of keratinocytes. Regular use of topical calcipotriene is associated with few adverse effects, such as skin irritation. Few systemic side effects have been reported, but rare cases of hypercalcemia have been reported in patients who use excess quantities for a significant period.[69] As monotherapy, the efficacy of calcipotriene is thought to be similar to that of a class two or three topical corticosteroid, and its efficacy improves significantly when used in combination with certain types of high-potency topical steroids.

Topical retinoids, such as tazarotene, are vitamin A derivatives that selectively bind to retinoic acid receptors. Retinoids are thought to exert their effects by modulating the cellular differentiation of the epidermis, which results in decreased scaling, erythema, and thickness of the plaques.[70] Topical retinoids have a slower onset of action compared with high potency corticosteroids; however, their use as a monotherapy resulted in an excellent response or complete clearing of target lesions, as evaluated by the investigators, in 70% of patients treated for 3 months in one clinical study.[71] Adverse side effects of topical retinoids include

irritation, burning, itching, stinging, and erythema, and they can occur in 20% to 40% of patients. Of note, tazarotene is labeled as pregnancy category X and, therefore, it should not be used in women of childbearing age.

Other topical agents include tacrolimus, salicylic acid, and emollients. Tacrolimus is a calcineurin inhibitor and functions as an immunosuppressant. Initial studies did not demonstrate significant efficacy of topical tacrolimus in treating plaque-type psoriasis, which may be related to poor penetration of the active ingredients into thick psoriatic plaques.[72-74] However, tacrolimus seems to be modestly efficacious in treating areas where skin is thinner, such as in the face and groin areas.[75] Salicylic acid is commonly used in combination with corticosteroids to improve penetration of topical steroids. Emollients are used to relieve dryness, scaling, and pruritus.

Phototherapy

Phototherapy has been used for decades to treat generalized psoriasis. PUVA and UV-B are effective in achieving significant clearance of psoriatic lesions. A main contraindication of phototherapy is having a photosensitive skin disease, such as lupus erythematosus.

PUVA phototherapy consists of emission of UVA wavelengths (320–400 nm) after patients have ingested psoralen. Compared with UV-B, PUVA penetrates deeper into the skin because of its longer wavelengths. Patients undergoing PUVA therapy require fewer treatment sessions than UV-B phototherapy to achieve clearance. However, PUVA is associated with greater short-term and long-term adverse effects. Short-term adverse reactions of PUVA include nausea, headache, depression, hyperkinesis, and phototoxicity. Long-term use of PUVA is associated with significant photoaging and an increased risk of squamous cell carcinomas and melanomas in patients exposed to high cumulative doses.[46,76-79] PUVA can be combined with other topical and systemic treatments to achieve greater clearance. Specifically, combination PUVA-acitretin regimen seems to reduce the risk of cutaneous malignancy through reduced number of phototherapy sessions and, thereby, lower cumulative dose.[80]

Broadband UV-B therapy (290–320 nm) remains one of the mainstay treatments for moderate-to-severe psoriasis. Broadband UV-B therapy can be combined with other topical and systemic therapies to improve patient response. A recent literature review of studies on the use of UV-B phototherapy for psoriasis from 1966 to 2002 found no increased incidence of skin cancer risk with the use of monotherapy or combined UV-B phototherapy.[81] The most important contributing factor to skin cancer seemed to be prior exposure to ionizing radiation.[82]

Narrowband UV-B is another subtype of UV-B phototherapy that consists of specific wavelengths in the range of 311 to 313 nm. Narrowband UV-B is effective in treating moderate-to-severe psoriasis while limiting wavelengths responsible for premature aging and burning. In a studying comparing narrow to broadband UV-B, narrowband seems to achieve greater clearance of psoriatic lesions but often with longer treatment periods.[83]

Oral Systemic Agents

Common oral agents used in the treatment of moderate-to-severe psoriasis include methotrexate, acitretin, and cyclosporine. These agents are effective in achieving initial clearance as well as long-term maintenance therapy. However, adverse effects of these agents must be carefully considered and monitored during treatment.

Methotrexate inhibits DNA synthesis, thereby directly inhibiting epidermal cell proliferation and slowing cell turnover rates. Methotrexate is effective in treating various subtypes of psoriasis, including plaque-type, erythrodermic, and pustular psoriasis as well as psoriatic arthritis. Adverse effects of methotrexate include bone marrow suppression, pneumonitis, infectious complications, and spontaneous abortion.[84] Preexisting liver and kidney diseases may enhance methotrexate toxicity. Liver and kidney function tests need to be obtained before the initiation of therapy as well as during therapy. The incidence of liver failure and cirrhosis can range from 3% with cumulative doses in the range of 1.5 to 2 g to as high as 26% with a cumulative dose of 4 g.[85] The risks of hepatotoxicity are greatest among those who are obese, have a history of viral hepatitis or diabetes, and have heavy alcohol consumption.[86]

Systemic retinoids, such as acitretin, modulate the cellular differentiation of the epidermis and lead to reduced scaling, erythema, and thickness of psoriatic plaques.[70] Acitretin can be used as a monotherapy or in combination with other agents to increase treatment efficacy. Acitretin is classified as pregnancy category X and can be associated with liver function test abnormalities in as many as 25& to 30% of patients, especially in those on high-dose therapy.[87] Of note, acitretin remains the only systemic therapy that is not immunosuppressive and, as such, it can be considered in patients with comorbid chronic conditions such as HIV and hepatitis B and C, with appropriate monitoring of liver function tests.

Cyclosporine is usually reserved for short-term, rapid control of psoriasis flares. Most studies recommend that the duration of cyclosporine administration not exceed 1 year.[88–91] Short-term use of cyclosporine is associated with side effects such as nausea, headache, malaise, and tremor that resolve in weeks to months. Long-term use is associated with adverse effects such as impaired kidney function, hypertension, hyperlipidemia, elevated creatinine, and elevated urea nitrogen. Cyclosporine is classified as pregnancy category B by the US Food and Drug Administration.

Biologic Therapy

Biologic treatments in psoriasis typically act through immunomodulation. To date, several classes of biologics exist for psoriasis treatment, including anti-tumor necrosis factor (anti-TNF) agents, anti-T cell agents, and anti-IL12/23p40 agents. TNF is a key pro-inflammatory cytokine involved in the pathogenesis of psoriasis. Tumor necrosis factor (TNF) levels have been found to be higher in psoriatic lesions compared with nonlesional skin.[92] Among the anti-TNF agents, etanercept is a dimeric fusion protein that joins the extracellular ligand-binding domain of human TNF receptor with the Fc component of the IgG1. Etanercept binds and inhibits TNF activity, thereby inhibiting downstream inflammatory events. Studies have suggested that etanercept has greater affinity for TNF than the endogenous receptors.[93]

Adalimumab is another member of the anti-TNF family; it is a fully humanized anti-TNF monoclonal IgG1 antibody that prevents binding of TNF to its receptor. Adalimumab has been found to be effective in the treatment of moderate-to-severe psoriasis in phase III trials.[94] Specifically, after the first 16 weeks of treatment, 71% of patients receiving adalimumab achieved greater than 75% improvement in PASI score, compared with 7% of patients receiving placebo.[94]

Infliximab is a chimeric anti-TNF monoclonal IgG antibody. It consists of both mouse and human constant and variable regions. It is able to bind with high affinity and specificity to membrane-bound TNF. The infliximab-TNF complex has a higher binding affinity than the etanercept-TNF complex.[95] A meta-analysis of reviews published on psoriasis from 2007 to 2008 found that, among biologic agents, infliximab is highly effective in achieving 75% reduction in the PASI in moderate-to-severe psoriasis after 10 to 14 weeks of treatment.[57]

Contraindications to the use of anti-TNF biologics include active, serious, and recurrent infections; active tuberculosis; history of demyelinating disease; or congestive heart failure.[92,96] Rarely,

TNF inhibitors have been associated with more severe systemic complications, such as congestive heart failure, cytopenia, increased liver function tests, malignancy, lupus-like syndrome, thrombocytopenia, and demyelinating disorders, although their role in these diseases is not fully understood.[97] However, a recent analysis of the safety of tumor necrosis factor antagonists found that, during the initial year of treatment, the rate of success with anti-TNF therapy was at least two orders of magnitude greater than the likelihood of serious toxicity.[98]

Another class of biologics is directed specifically against T-cells. Alefacept is an antibody that blocks the interaction between costimulatory molecules leukocyte function antigen-3 (LFA-3) and CD2. Inhibition of binding between LFA3 and CD2 mitigates T cell response.[92] Alefacept selectively inhibits the memory-effector T cells, which compose more than 75% of the T cells found in psoriatic plaques.[92] Controlled studies have shown that alefacept was associated with significant improvements in PASI. Specifically, the mean reductions in PASI in the 15 mg alefacept, 10 mg alefacept, and placebo were 46%, 41%, and 25%, respectively.[99] Although side effects are generally mild and well-tolerated, alefacept has been associated with reduced immunity. Because of its mechanism of action, alefacept can cause a dose-dependent reduction in the total number of circulating lymphocytes, which places the patient at greater risk for infection, such as upper respiratory infections and the common cold.[100]

Ustekinumab is a monoclonal antibody directed against the p40 subunit of IL12 and IL23. Specifically, ustekinumab binds with high affinity to the p40 subunit common to both IL12 and IL23. In a 12-week comparison study of ustekinumab (45 mg or 90 mg) and high-dose etanercept (50 mg twice weekly) for moderate-to-severe psoriasis, ustekinumab was found to have statistically significant greater efficacy.[101] As with all currently available biologics for the treatment of psoriasis, although safety data beyond 3 years have not been reported with ustekinumab, clinicians need to exercise caution when prescribing ustekinumab to immunosuppressed patients and those with a history of malignancy.[102] Common adverse effects include nasopharyngitis, upper respiratory tract infections, and headaches.

Combination Therapy

Combination therapy has been used to increase efficacy and minimize toxicity by leveraging synergism among different medications. Combination

therapy may also be necessary when a single agent is insufficient to adequately control disease severity.

Phototherapy is often used in combination with oral retinoids, such as acitretin, to decrease the total amount of phototherapy sessions necessary to achieve clearance.[103–105] A retrospective study of 40 patients with recalcitrant plaque psoriasis treated with a combination of acitretin and broad-band UV-B three times a week resulted in at least 75% improvements in 29 of the patients examined.[106] A randomized, double-blinded comparison of PUVA with and without acitretin found that 96% of patients receiving combination therapy (PUVA and acitretin) achieved complete or near clearance of psoriasis compared with 80% of patients who received PUVA alone ($P<.05$).[107] The side-effect profiles were also favorable with combination therapy because the cumulative dose of administered PUVA was 42% less with combination therapy compared with monotherapy with PUVA.

Certain combinations of topical therapies have been developed with the goal of achieving greater synergistic efficacy than either agent alone achieves. For example, the efficacy of calcipotriene is enhanced when used in combination with a selected number of agents. In a randomized, double-blinded, phase III clinical trial examining the combined use of calcipotriene with betamethasone compared with monotherapy of each component, the combination of calcipotriene and betamethasone resulted in PASI of 65% to 72% compared with a PASI of 46% to 57% in patients treated with monotherapy alone.[108] A separate study examining combination calcipotriol and acitretin found that 40% of patients achieved complete clearance with the combination therapy compared with 15% in the acitretin monotherapy group after 12 weeks.[109]

Economic Considerations of Treatment Costs

The costs of health care and medications for the treatment of psoriasis continue to climb for patients and society at-large. One study estimated that outpatient cost for treating psoriasis ranged from $1400 to $6000 per year.[4] A 2008 study comparing direct medical costs of 12,280 patients with psoriasis to 36,840 control participants showed that psoriatic patients spend $366 more per month in medical costs compared with the control population.[8] Pearce and colleagues[110] examined the cost-effectiveness of psoriasis treatments over a 12-week period comparing methotrexate, acitretin, cyclosporine, narrow band UV-B, PUVA, etanercept, and efalizumab. The total cost per completed treatment regimen was calculated based on drug acquisition costs, dosing and cost of physician visits, laboratory testing, phototherapy treatment charges, liver biopsy, and infusions charges. The total cost for a 12-week completed treatment was $3921 for PUVA, $2658 for UV-B, $436 for methotrexate, $1419 for acitretin, $2464 for cyclosporine, $4299 for efalizumab, and $7993 for etanercept. The cost-effectiveness for a 12-week completed treatment was $623 for methotrexate, $2729 for acitretin, $3692 for narrow band UV-B, $4668 for PUVA, $16,323 for etanercept, and $17,196 for efalizumab.[110]

SERVICES AVAILABLE
National Resources

Patients with psoriasis and their families can seek educational resources, along with support and advocacy groups, from a variety of national resource organizations. Online educational resources exist on Web sites from the American Academy of Dermatology (www.aad.org), the National Psoriasis Foundation (www.psoarisis.org), and the National Institute of Arthritis and Musculoskeletal and Skin Diseases (www.niams.nih.gov). Psoriasis Cure Now! is a nonprofit patient advocacy group aimed to increase federal funding for psoriasis research and increase access to safe, effective treatments for all psoriasis patients.

One challenge for many psoriasis patients who are uninsured or underinsured is gaining access to the wide range of available treatments. Patients who need assistance on learning how to obtain insurance approval or health care access can find helpful information at Patient Advocate Foundation (www.patientadvocate.org). For patients interested in helping to advance research in psoriasis, patients can search the Web site of the US National Institutes of Health for clinical research studies on psoriasis and psoriatic arthritis (http://clinicaltrials.gov).

Primary Care and Specialty Care of Psoriasis Patients

A recent survey found that psoriasis was more likely to be diagnosed by a dermatologist than by a primary care physician.[111] Eighty-five percent of patients with mild psoriasis were diagnosed during an initial visit with the dermatologist compared with 55% initially seen by a primary care physician. In comparison, 78% and 60% of patients with moderate-to-severe psoriasis were diagnosed by dermatologists and primary care physicians, respectively.[111] Referral to dermatologists need to be considered for patients who had unsatisfactory treatment response to topical

therapy, greater than 10% affected TBSA, presence of pustular lesions, and are candidates for systemic therapy.[112] Patients with moderate-to-severe psoriasis will likely benefit from a multidisciplinary team of dermatologists and other physicians for management of psoriasis and associated co-morbid conditions.

SUMMARY

As basic and translational research efforts continue to expand, researchers are developing novel agents to treat psoriasis, especially for those with moderate-to-severe disease. However, access and affordability of current treatments often present a challenge for segments of the patient population, such as those who are uninsured or underinsured. As previously discussed, the average cost of outpatient treatment can range from $1600 to $6000 per year, which can be prohibitively high for patients without a comprehensive insurance plan.[4] For patients with moderate-to-severe psoriasis who would benefit from biologic therapy, costs often influence the therapeutic decision-making process.[110] Advocacy groups, such as Psoriasis Cure Now!, are working to increase access to safe, effective treatments for all psoriasis patients. The pharmaceutical industry, which produces biologic agents, has begun concerted efforts to offer programs for drug access for underinsured patients. Continued efforts to reduce treatment disparity are necessary in the coming years.

As our understanding of psoriasis evolve from a skin-limited condition to a systemic condition, greater research efforts are necessary in the dermatoepidemiology of psoriasis. Specifically, exploring psoriasis comorbidities will have significant implications on improving the overall health status of psoriasis patients. Although literature is growing on the association between psoriasis and cardiovascular, rheumatologic, and psychiatric comorbidities, we will need to dissect the degree to which these comorbid conditions interact with psoriasis disease process. Future translational research will be necessary to understand common pathophysiological mechanisms that underlie psoriasis and its comorbidities.

In addition to elucidating which comorbid conditions are associated with psoriasis, increased clinical and translational research efforts may be directed at (1) predicting the development of co-morbid conditions, and (2) whether systemic treatment of psoriasis impact health outcomes of comorbid conditions. This scrupulous approach to translational and clinical research will allow us to improve overall wellboing of psoriasis patients.

List of Acronyms

AAD	American Academy of Dermatology
AHA	American Heart Association
CD2	Cluster of differentiation 2
FDA	US Food and Drug Administration
HPA	Hypothalamic-pituitary-adrenal axis
HRQoL	Health-related quality of life
IL12	Interleukin 12
LFA-3	Leukocyte function antigen 3
MI	Myocardial infarction
NAIMS	National Institute of Arthritis and Musculoskeletal and Skin Diseases
NBUVB	Narrow band ultraviolet B
NPF	National Psoriasis Foundation
PASI	Psoriasis Area and Severity Index
PASI75	75% Reduction in the Psoriasis Area and Severity Index
PUVA	Psoralen plus ultraviolet A
RR	Relative risk
TBSA	Total body surface area
TNF	Tumor-necrosis factor
UVB	Ultraviolet B

REFERENCES

1. Neimann AL, Gelfand JM. The epidemiology of psoriasis. Expert Rev Dermatol 2006;1(1):63–75.
2. Freedberg I. Fitzpatrick's dermatology in general medicine. 6th edition. New York: McGraw-Hill; 2003.
3. Schon BW. Psoriasis. N Engl J Med 2005;352:1899–912.
4. Sander HM, Morris LF, Phillips CM, et al. The annual cost of psoriasis. J Am Acad Dermatol 1993;28:422–5.
5. Ferrandiz C, Pujol RM, Garcia-Patos V, et al. Psoriasis of early and late onset: a clinical and epidemiologic study from Spain. J Am Acad Dermatol 2002;46(6):867–73.
6. De Korte J, Sprangers MA, Mombers FM, et al. Quality of life in patients with psoriasis: a systemic literature review. J Investig Dermatol Symp Proc 2004;9(2):140–7.
7. Stern RS, Nijsten T, Feldman SR, et al. Psoriasis is common, carries a substantial burden even when not extensive and is associated with widespread treatment dissatisfaction. J Investig Dermatol Symp Proc 2004;9:136–9.
8. Fowler JF, Duh MS, Rovba L, et al. The impact of psoriasis on health care costs and patient work loss. J Am Acad Dermatol 2008;59(5):772–80.
9. Javitz HS, Ward MM, Farber E, et al. The direct cost of care for psoriasis and psoriatic arthritis in the United States. J Am Acad Dermatol 2002;46(6):850–60.
10. Yu AP, Tang J, Xie J, et al. Economic burden of psoriasis compared to the general population and stratified by disease severity. Curr Med Res Opin 2009;25(10):2429–38.
11. Koo J. Population based epidemiologic study of psoriasis with emphasis on quality of life assessment. Dermatol Clin 1996;14(3):485–96.
12. Gelfand JM, Feldman SR, Stern RS, et al. Determinants of quality of life in patients with psoriasis: a study from the US population. J Am Acad Dermatol 2004;51(5):704–8.
13. Kreuger GK, Koo J, Lebwohl M, et al. The impact of psoriasis on quality of life: results of a 1998 National Psoriasis Foundation patient-membership survey. Arch Dermatol 2001;137(3):280–4.
14. McHenry PM, Doherty V. Psoriasis: an audit of patients' views on the disease and its treatment. Br J Dermatol 1992;127(1):13–7.
15. Gupta MA, Gupta AK, Watteel GN. Perceived deprivation of social touch in psoriasis is associated with greater psychologic morbidity: an index of the stigma experience in dermatologic disorders. Cutis 1998;61(6):339–42.
16. Horn EJ, Fox KM, Patel V, et al. Association of patient-reported psoriasis severity with income and employment. J Am Acad Dermatol 2007;57(6):963–71.
17. Gupta MA, Gupta AK. Psoriasis and sex: a study of moderately to severely affected patients. Int J Dermatol 1997;36(4):259–62.
18. Ramsay B, O'Reagan M. A survey of the social and psychological effects of psoriasis. Br J Dermatol 1988;118(2):195–201.
19. Gottlieb A, Chao C, Dann F. Psoriasis comorbidities. J Dermatolog Treat 2008;19:5–21.
20. Kimball AB, Gladman D, Gelfand JM, et al. National psoriasis foundation clinical consensus on psoriasis comorbidities and recommendations for screening. J Am Acad Dermatol 2008;58:1031–42.
21. Schiepers OJ, Wichers MC, Maes M. Cytokines and major depression. Prog Neuropsychopharmacol Biol Psychiatry 2005;29:201–17.
22. Chodorowska G, Wojnowska D, Juszkiewicz-Borowiec M. Reactive protein and alpha2-macroglobulin plasma activity in medium-severe and severe psoriasis. J Eur Acad Dermatol Venereol 2004;18:180–3.
23. Gupta MA, Gupta AK. Depression and suicidal ideation in dermatology patients with acne, alopecia areata, atopic dermatitis and psoriasis. Br J Dermatol 1998;139(5):846–50.

24. Esposito M, Saraceno R, Guinta A, et al. An Italian study on psoriasis and depression. Dermatology 2006;212:123–7.

25. Van Voorhees AS, Fried R. Depression and quality of life in psoriasis. Postgrad Med 2009;121(4):154–61.

26. Kurd SK, Troxel AB, Crtis-Chritsoph P, et al. The risk of depression, anxiety and suicidality in patients with psoriasis. Arch Dermatol 2010;146(8):891–5.

27. Schmitt J, Ford DE. Psoriasis is independently associated with psychiatric morbidity and adverse cardiovascular risk factors, but not with cardiovascular events in a population-based sample. J Eur Acad Dermatol Venereol 2010;24(8):885–92.

28. Gladman DD. Psoriatic arthritis. Dermatol Ther 2004;17:350–63.

29. Torre Alono JC, Rodriguez Perez A, Arribas Castrillo JM. Psoriatic arthritis (PA): a clinical, immunological and radiological study of 180 patients. Br J Dermatol 1991;30:245–50.

30. McDonald CJ, Calabresi P. Complication of psoriasis. JAMA 1973;224:629.

31. Henseler T, Christophers E. Disease concomitance in psoriasis. J Am Acad Dermatol 1995;32:982–6.

32. Mallbris L, Akre O, Granath F, et al. Increased risk for cardiovascular mortality in psoriasis inpatients but not in outpatients. Eur J Epidemiol 2004;19:225–30.

33. Herron MD, Hinckley M, Hoffman MS, et al. Impact of obesity and smoking on psoriasis presentation and management. Arch Dermatol 2005;141(1):1527–34.

34. Gelfand JM, Neimann AI, Shin DB, et al. Risk of myocardial infarction in patients with psoriasis. JAMA 2006;296(14):1735–41.

35. Neimann AL, Shin DB, Wang X. Prevalence of cardiovascular risk factors in patients with psoriasis. J Am Acad Dermatol 2006;55:829–35.

36. Mallbris L, Granath F, Hamsten A, et al. Psoriasis is associated with lipid abnormalities at the onset of skin disease. J Am Acad Dermatol 2006;54:614–21.

37. Akhyani M, Ehsani AH, Robati RM, et al. The lipid profile in psoriasis: a controlled study. J Eur Acad Dermatol Venereol 2007;21:1330–2.

38. Grundy SM, Cleeman JI, Daniels SR, et al. Diagnosis and management of the metabolic syndrome: an American Heart Association/National Heart, Lung and Blood Institute Scientific Statement. Circulation 2005;112:2735–52.

39. Love TJ, Qureshi AA, Karlson EW, et al. Prevalence of the metabolic syndrome in psoriasis: results from the National Health and Nutrition Examination Survey, 2003-2006. Arch Dermatol 2011;147(4):419–24.

40. Laaksonen DE, Laaka HM, Niskanen LK, et al. Metabolic syndrome and development of diabetes mellitus: application and validation of recently suggested definitions of the metabolic syndrome in a prospective cohort study. Am J Epidemiol 2002;156:1070–7.

41. Isomaa B, Almgren P, Tuomi T, et al. Cardiovascular morbidity and mortality associated with the metabolic syndrome. Diabetes Care 2001;24:683–9.

42. Margolis D, Biker W, Hennessy S, et al. The risk of malignancy associated with psoriasis. Arch Dermatol 2001;137:778–83.

43. Frentz G, Olsen JH. Malignant tumours and psoriasis: a follow-up study. Br J Dermatol 1999;140:237–42.

44. Boffetta P, Gridley G, Lindelof B. Cancer risk in a population-based cohort of patients hospitalized for psoriasis in Sweden. J Invest Dermatol 2001;117:1531–7.

45. Paul CF, Ho VC, McGeown C, et al. Risk of malignancies in psoriasis patients treated with cyclosporine: a 5 y cohort study. J Invest Dermatol 2003;120:211–6.

46. Stern RS, Nichols KT, Vakeva LH. Malignant melanoma in patients treated for psoriasis with methoxsalen (psoralen) and ultraviolet A radiation (PUVA). The PUVA Follow-up Study. N Engl J Med 1997;336(15):1041–5.

47. Gerdes S, Mrowietz U. Impact of comorbidities on the management of psoriasis. In: Yawalkar N, editor, Management of psoriasis, vol. 38. Basel (Switzerland): Karger; 2009. p. 21–6.

48. Farber EM, Nall L. Psoriasis and alcoholism. Cutis 1994;53(1):21–7.

49. Higgins EM, Du Vivier AW. Alcohol abuse and treatment resistance in skin disease. J Am Acad Dermatol 1994;30(6):1048.

50. Wolf R, Wolf D, Ruocco V. Alcohol intake and psoriasis. Clin Dermatol 1999;17(4):423–30.

51. Qureshi AA, Dominguez PL, Choi HK, et al. Alcohol intake and risk of incident psoriasis in US women: a prospective study. Arch Dermatol 2010;146(12):1364–9.

52. Fortes C, Mastroeni S, Leffondre K, et al. Relationship between smoking and clinical severity of psoriasis. Arch Dermatol 2005;141(12):1580–4.

53. Hayes J, Koo J. Psoriasis: depression, anxiety, smoking and drinking habits. Dermatol Ther 2010;23(2):174–80.

54. Fortune DG, Richards HL, Kirby B, et al. A cognitive-behavioural symptom management programme as an adjunct in psoriasis therapy. Br J Dermatol 2002;146(3):458–65.

55. Weinsterin GD, Menter MA. An overview of psoriasis. In: Weinstein GD, Gottlieb AB, editors. Therapy of moderate-to-severe psoriasis. New York: Mercel Dekker, Inc; 2003. p. 1–28.

56. Drake LA, Ceilley RI, Cornelison RL, et al. Guidelines of care for psoriasis. J Am Acad Dermatol 1993;28:632–7.

57. Brown BC, Warren RB, Grindlay DJ, et al. What's new in psoriasis? Analysis of the clinical

significance of systematic reviews on psoriasis published in 2007 and 2008. Clin Exp Dermatol 2009;34:664–7.

58. Koo J. Sequential therapy of psoriasis. Introducing a new therapeutic paradigm for better clinical results. J Am Acad Dermatol 1999;41:S25–8.

59. Kreuger G. Current concepts and review of alefacept in the treatment of psoriasis. Dermatol Clin 2004;22:407–26.

60. Wahl A, Loge JH, Wiklund I, et al. The burden of psoriasis: a study concerning health-related quality of life among Norwegian adult patients with psoriasis compared with general population norms. J Am Acad Dermatol 2000;43(5 Pt 1):803–8.

61. Katz HI, Hien NT, Prawer SE, et al. Superpotent topical steroid treatment of psoriasis vulgaris—clinical efficacy and adrenal function. J Am Acad Dermatol 1987;16(4):804–11.

62. Tristani-Firouzi P, Kreuger GG. Efficacy and safety of treatment modalities for psoriasis. Cutis 1998;61(Suppl 2):11–21.

63. Pariser DM, Bagel J, Gelfand JM, et al. National Psoriasis Foundation clinical consensus on disease severity. Arch Dermatol 2007;143:239–42.

64. Kreuger CG, Feldman SR, Camisa C. Two considerations for patients with psoriasis and their clinicians: what defines mild, moderate, and severe psoriasis? J Am Acad Dermatol 2000;43(2 Pt 1):281–5.

65. Gower WR Jr. Mechanism of glucocorticoid action. J Fla Med Assoc 1993;80(10):697–700.

66. Cornell RC. Clinical trials of topical corticosteroids in psoriasis: correlations with the vasoconstrictor assay. Int J Dermatol 1992;31(Suppl 1):38–40.

67. Gibson JR, Kirsch JM, Darley CR, et al. An assessment of the relationship between vasoconstrictor assay findings, clinical efficacy and skin thinning effects of a variety of undiluted and diluted corticosteroid preparations. Br J Dermatol 1984;111(Suppl 27):204–12.

68. Levin C, Maibach HI. Topical corticosteroid-induced adrenocortical insufficiency: clinical implications. Am J Clin Dermatol 2002;3(3):141–7.

69. Georgiou S, Tsambaos D. Hypercalcaemia and hypercalciuria after topical treatment of psoriasis with excessive amounts of calcipotriol. Acta Derm Venereol 1999;79(1):86.

70. Yamauchi PS, Rizk D, Kormili T, et al. Systemic retinoids. In: Weinstein GD, Gottlieb AB, editors. Therapy of moderate-to-severe psoriasis. New York: Marcel Dekker, Inc; 2003. p. 137–50.

71. Lebwohl M, Ast E, Callen JP, et al. Once-daily tazarotene gel versus twice-daily fluocinonide cream in the treatment of plaque psoriasis. J Am Acad Dermatol 1998;38(5 Pt 1):705–11.

72. Vissers WH, Van Vlijmen I, Van Erp PE, et al. Topical treatment of mild to moderate plaque psoriasis with 0.3% tacrolimus gel and 0.5% tacrolimus cream: the effect on SUM score, epidermal proliferation, keratinization, T-cell subsets and HLA-DR expression. Br J Dermatol 2008;158(4):705–12.

73. Zonneveld IM, Rubins A, Jablonska S, et al. Topical tacrolimus is not effective in chronic plaque psoriasis: a pilot study. Arch Dermatol 1998;134:1101–2.

74. Remitz A, Reitamo S, Erkko P, et al. Tacrolimus ointment improves psoriasis in microplaque assay. Br J Dermatol 1999;141:103–7.

75. Clayton TH, Harrison PV, Nicholls R, et al. Topical tacrolimus for facial psoriasis. Br J Dermatol 2003;149:419–20.

76. Stern RS. The risk of melanoma in association with long-term exposure to PUVA. J Am Acad Dermatol 2001;44:755–61.

77. Hanseler T, Christophers E, Honigsmann H, et al. Skin tumors in the European PUVA study. J Am Acad Dermatol 1987;16:108–16.

78. Stern RS, Thibodeau LA, Kleinerman RA, et al. Risk of cutaneous carcinoma in patients treated with oral methoxsalen photochemotherapy for psoriasis. N Engl J Med 1979;300:809–13.

79. Marcil I, Stern RS. Squamous cell cancer of the skin in patients given PUVA and cyclosporin: nested cohort crossover study. Lancet 2001;358:1042–5.

80. Lindelof B, Siguirgeirsson B, Tegner E, et al. PUVA and cancer: a large-scale epidemiological study. Lancet 1991;338(8759):91–3.

81. Lee E, Koo J, Berger T. UVB phototherapy and skin cancer risk: a review of the literature. Int J Dermatol 2005;44(5):355–60.

82. Torinuki W, Tagami H. Incidence of skin cancer in Japanese psoriatic patients treated with either methoxsalen phototherapy, Goeckerman regimen, or both therapies. A 10-year follow-up study. J Am Acad Dermatol 1988;18(6):1278–81.

83. Coven TR, Burack LH, Gillaeudeau P, et al. Narrow-band UVB produces superior clinical and histopathological resolution of moderate-to-severe psoriasis in patients compared with broadband UVB. Arch Dermatol 1997;133:1514–22.

84. Van Dooren-Greebe RJ, Kiujpers AL, Mulder J, et al. Methotrexate revisited: effects of long-term treatment in psoriasis. Br J Dermatol 1994;130(2):204–10.

85. Roenigk HH, Auerbach R, Maibach HI, et al. Methotrexate guidelines revised. J Am Acad Dermatol 1982;6:145–55.

86. Roenigk HH, Auerbach R, Maibach HI, et al. Methotrexate in psoriasis: consensus conference. J Am Acad Dermatol 1998;38:478–85.

87. Otley CC, Stasko T, Tope WD, et al. Chemoprevention of nonmelanoma skin cancer with systemic

retinoids: practical dosing and management of adverse effects. Dermatol Surg 2006;32:562–8.

88. Ellis CN, Fradin MS, Messana JM, et al. Cyclosporine for plaque-type psoriasis. Results of a multidose, double-blind trial. N Engl J Med 1991;324(5):277–84.

89. Shupack J, Abel E, Bauer E, et al. Cyclosporine as maintenance therapy in patients with severe psoriasis. J Am Acad Dermatol 1997;36:423–32.

90. Mahrle G, Schulze HJ, Farber L, et al. Low-dose short-term cyclosporine versus etretinate in psoriasis: improvement of skin, nail and join involvement. J Am Acad Dermatol 1995;32:78–88.

91. Ho VC, Griffiths CE, Berth-Jones J, et al. Intermittent short courses of cyclosporine microemulsion for the long-term management of psoriasis: a 2-year cohort study. J Am Acad Dermatol 2001;44:643–51.

92. Bahner JD, Cao LY, Korman NJ. Biologics in the management of psoriasis. Clin Cosmet Investig Dermatol 2009;2:111–28.

93. Weinberg JM. An overview of infliximab, etanercept, efalizumab, and alefacept as biologic therapy for psoriasis. Clin Ther 2003;25(10): 2487–505.

94. Menter A, Tyring SK, Gordon K, et al. Adalimumab therapy for moderate to severe psoriasis: a randomized, controlled phase III trial. J Am Acad Dermatol 2008;58(1):106–15.

95. Scallon B, Cai A, Solowski N, et al. Binding and functional comparisons of two types of tumor necrosis factor antagonists. J Pharmacol Exp Ther 2002;301(2):418–26.

96. Schmitt J, Zhang Z, Wozel G, et al. Efficacy and tolerability of biologic and nonbiologic systemic treatments for moderate-to-severe psoriasis: meta-analysis of randomized controlled trials. Br J Dermatol 2008;159(3):513–26.

97. Desai SB, Furst DE. Problems encountered during anti-tumor necrosis factor therapy. Best Pract Res Clin Rheumatol 2006;20(4):757–90.

98. Langley RG, Strober BE, Gu Y, et al. Benefit-risk assessment of tumour necrosis factor antagonists in the treatment of psoriasis. Br J Dermatol 2010; 162(6):1349–58.

99. Lebwohl M, Christophers E, Langley R, et al. An international, randomized, double-blind, placebo-controlled phase 3 trial of intramuscular alefacept in patients with chronic plaque psoriasis. Arch Dermatol 2003;139(6):719–27.

100. Ellis CN, Krueger GG. Alefácept Clinical Study Group. Treatment of chronic plaque psoriasis by selective targeting of memory effector T lymphocytes. N Engl J Med 2001;345(4):248–55.

101. Griffiths CEM, Stroker BE, Van de Kerkhof P, et al. Comparison of Ustekinumab and Etanercept for Moderate-to-Severe Psoriasis. N Engl J Med 2010;362:118–28.

102. Stelara safety information. Available at: www.stelarainfo.com. 2010. Accessed February 10, 2011.

103. Iest J, Boer J. Combined treatment of psoriasis with acitretin and UVB phototherapy compared with acitretin alone and UVB alone. Br J Dermatol 1989; 120:665–70.

104. Lebwohl M. Acitretin in combination with UVB or PUVA. J Am Acad Dermatol 1999;41(3 Pt 2): S22–4.

105. Lowe N, Prystowsky JH, Bourget T, et al. Acitretin plus UVB therapy for psoriasis: comparisons with placebo plus UVB and acitretin alone. J Am Acad Dermatol 1991;24:591–4.

106. Spuls PI, Lebwohl M. Retrospective study of the efficacy of narrowband UVB and acitretin. J Dermatolog Treat 2003;14(Suppl 2):17–20.

107. Tanew A, Guggenbichler A, Honigsmann H, et al. Photochemotherapy for severe psoriasis without or in combination with acitretin: a randomized, double-blind comparison study. J Am Acad Dermatol 1991;26:682–4.

108. Kragballe K, Van de Kerhof PC. Consistency of data in six phase III clinical studies of a two-compound product containing calcipotriol and betamethasone dipropionate ointment for the treatment of psoriasis. J Eur Acad Dermatol Venereol 2006;20(1):39–44.

109. Rim JH, Paark JY, Choe YB, et al. The efficacy of calcipotriol and acitretin combination therapy for psoriasis. Am J Clin Dermatol 2003;4(7):507–10.

110. Pearce DJ, Nelson AA, Fleischer AB, et al. The cost-effectiveness and cost of treatment failures associated with systemic psoriasis therapies. J Dermatolog Treat 2006;17:29–37.

111. Available at: www.decisionresources.com. 2010. Accessed February 15, 2011.

112. Referral Guide. Psoriasis. In: Dermatology AAO, editor. Indications for dermatology referrals in a managed care setting. Schaumburg (IL): American Academy of Dermatology; 2009.

Health Outcomes in Atopic Dermatitis

Balvinder Rehal, BS[a], April W. Armstrong, MD, MPH[b],*

KEYWORDS

- Atopic dermatitis • Health outcomes • Disease severity
- Quality of life

Atopic dermatitis or eczema is a chronic inflammatory skin disease characterized by itchy, scaly lesions. The Hanifin and Rajka criteria require that three or more major criteria and three or more minor criteria be present for diagnosis (**Box 1**).[1] Major criteria include pruritus, a typical morphology and distribution, a chronic relapsing dermatitis, and a personal or family history of atopy.[1] Examples of minor criteria include xerosis, raised serum IgE, and an early age of onset.[1]

PREVALENCE AND INCIDENCE OF ATOPIC DERMATITIS

Atopic dermatitis is a common skin disease that affects up to 25% of children worldwide.[2] The condition begins in infancy in 60% of cases.[3] Data from the 2003 National Survey of Children's Health estimated an overall prevalence rate of 10.7% for atopic dermatitis in children younger than 17 years in the United States, with a range from 8.7% to 18.1%.[4]

ASSESSMENT OF HEALTH OUTCOMES IN ATOPIC DERMATITIS

Although primarily focused on disease severity and quality of life, the range of potential measurable health outcomes in atopic dermatitis is wide. Disease-severity measurements can include objective clinical parameters that assess degree of erythema, exudation, and excoriations; they can also include subjective criteria such as itching and sleep disturbance. Quality of life is defined as the perception of disease impact on physical, psychological, and social well-being.[5,6]

Disease-severity scales in atopic dermatitis include disease-specific and non–disease-specific scales. Examples of disease-specific scales include the Severity Scoring of Atopic Dermatitis (SCORAD), Eczema Area and Severity Index (EASI), and Six Area, Six Sign Atopic Dermatitis (SASSAD), while non–disease-specific scales include the Investigators' Global Assessment (IGA), Total Body Severity Assessment (TBSA), and Visual Analog Scale (VAS). Since the number and type of assessed clinical features vary between scales, a lack of standardization of objective severity scales exists for atopic dermatitis. With some scales assessing multiple body sites while other scales assess only the most severely affected site, diversity exists in the methods of measuring disease extent. Disease-severity scales commonly used in randomized controlled trials (RCTs) of atopic dermatitis treatment include SCORAD, EASI, and IGA. The characteristic features, validity, and reliability of these scales are discussed in the following section.

The SCORAD was developed in 1993 by the European Task Force on Atopic Dermatitis.[7] This scale uses the "rule of nines" to assess disease

Funding sources: None.

Disclosures: The authors have no disclosures relevant to this article.

[a] Department of Dermatology, University of California Davis Health System, University of California Davis, 3301 C Street, Suite 1400, Sacramento, CA 95816, USA

[b] Dermatology Clinical Research Unit, Teledermatology Program, Department of Dermatology, University of California Davis Health System, University of California Davis School of Medicine, 3301 C Street, Suite 1400, Sacramento, CA 95816, USA

* Corresponding author.

E-mail address: aprilarmstrong@post.harvard.edu

Dermatol Clin 30 (2012) 73–86

doi:10.1016/j.det.2011.08.007

0733-8635/12/$ – see front matter Published by Elsevier Inc.

Box 1
Atopic dermatitis diagnosis criteria

Major Criteria

Pruritus, a typical morphology and distribution, a chronic relapsing dermatitis, and a personal or family history of atopy

Minor Criteria

Xerosis; ichthyosis, palmar hyperlinearity, or keratosis pilaris; immediate (type 1) skin-test reactivity; elevated serum IgE; early age of onset; tendency toward cutaneous infections (especially *Staphylococcus aureus* and herpes simplex) or impaired cell-mediated immunity; tendency toward nonspecific hand or foot dermatitis; nipple eczema; cheilitis; recurrent conjunctivitis; Dennie-Morgan infraorbital fold; keratoconus; anterior subcapsular cataracts; orbital darkening; facial pallor or facial erythema; pityriasis alba; anterior neck folds; itch when sweating; intolerance to wool and lipid solvents; perifollicular accentuation; food intolerance; course influenced by environmental or emotional factors; white dermographism or delayed blanch

Data from Hanifin J, Rajka G. Diagnostic features of atopic dermatitis. Acta Derm Venereol 1980;92:44–7.

---

extent and evaluates 5 clinical characteristics to determine disease severity: (1) erythema, (2) edema/papulation, (3) oozing/crusts, (4) excoriation, and (5) lichenification. The SCORAD also assesses subjective symptoms of pruritus and sleep loss with VAS.[7] Extent of disease, disease severity, and subjective symptoms combine to give a maximum possible score of 103. Although it is a combined score, the three aspects can be separated and used individually if necessary. Of all the severity scales used in atopic dermatitis, the SCORAD is the most widely validated disease-severity instrument.[8] The SCORAD is valid and reliable and has shown excellent agreement with global assessments of disease severity.[7–9] However, some studies have shown interobserver variation in scoring lichenification and extent of disease.[7–12]

The EASI was developed by modifying the PASI (Psoriasis Area and Severity Index), a widely accepted and standardized scoring system for psoriasis.[13] The EASI assesses extent of disease at four body sites and measures four clinical signs on a scale of 0 to 3: (1) erythema, (2) induration/papulation, (3) excoriation, and (4) lichenification. The EASI confers a maximum score of 72[14] and

evaluates two dimensions of atopic dermatitis: disease extent and clinical signs. Although some investigators contend that subjective symptoms may be the most important marker for assessing patient morbidity and may act as a good indicator for disease severity, unlike the SCORAD, the EASI does not assess symptoms such as pruritus and sleep loss. In a large validation study with a cohort of 1550 pediatric patients, the EASI was found to have excellent validity, internal consistency, and sensitivity to change.[15] While the EASI is a valid and reliable instrument, most interobserver variability lies in the dimension of induration/papulation.[14–18]

The IGA allows investigators to assess overall disease severity at one given time point, and it consists of a 6-point severity scale from "clear" to "very severe" disease (0 = clear, 1 = almost clear, 2 = mild disease, 3 = moderate disease, 4 = severe disease, and 5 = very severe disease).[19] The IGA uses clinical characteristics of erythema, infiltration, papulation, oozing, and crusting as guidelines for the overall severity assessment.[19] To the authors' knowledge, the IGA has not been validated as an outcome measure.[20] However, the IGA has been used to validate other outcome scales.[8,15] Potential weaknesses of the IGA include lack of responsiveness and discrimination for disease severity and lack of subjective symptoms.

Quality-of-life scales also include both disease-specific and non–disease-specific scales. Instruments specific to atopic dermatitis include the Dermatitis Family Impact (DFI), Parent's Index of Quality of Life in Atopic Dermatitis (PIQoL-AD), and Quality of Life Index for Atopic Dermatitis (QoLIAD). Non–disease-specific scales include the Dermatology Life Quality Index (DLQI), Children's Dermatology Life Quality Index (CDLQI), and Infants' Dermatitis Quality of Life Index (ID-QOL). Quality-of-life measurements are increasingly being recognized as important outcome measures but currently are primarily used to supplement existing measurement tools in dermatology. Quality-of-life scales commonly used in RCTs of the treatment of atopic dermatitis are the CDLQI, DFI, and DLQI. The features and validity of these scales are reviewed in the following section.

The CDLQI, which purposes to measure the quality of life in children with skin disease, was developed by Lewis-Jones and Finlay[21] and validated in 1995. The questionnaire was designed for children of ages 4 through 16 years. The CDLQI is completed by the child with assistance from an adult if necessary. The survey consists of 10 questions that evaluate the aspects of a child's life that could be affected by their skin disease. The instrument includes physical symptoms such as itching and sleep loss and psychosocial questions regarding friendships, bullying, school performance, sports participation, and enjoyment of vacation. The questions are individually graded from 0 to 3 with a maximum possible combined score of 30; the higher scores represent worse quality of life.[21] In the initial validation study, children with atopic eczema accounted for 20% of all patients.[21] To determine test-retest repeatability, the CDLQI was used in a population of children without skin disease.[21]

Since its validation, the CDLQI has been used in numerous studies to determine the effectiveness of interventions in children with atopic dermatitis.[22,23] The CDLQI has been translated and validated in Cantonese.[24–26] A cartoon version of the CDLQI, which appears to be quicker and preferred by children, was validated in 2003.[27]

The DFI questionnaire was developed in 1998 by Lawson, Lewis-Jones, Finlay, Reid, and Owens to help measure how family life is affected by a child suffering from atopic dermatitis.[28] The DFI is designed to be completed by a caretaker of the child, who is often the parent. It consists of 10 questions related to housework, food preparation and feeding, sleep, family leisure activity, shopping, fatigue, emotional distress, and relationships.[28] Each question is graded from 0 to 3 with a maximum combined score of 30. The DFI was deemed valid, reliable, and sensitive to change in multiple studies.[24,28–34] Two of the studies assessing validity of the instrument used the separate components of the DFI instead of the total score as was originally intended.[28,31] The DFI has also been validated in Malay and Portuguese.[24,29,30,34]

The DLQI was developed in 1994 by Finlay and Khan[35] to measure quality of life in adults older than 18 years in routine clinical-practice settings. The DLQI is a 10-item questionnaire that evaluates skin symptoms, feelings of embarrassment, and how skin disease has affected day-to-day activities, working life, and social life. Similar to the CDLQI, each question on DLQI is scored from 0 to 3 with a maximum score of 30 indicating the worst quality of life. In the original article by Finlay and Khan, scores of those patients with atopic dermatitis indicated poorer quality of life than the scores of patients with other skin diseases assessed by the DLQI.[35] The DLQI has been extensively validated in multiple studies.[35–37] A 10-year review of the literature found that the DLQI is highly specific for assessing decrements in quality of life in patients with atopic dermatitis.[37] Specifically, patients with atopic eczema had a mean score of 4.2 compared with 0.3 in the disease-free population. The DLQI has high repeatability, internal consistency, and sensitivity to change.[37]

RESULTS OF HEALTH OUTCOMES IN ATOPIC DERMATITIS

Atopic dermatitis makes a significant impact on patients' quality of life given its potential long-term physical, social, and psychological impairments.[38–42] In children suffering from atopic dermatitis, 60% of the parents reported that their child had difficulties with school performance and with social and leisure activities.[43] Scratching has been associated with disturbed sleep patterns, including difficulty in getting to sleep, frequent night-time wakening, reduced total sleep, and difficulty awakening for school.[44–47] Children rate itching and sleep loss as the most bothersome aspect of their disease.[21,32,44] Sleep loss can lead to daytime behavior and discipline problems.[45] Daud and colleagues[48] showed that 23% of preschool children had a significant increase in behavioral symptoms compared with 5% of controls. Children also experience teasing and bullying from the appearance of atopic dermatitis lesions, which may lead to embarrassment, loss of confidence, mood changes, and depression.[21]

The family members of children with atopic dermatitis can likewise suffer decrements in quality of life. Parents may lose an average of 2.5 hours of sleep per night, while 38% of siblings of children with atopic dermatitis experienced disturbed sleep.[44,49] Physical and mental exhaustion from sleep loss causes mood changes and impaired performance at school or work for family members.[45,49] Caring for a child with atopic dermatitis can cause parents to miss work and suffer financial losses.[49,50] When a child in the family is diagnosed with atopic dermatitis, families may experience lifestyle restrictions, including dietary limitations, vacation choices, and pet ownership.[49] Ninety percent of families reported problems with household issues such as laundry, cleaning, and food preparation.[49] Parents may also suffer psychological distress from hearing others comment negatively about their child's appearance.[51]

In a study using the DLQI and another quality-of-life instrument, the SF-36 (Short Form Health Survey), adult patients with atopic dermatitis were found to have significantly impaired quality of life in comparison with the general United States population in the vitality, social functioning, and mental health dimensions of the SF-36.[38] Atopic dermatitis patients had similar DLQI scores to patients with other chronic dermatologic diseases.[38] When compared specifically with psoriasis, atopic dermatitis patients had lower scores in vitality, social functioning, role-emotional, role-physical, and mental health.[38] When compared with other nondermatologic chronic diseases such as diabetes and hypertension, atopic dermatitis patients had lower mental health scores. A correlation also existed between increased severity of atopic dermatitis and greater impairments in quality of life.[52]

Gender differences appear to play a role in the psychological impact of atopic dermatitis. With similar levels of disease severity, women with atopic dermatitis report a poorer quality of life than men.[53–55] Women with visible skin lesions report more social anxiety, helplessness, and anxious-depressive symptoms than men.[56]

Atopic dermatitis can also have an impact on patient-partner relationships. In a study investigating the sexual life of atopic dermatitis patients and their partners, 57.5% of patients reported a decrease in sexual desire due to atopic dermatitis, with 36.5% reporting that the appearance of eczema had an impact on their sex life.[57]

TREATMENT OF ATOPIC DERMATITIS AND ITS EFFECT ON HEALTH OUTCOMES

The symptoms of atopic dermatitis can be controlled with both topical and oral medications. Treatment is aimed at reducing skin inflammation and controlling pruritus. The general categories of therapy for mild to moderate atopic dermatitis include emollients, topical steroids, topical calcineurin inhibitors, oral antihistamines, phototherapy, probiotics, and educational support. The most common treatment is a combination of an emollient and corticosteroid. The following section presents the most common treatment options for atopic dermatitis, the evidence for their efficacy, and the effect of treatment on health outcome measures.

Emollients

Skin hydration is an important component of the treatment of atopic dermatitis, as xerosis is a hallmark of the disease. Maintaining hydration is often achieved by ample lubrication of the skin with emollients. Emollients also have a steroid-sparing effect in the treatment of atopic dermatitis. In a study done in infants with atopic dermatitis, emollients decreased the need for moderate-potency or high-potency topical corticosteroids.[31] The study evaluated the effect of an oat extract–containing emollient on the amount of topical steroid used; the intervention group decreased steroid use by 42%, while the control group decreased use by 7.5%. In addition to comparing the amount of corticosteroid used, disease severity and quality of life

of the infant and parent was evaluated. Disease severity was assessed with the SCORAD. Infant's and parent's quality of life was assessed using the IDQOL and DFI, respectively. All aspects of the SCORAD significantly improved for both treatment groups. However, the only significant difference in symptom relief between treatment groups was dryness, which was decreased in the emollient group. Both groups showed highly significant improvement in the quality of life for infants and parents. Comparing the two treatment groups, the only significant difference included the sleep item in the DFI score, which was better in the emollient group than in the control group.

In another study, a new emollient containing 2% Sunflower oil Oleodistillate (SO) was tested for its steroid-sparing effect.[58] Disease severity and quality of life were also assessed with the SCORAD and IDQOL/DFI, respectively. The components of the SCORAD that improved significantly among all groups were lichenification and excoriation.[58] The study showed that application of steroid every other day with the SO cream was as effective as once or twice daily application of the steroid alone; these findings suggest that the new emollient provided a steroid-sparing effect. According to the IDQOL, parents reported a large improvement in quality of life for children who were treated with SO cream and any dose of steroid. Furthermore, parents of children receiving SO cream in combination with topical steroids reported a greater improvement in DFI scores compared with parents of children receiving steroid cream without SO cream.

Topical Corticosteroids

Topical corticosteroids are a mainstay of treatment in atopic dermatitis. Steroids of different potency are used based on the severity of disease. Low-potency topical steroids are effective for mild disease, whereas high-potency topical corticosteroids can be in used in patients with acute flares. High-potency corticosteroids are avoided in sensitive areas such as the face and skin folds. Topical steroids can be used multiple times a day, but no clear benefit has been shown for more frequent use than once daily.[59–62]

Various formulations of corticosteroids have been shown to be efficacious in the treatment of atopic dermatitis. For example, a review of two RCTs using 0.05% halobetasol propionate (HP) ointment twice daily for 2 weeks showed an improvement in symptoms scores in the HP group compared with the placebo group.[63] One RCT used the Physician's Global Assessment (PGA) to evaluate overall disease severity and showed a significant improvement in the HP group over the placebo group, with 38% of patients in the HP group completely resolving their lesions compared to 6.5% in the placebo group. Another study that also used the PGA to assess disease severity tested clobetasol propionate (CP) emollient cream 0.05% in a 4-week RCT.[64] Patients with moderate to severe atopic dermatitis were treated with CP cream twice daily for 4 weeks. PGA scores were improved in the treatment group in comparison with the placebo group by day 4 and remained improved throughout the treatment period.

Topical steroids can also be used in maintenance therapy to help prevent relapse. In a study in adults with atopic dermatitis, long-term management for recurring atopic dermatitis was studied using fluticasone propionate (FP) ointment.[65] All patients were initially treated with FP 0.005% ointment. Those who achieved clearance or near clearance then entered one of two long-term treatment categories: either FP or placebo ointment once daily, twice a week for 16 weeks to healed lesions. Efficacy was measured using the SCORAD. At the end of the initial treatment, SCORAD values were significantly improved. After the maintenance phase, the FP group maintained their improvement from baseline, but the placebo group deteriorated.

FP 0.005% ointment was also tested in children for maintenance therapy.[66] Children with moderate to severe atopic dermatitis were treated initially with FP ointment. Those who entered remission were subsequently treated twice weekly with either FP or placebo ointment for 16 weeks to test prevention of exacerbations. A decrease in disease severity was observed at the end of the initial treatment phase. SCORAD values increased in both the FP and placebo group after the maintenance phase. However, the scores from the FP group increased to a lesser degree than the placebo group's scores. The risk of exacerbation was also calculated with hazard ratios using a target lesion score, and the risk was found to be more than twice as high in the placebo group than in the FP group, which demonstrates that FP maintenance therapy reduces the risk of disease relapse in children with atopic dermatitis.

Maintenance therapy with topical corticosteroids has also been shown to improve quality of life in patients with atopic dermatitis.[67] In a study testing methylprednisolone aceponate (MPA) cream twice weekly for 16 weeks in patients 12 years of age or older, investigators examined intensity of itch, quality of sleep, and overall quality of life.[67] The total DLQI and CDLQI scores improved with MPA treatment and worsened in all categories in the placebo group. While intensity of itch decreased in both groups, the improvement was more substantial in the MPA group than in the placebo group.

Topical Calcineurin Inhibitors

Topical calcineurin inhibitors are a class of steroid-sparing medications effective for the treatment of atopic dermatitis.[68–70] One advantage of calcineurin inhibitors is that they do not cause skin atrophy, a side effect which can be observed with long-term topical steroid use. Two calcineurin inhibitors approved by the Food and Drug Administration for use in children older than 2 years are tacrolimus and pimecrolimus. These two topical calcineurin inhibitors are considered equivalent in strength to low-potency topical steroids and are both applied twice a day.[71] Calcineurin inhibitors are second-line agents; mid-potency to high-potency topical steroids exhibit greater clinical efficacy and are therefore preferred as first-line agents.[71] In a study comparing the efficacy of MPA ointment 0.1% with that of tacrolimus 0.03% in children and adolescents with an acute atopic dermatitis flare, a significantly greater mean percentage improvement from baseline was found in the MPA group compared with tacrolimus, as measured by the EASI.[72] Results for the CDLQI also showed greater improvement in the MPA group in comparison with the tacrolimus group in the categories of "symptoms and feelings" and "sleep."

Topical tacrolimus has been shown to be an effective alternative to topical steroids, and its efficacy has been shown in several RCTs.[73–80] Specifically, studies measuring disease severity by the EASI in both adult and pediatric patients have shown significantly greater improvement in tacrolimus treatment groups compared with placebo groups.[79,81,82] Tacrolimus has also been shown to improve quality of life in patients with atopic dermatitis.[83–85] In a study comparing two concentrations of tacrolimus ointment (0.03% and 0.1%) versus placebo, both adult and pediatric quality of life was evaluated. Adult quality of life was evaluated using the DLQI, and pediatric quality of life was evaluated using the CDLQI.[83] Quality of life was assessed at baseline, 3 weeks, and at the end of the trial at 12 weeks. Results showed a significant improvement among adults in both tacrolimus groups in comparison with the placebo group and in all aspects of quality of life. In the pediatric patients, both tacrolimus groups demonstrated significant improvements in quality of life in all aspects, except for personal relationships. In a long-term study of maintenance treatment with 0.1% tacrolimus ointment in adults, quality of life was measured using the EQ-5D.[84] Patients were treated twice daily with tacrolimus ointment for 6 weeks and were subsequently treated with either tacrolimus ointment or emollient vehicle twice weekly for 1 year. Results showed initial treatment with tacrolimus ointment significantly improved quality of life for adults with moderate and severe atopic dermatitis. The improvement was sustained over the 1-year maintenance period.

Pimecrolimus has a similar mechanism of action to tacrolimus. Pimecrolimus is effective in treating atopic dermatitis but does not have systemic immune effects.[86] Pimecrolimus is also effective in reducing the need for topical steroids and preventing atopic dermatitis flares.[87,88] Several studies have assessed the effects of pimecrolimus treatment on disease severity and quality of life in patients with atopic dermatitis. In adolescents and adults, disease severity was measured using the EASI and IGA in two studies.[89,90] The first study investigated the efficacy of pimecrolimus cream 1%, twice daily and four times daily to all affected areas in patients with moderate to severe atopic dermatitis.[90] Both groups improved in IGA and EASI scores, with no statistical difference between groups. In the second study, pimecrolimus cream 1% was tested in the head and neck of patients older than 12 years with mild to moderate atopic dermatitis. Results showed a significant improvement in IGA and head and neck EASI scores. Of note, compared to those patients treated with placebo, significantly more patients treated with pimecrolimus achieved clearance of their eyelid dermatitis. Studies in children and infants have also shown greater improvement in the EASI and IGA scores of patients using pimecrolimus than those using placebo.[91–95]

In quality-of-life studies, pimecrolimus has been shown to improve parents' quality of life.[18,96,97] In two studies, the PIQoL-AD was used to assess parents' quality of life after treatment with pimecrolimus cream.[96,97] In the first study, pediatric patients were treated with pimecrolimus cream 1% for 24 weeks. Results showed a significant improvement in parents' quality of life compared with the control group after acute and after long-term treatment.[96] In the second study, also done in a pediatric population, pimecrolimus cream 1% was given for 26 weeks. Parents' quality of life was assessed at baseline, 6 weeks, and 6 months.[97] Results showed a statistically significant improvement in PIQoL-AD scores at 6 weeks and 6 months. In a study in infants with mild to severe atopic dermatitis, parents' quality of life was measured by the PQoL-AD after 4 weeks of treatment with pimecrolimus.[18] Results showed

an improvement in all 5 areas of the questionnaire, including psychosomatic well-being, effects on social life, confidence in medical treatment, emotional coping, and acceptance of disease.

Oral Antihistamines

Oral antihistamines are often used in the treatment of atopic dermatitis as an adjunctive therapy for pruritus.[98] However, the studies testing antihistamines have shown conflicting results.[99] In a study in 2006, 20 adult patients with moderate atopic dermatitis who had not received any treatment for two weeks were randomized to the second-generation antihistamine, fexofenadine, and either emollient treatment or steroid treatment for 1 week.[100] Disease severity was assessed with the SCORAD and VAS for pruritus before and after treatment. Results showed a significant improvement in both instruments for both treatment groups, suggesting antihistamine therapy reduces pruritus in adult atopic dermatitis patients.

Other antihistamines have been shown in small trials to be effective in atopic dermatitis patients complaining of pruritus.[101,102] Langeland and colleagues[101] conducted a study of loratadine in 16 adult patients with moderate or severe atopic dermatitis. Patients were randomized to either 10 mg loratadine or placebo once daily, alternating between loratadine and placebo every 2 weeks. Pruritus was assessed twice a day by the patients using a VAS. Results showed a significant improvement in pruritus during loratadine treatment during the day and at the end of each treatment period. However, the effect of loratadine on pruritus during the night was not statistically significant. Doherty and colleagues[102] conducted a study in 49 adult atopic dermatitis patients who were randomized to 10-day courses of 8 mg acrivastine, 60 mg terfenadine, or placebo. Both drugs are selective H1 histamine receptor blockers with no major sedative effects. Results showed a statistically significant improvement in pruritus with both acrivastine and terfenadine and no significant differences between groups. However, it is difficult to compare these two interventions because acrivastine was measured using a doctor's assessment and terfenadine was measured using a VAS.

Multiple studies show the ineffectiveness of antihistamines in treating pruritus in patients with atopic dermatitis.[103,104] Wahlgren and colleagues[103] conducted an RCT using both a sedative (clemastine) and nonsedative (terfenadine) antihistamine in 25 adult patients with atopic dermatitis. Itch was assessed using a VAS after 3 days of treatment with either clemastine 2 mg twice a day, terfenadine 60 mg twice a day, or placebo. Results showed no significant differences in itch intensity between groups. Berth-Jones and Graham-Brown[104] conducted a RCT using terfenadine 120 mg twice a day for 1 week for the treatment of pruritus in patients with chronic atopic dermatitis. Patient-recorded VAS scores showed no improvement in severity of pruritus. To determine whether antihistamines are effective in the treatment of pruritus in atopic dermatitis patients, large randomized placebo-controlled trials are needed.

Phototherapy

Phototherapy has been shown to be effective in the treatment of atopic dermatitis.[105–107] Multiple types of ultraviolet (UV) light therapy are effective, including psoralen-UVA, broadband UVA, broadband UVB, combined UVA and UVB, narrowband UVB, and UVA1.[108–110] In a study comparing high-dose UVA1 therapy with UVA-UVB or topical glucocorticoid therapy in patients with acute, severe atopic dermatitis, significantly greater improvement in Costa scores was observed with the UVA1 and glucocorticoid group compared with the UVA-UVB group after 10 days of treatment.[108] Another study comparing the efficacy of medium-dose UVA1 versus narrow-band UVB assessed clinical disease and quality of life using the SASSAD and the Skindex-29 (a 29-item self-administered questionnaire), respectively.[109] Twenty-eight patients completed the 6-week study. Results showed a significant improvement in SASSAD scores in both groups with no significant difference between groups. No significant improvement in Skindex-29 scores was seen in either treatment group. Majoie and colleagues[110] also conducted a study in 13 adult patients comparing medium-dose UVA1 and narrow-band UVB. Results from that study showed a significant improvement in disease severity in both treatment groups using the Leicester Sign Score (LSS). In a study of UVB-only phototherapy, 20 patients were treated with either a conventional fixed dosing regimen or varying dosages based on skin pigmentation and erythema.[111] Results showed a decrease in clinical severity of disease as measured by the SCORAD in both groups, but no significant difference existed between treatment groups. However, final UVB dosage and cumulative UVB dosage was significantly lower in the group receiving the optimized dose. Phototherapy can also be used in combination with other forms of therapy for atopic dermatitis, such as corticosteroids. In a study comparing the efficacy of UVA/UVB treatment with UVA/UVB plus topical corticosteroid therapy,[112] Costa scores showed significant improvement in both groups. Although no significant difference was noted between groups, improvement appeared earlier in the UVA/UVB plus corticosteroid group, which reduced the total UVB dose and duration of treatment. Although UV light therapy is effective, this treatment modality is limited to severe cases of atopic dermatitis because of the cost and increased risk of skin cancer.[113–115]

Probiotics

Probiotic therapy with *Lactobacillus* and other live strains has been studied for the treatment of atopic dermatitis, since patients with atopic dermatitis possess different gut bacteria than patients without the disease.[116] Suggested mechanisms of action include a reduction of intestinal inflammation and permeability, which leads to a decrease in antigen presentation in gut lymphoid tissue.[117] In two recent reviews of probiotic therapy in the treatment of atopic dermatitis, evidence to support probiotic therapy was lacking.[118,119] In a Cochrane review by Boyle and colleagues,[118] 12 RCTs examining the efficacy of probiotics compared to placebo showed no statistically significant improvements in disease severity based on measurements by SCORAD. Three studies using *Lactobacillus rhamnosus* strain GG demonstrated an increase in disease severity, but results for all other *Lactobacillus* strains showed a decrease in disease severity. Therefore, it is possible that specific probiotic strains might show benefit. In another systematic review by Michail and colleagues,[119] 11 of the 12 studies from the review by Boyle and colleagues were included. However, Michail and colleagues were able to obtain unpublished SCORAD values for 10 of the studies previously reviewed by Boyle and colleagues. Although Michail and colleagues reported a statistically significant reduction in mean SCORAD values in the probiotic group compared with the placebo group, the small difference may be of limited clinical significance.

Two studies assessed quality of life during treatment with probiotics.[120,121] Weston and colleagues[120] used the DFI to assess quality of life in families of children with atopic dermatitis. Fifty-six children with moderate or severe atopic dermatitis were randomized to receive either *Lactobacillus fermentum* twice daily for 8 weeks or placebo. Quality of life was assessed at the end of intervention (8 weeks) and after an 8-week follow-up period (16 weeks). Median DFI scores improved in both groups at both time periods, but the statistical significance was not mentioned. No differences existed between groups at 8 weeks, but at 16 weeks the median DFI score was −2.5 in the probiotic group versus −3.0 in the placebo group. Fölster-Holst and colleagues[121] used a different published scale to assess quality of life in patients treated with probiotics. The scale assessed different aspects of quality of life including psychosomatic well-being, effects on social life, satisfaction with medical care, dealing emotionally with the illness, and acceptance of the disease. Fifty-four infants with moderate to severe atopic dermatitis were randomized to daily L rhamnosus strain (GG) or placebo for 8 weeks. Results showed no significant difference in quality-of-life scores from baseline to 8 weeks in either treatment group. In addition, no statistical difference existed between treatment groups.

Psychological and Educational Interventions

Multiple studies have shown that psychological treatment of atopic dermatitis can reduce the anxiety level for both patients and families and decrease the amount of medications necessary to control the disease.[122–129] Specifically, individual psychotherapy, group therapy, and educational programs have shown benefit in atopic dermatitis. Linnet and Jemec used the Spielberger State-Trait Anxiety Index (STAI) to assess anxiety levels in adult patients with mild to severe atopic dermatitis after 6 months of either brief dynamic psychotherapy or no treatment. After post hoc multiple regression, atopic dermatitis patients with a higher level of trait anxiety at baseline showed a greater improvement in anxiety level after psychotherapy.[130]

Group therapy not only can improve the quality of life of patients and their families, but can also improve disease severity and lead to better treatment adherence.[34] In a study by Weber and colleagues,[34] the quality of life of children with atopic dermatitis and their families was studied using the CDLQI and DFI after they had joined support groups. The patient-parent family unit was randomized to either 6 months of group therapy with one meeting every 2 weeks or no psychotherapy. Results showed a significant improvement in CDLQI scores in the intervention group in comparison with the control group. However, DFI scores showed no improvement after treatment.

Video-based education is another option for provision of educational counseling to patients. In a study by Armstrong and colleagues,[131] online video-based patient education was compared to written pamphlet education in a randomized control trial. Eighty adult atopic dermatitis patients were given identical information about atopic dermatitis and its management in either video format or written pamphlet form.[131] Knowledge of atopic dermatitis was assessed with standardized questionnaires and atopic dermatitis disease severity was measured by the Patient-Oriented Eczema Measure (POEM).[131] Results showed a significantly greater increase in atopic dermatitis knowledge in the video group over the pamphlet group, along with greater improvements in clinical outcome as measured by the POEM.[131]

Educational counseling has shown conflicting results. In a study of a single 15-minute educational session with an atopic dermatitis educator, Shaw and colleagues[132] showed no significant difference in CDLQI and IDQOL scores. In a study using a 30-minute session which included instruction and demonstration of techniques for applying medication by a trained dermatology nurse, no significant differences between intervention and control groups in CDLQI, IDQOL, or DFI mean scores were reported.[133] However, with more extensive interventions, improvement was seen with educational programs.[134,135] Grillo and colleagues[134] conducted a study of a 2-hour workshop, which included education and a practical session on wet wrapping and cream application. CDLQI, IDQOL, and DFI were assessed at 4 and 12 weeks after intervention. Results showed an improvement in all scores in both treatment groups. However, a significant difference between treatment and control group existed only for mean CDLQI scores at 12 weeks. More definitive results were shown by Staab and colleagues[135] in a study of an age-specific educational program for children and adolescents. The education program involved 6 2-hour sessions held once a week. The sessions covered medical, nutritional, and psychological issues. Quality of life was assessed with a German questionnaire called "Quality of life in parents of children with atopic dermatitis." The instrument included questions related to 5 different topics: psychosomatic well-being, effects on social life, confidence in medical treatment, emotional coping, and acceptance of the disease. Results showed that parents who had children younger than 7 years experienced a significant improvement in quality of life for all 5 subscales, and parents with children aged 8 to 12 years showed significant improvement in 3 of 5 subscales (including confidence in medical treatment, emotional coping, and acceptance of the disease).

SUMMARY

Atopic dermatitis is a common inflammatory skin disease affecting an estimated 31.6 million people in the United States.[136] Health outcomes in atopic dermatitis can be measured using both disease-severity and quality-of-life instruments.

List of Acronyms	
CDLQI	Children's Dermatology Life Quality Index
DFI	Dermatitis Family Impact
DLQI	Dermatology Life Quality Index
EASI	Eczema Area and Severity Index
EQ-5D	Standardized Questionnaire of Health Outcome
IDQOL	Infant's Dermatology Quality of Life Index
IGA	Investigators' Global Assessment
LSS	Leicester Sign Score
PASI	Psoriasis Area and Severity Index
PIQoL-AD	Parent's Index of Quality of Life in Atopic Dermatitis
POEM	Patient Oriented Eczema Measure
QoLIAD	Quality of Life Index for Atopic Dermatitis
SASSAD	Six Area, Six Sign Atopic Dermatitis
SCORAD	Severity Scoring of Atopic Dermatitis
SF-36	Short Form Health Survey
STAI	State-Trait Anxiety Index
TBSA	Total Body Severity Assessment
VAS	Visual Analog Scale

Atopic dermatitis has been shown to disrupt the lives of patients from daily activities such as work, school, and interpersonal relationships including intimacy. Treatment for atopic dermatitis includes medications, nutritional supplements, and psychotherapy. Researchers have evaluated efficacy, safety, and impact on health-related quality of life of these therapies. The authors anticipate that with the continued development of pertinent drugs and devices, safe and effective novel therapies will not only reduce disease severity but also significantly improve patients' quality of life. Further investigation, however, is needed to determine the efficacy of certain treatments in patients with atopic dermatitis. In atopic dermatitis specifically, large RCTs are needed for the treatment categories of oral antihistamines, probiotics, and psychological counseling. In addition, further assessment of the instruments used to measure disease severity and quality of life is needed. Numerous scales exist that measure disease severity and quality of life in atopic dermatitis, yet few have been validated. With increasing recognition of the importance of health outcomes research, the authors anticipate that more outcome measures will be developed not only for atopic dermatitis but also for other dermatologic diseases. Ultimately, carefully validated outcome measures are critical for clinical evaluation and assessment of interventions.

REFERENCES

1. Hanifin J, Rajka G. Diagnostic features of atopic dermatitis. Acta Derm Venereol 1980;92:44–7.
2. Williams HC. Is the prevalence of atopic dermatitis increasing? Clin Exp Dermatol 1992;17(6):385–91.
3. Hanifin JM. Atopic dermatitis in infants and children. Pediatr Clin North Am 1991;38(4):763–89.
4. Shaw TE, Currie GP, Koudelka CW, et al. Eczema prevalence in the United States: data from the 2003 National Survey of Children's Health. J Invest Dermatol 2011;131(1):67–73.
5. Eiser C, Morse R. Quality-of-life measures in chronic diseases of childhood. Health Technol Assess 2001;5(4):1–157.
6. Annett RD, Bender BG, Lapidus J, et al. Predicting children's quality of life in an asthma clinical trial: what do children's reports tell us? J Pediatr 2001;139(6):854–61.
7. Kunz B, Oranje AP, Labreze L, et al. Clinical validation and guidelines for the SCORAD index: consensus report of the European Task Force on Atopic Dermatitis. Dermatology 1997;195(1):10–9.
8. Charman C, Williams H. Outcome measures of disease severity in atopic eczema. Arch Dermatol 2000;136(6):763–9.
9. Severity scoring of atopic dermatitis: the SCORAD index. Consensus Report of the European Task Force on Atopic Dermatitis. Dermatology 1993;186(1):23–31.
10. Oranje AP, Stalder JF, Taieb A, et al. Scoring of atopic dermatitis by SCORAD using a training atlas by investigators from different disciplines. ETAC Study Group. Early Treatment of the Atopic Child. Pediatr Allergy Immunol 1997;8(1):28–34.
11. Schafer T, Dockery D, Kramer U, et al. Experiences with the severity scoring of atopic dermatitis in a population of German pre-school children. Br J Dermatol 1997;137(4):558–62.
12. Sprikkelman AB, Tupker RA, Burgerhof H, et al. Severity scoring of atopic dermatitis: a comparison of three scoring systems. Allergy 1997;52(9):944–9.
13. Fredriksson T, Pettersson U. Severe psoriasis—oral therapy with a new retinoid. Dermatologica 1978;157(4):238–44.

14. Hanifin JM, Thurston M, Omoto M, et al. The Eczema Area and Severity Index (EASI): assessment of reliability in atopic dermatitis. EASI Evaluator Group. Exp Dermatol 2001;10(1):11–8.

15. Barbier N, Paul C, Luger T, et al. Validation of the Eczema Area and Severity Index for atopic dermatitis in a cohort of 1550 patients from the pimecrolimus cream 1% randomized controlled clinical trials programme. Br J Dermatol 2004;150(1):96–102.

16. Belloni G, Pinelli S, Veraldi S. A randomised, double-blind, vehicle-controlled study to evaluate the efficacy and safety of MAS063D (Atopiclair) in the treatment of mild to moderate atopic dermatitis. Eur J Dermatol 2005;15(1):31–6.

17. Breuer K, Braeutigam M, Kapp A, et al. Influence of pimecrolimus cream 1% on different morphological signs of eczema in infants with atopic dermatitis. Dermatology 2004;209(4):314–20.

18. Staab D, Kaufmann R, Brautigam M, et al. Treatment of infants with atopic eczema with pimecrolimus cream 1% improves parents' quality of life: a multicenter, randomized trial. Pediatr Allergy Immunol 2005;16(6):527–33.

19. Siegfried E, Korman N, Molina C, et al. Safety and efficacy of early intervention with pimecrolimus cream 1% combined with corticosteroids for major flares in infants and children with atopic dermatitis. J Dermatolog Treat 2006;17(3):143–50.

20. Schmitt J, Langan S, Williams HC. What are the best outcome measurements for atopic eczema? A systematic review. J Allergy Clin Immunol 2007;120(6):1389–98.

21. Lewis-Jones MS, Finlay AY. The Children's Dermatology Life Quality Index (CDLQI): initial validation and practical use. Br J Dermatol 1995;132(6):942–9.

22. Emerson RM, Lawson S, Williams HC. Do specialist eczema clinics benefit children with atopic dermatitis? Br J Dermatol 1998;139(Suppl 51):46.

23. Harper JI, Ahmed I, Barclay G, et al. Cyclosporin for severe childhood atopic dermatitis: short course versus continuous therapy. Br J Dermatol 2000;142(1):52–8.

24. Aziah MS, Rosnah T, Mardziah A, et al. Childhood atopic dermatitis: a measurement of quality of life and family impact. Med J Malaysia 2002;57(3):329–39.

25. Chuh AA. Validation of a Cantonese version of the Children's Dermatology Life Quality Index. Pediatr Dermatol 2003;20(6):479–81.

26. Clayton TH, Clark SM, Britton J, et al. A comparative study of the Children's Dermatology Life Quality Index (CDLQI) in paediatric dermatology clinics in the UK and Bulgaria. J Eur Acad Dermatol Venereol 2007;21(10):1436–7.

27. Holme SA, Man I, Sharpe JL, et al. The Children's Dermatology Life Quality Index: validation of the cartoon version. Br J Dermatol 2003;148(2):285–90.

28. Beattie PE, Lewis-Jones MS. An audit of the impact of a consultation with a paediatric dermatology team on quality of life in infants with atopic eczema and their families: further validation of the Infants' Dermatitis Quality of Life Index and Dermatitis Family Impact score. Br J Dermatol 2006;155(6):1249–55.

29. Lewis-Jones M, Finlay A. Quality of life research. 2006. Available at: http://www.dermatology.org.uk. Accessed May, 2011.

30. Alvarenga TM, Caldeira AP. Quality of life in pediatric patients with atopic dermatitis. J Pediatr (Rio J) 2009;85(5):415–20.

31. Grimalt R, Mengeaud V, Cambazard F. The steroid-sparing effect of an emollient therapy in infants with atopic dermatitis: a randomized controlled study. Dermatology 2007;214(1):61–7.

32. Lewis-Jones MS, Finlay AY, Dykes PJ. The Infants' Dermatitis Quality of Life Index. Br J Dermatol 2001;144(1):104–10.

33. McKenna SP, Doward LC. Quality of life of children with atopic dermatitis and their families. Curr Opin Allergy Clin Immunol 2008;8(3):228–31.

34. Weber MB, Fontes Neto Pde T, Prati C, et al. Improvement of pruritus and quality of life of children with atopic dermatitis and their families after joining support groups. J Eur Acad Dermatol Venereol 2008;22(8):992–7.

35. Finlay AY, Khan GK. Dermatology Life Quality Index (DLQI)—a simple practical measure for routine clinical use. Clin Exp Dermatol 1994;19(3):210–6.

36. Badia X, Mascaro JM, Lozano R. Measuring health-related quality of life in patients with mild to moderate eczema and psoriasis: clinical validity, reliability and sensitivity to change of the DLQI. The Cavide Research Group. Br J Dermatol 1999;141(4):698–702.

37. Lewis V, Finlay AY. 10 years experience of the Dermatology Life Quality Index (DLQI). J Investig Dermatol Symp Proc 2004;9(2):169–80.

38. Kiebert G, Sorensen SV, Revicki D, et al. Atopic dermatitis is associated with a decrement in health-related quality of life. Int J Dermatol 2002;41(3):151–8.

39. Kurwa HA, Finlay AY. Dermatology in-patient management greatly improves life quality. Br J Dermatol 1995;133(4):575–8.

40. Schmid-Ott G, Kuensebeck HW, Jaeger B, et al. Validity study for the stigmatization experience in atopic dermatitis and psoriatic patients. Acta Derm Venereol 1999;79(6):443–7.

41. Linnet J, Jemec GB. An assessment of anxiety and dermatology life quality in patients with atopic dermatitis. Br J Dermatol 1999;140(2):268–72.

42. Beattie PE, Lewis-Jones MS. A comparative study of impairment of quality of life in children with skin disease and children with other chronic childhood diseases. Br J Dermatol 2006;155(1):145–51.

43. Paller AS, McAlister RO, Doyle JJ, et al. Perceptions of physicians and pediatric patients about

atopic dermatitis, its impact, and its treatment. Clin Pediatr (Phila) 2002;41(5):323–32.

44. Reid P, Lewis-Jones MS. Sleep difficulties and their management in preschoolers with atopic eczema. Clin Exp Dermatol 1995;20(1):38–41.

45. Dahl RE, Bernhisel-Broadbent J, Scanlon-Holdford S, et al. Sleep disturbances in children with atopic dermatitis. Arch Pediatr Adolesc Med 1995;149(8):856–60.

46. Stores G, Burrows A, Crawford C. Physiological sleep disturbance in children with atopic dermatitis: a case control study. Pediatr Dermatol 1998;15(4):264–8.

47. Long CC, Funnell CM, Collard R, et al. What do members of the National Eczema Society really want? Clin Exp Dermatol 1993;18(6):516–22.

48. Daud LR, Garralda ME, David TJ. Psychosocial adjustment in preschool children with atopic eczema. Arch Dis Child 1993;69(6):670–6.

49. Lawson V, Lewis-Jones MS, Finlay AY, et al. The family impact of childhood atopic dermatitis: the Dermatitis Family Impact Questionnaire. Br J Dermatol 1998;138(1):107–13.

50. Su JC, Kemp AS, Varigos GA, et al. Atopic eczema: its impact on the family and financial cost. Arch Dis Child 1997;76(2):159–62.

51. Chamlin SL, Frieden IJ, Williams ML, et al. Effects of atopic dermatitis on young American children and their families. Pediatrics 2004;114(3):607–11.

52. Wittkowski A, Richards HL, Griffiths CE, et al. The impact of psychological and clinical factors on quality of life in individuals with atopic dermatitis. J Psychosom Res 2004;57(2):195–200.

53. Holm EA, Wulf HC, Stegmann H, et al. Life quality assessment among patients with atopic eczema. Br J Dermatol 2006;154(4):719–25.

54. Whalley D, McKenna SP, Dewar AL, et al. A new instrument for assessing quality of life in atopic dermatitis: international development of the Quality of Life Index for Atopic Dermatitis (QoLIAD). Br J Dermatol 2004;150(2):274–83.

55. Holm EA, Esmann S, Jemec GB. Does visible atopic dermatitis affect quality of life more in women than in men? Gend Med 2004;1(2):125–30.

56. Stangier U, Ehlers A, Gieler U. Measuring adjustment to chronic skin disorders: validation of a self-report measure. Psychol Assess 2003;15(4):532–49.

57. Misery L, Finlay AY, Martin N, et al. Atopic dermatitis: impact on the quality of life of patients and their partners. Dermatology 2007;215(2):123–9.

58. Msika P, De Belilovsky C, Piccardi N, et al. New emollient with topical corticosteroid-sparing effect in treatment of childhood atopic dermatitis: SCORAD and quality of life improvement. Pediatr Dermatol 2008;25(6):606–12.

59. Bleehen SS, Chu AC, Hamann I, et al. Fluticasone propionate 0.05% cream in the treatment of atopic eczema: a multicentre study comparing once-daily treatment and once-daily vehicle cream application versus twice-daily treatment. Br J Dermatol 1995;133(4):592–7.

60. Jones SM, Sampson HA. The role of allergens in atopic dermatitis. Clin Rev Allergy 1993;11(4):471–90.

61. Koopmans B, Lasthein Andersen B, Mork N. Multicentre randomized double-blind study of locoid lipocream fatty cream twice daily versus locoid lipocream once daily and locobase once daily. J Dermatol Treat 1995;6:103.

62. Green C, Colquitt JL, Kirby J, et al. Topical corticosteroids for atopic eczema: clinical and cost effectiveness of once-daily vs. more frequent use. Br J Dermatol 2005;152(1):130–41.

63. Guzzo CA, Weiss JS, Mogavero HS, et al. A review of two controlled multicenter trials comparing 0.05% halobetasol propionate ointment to its vehicle in the treatment of chronic eczematous dermatoses. J Am Acad Dermatol 1991;25(6 Pt 2):1179–83.

64. Maloney JM, Morman MR, Stewart DM, et al. Clobetasol propionate emollient 0.05% in the treatment of atopic dermatitis. Int J Dermatol 1998;37(2):142–4.

65. Van Der Meer JB, Glazenburg EJ, Mulder PG, et al. The management of moderate to severe atopic dermatitis in adults with topical fluticasone propionate. The Netherlands Adult Atopic Dermatitis Study Group. Br J Dermatol 1999;140(6):1114–21.

66. Glazenburg EJ, Wolkerstorfer A, Gerretsen AL, et al. Efficacy and safety of fluticasone propionate 0.005% ointment in the long-term maintenance treatment of children with atopic dermatitis: differences between boys and girls? Pediatr Allergy Immunol 2009;20(1):59–66.

67. Peserico A, Stadtler G, Sebastian M, et al. Reduction of relapses of atopic dermatitis with methylprednisolone aceponate cream twice weekly in addition to maintenance treatment with emollient: a multicentre, randomized, double-blind, controlled study. Br J Dermatol 2008;158(4):801–7.

68. Ashcroft DM, Dimmock P, Garside R, et al. Efficacy and tolerability of topical pimecrolimus and tacrolimus in the treatment of atopic dermatitis: meta-analysis of randomised controlled trials. BMJ 2005;330(7490):516.

69. Ashcroft DM, Chen LC, Garside R, et al. Topical pimecrolimus for eczema. Cochrane Database Syst Rev 2007;4:CD005500.

70. El-Batawy MM, Bosseila MA, Mashaly HM, et al. Topical calcineurin inhibitors in atopic dermatitis: a systematic review and meta-analysis. J Dermatol Sci 2009;54(2):76–87.

71. Nakagawa H. Comparison of the efficacy and safety of 0.1% tacrolimus ointment with topical corticosteroids in adult patients with atopic

dermatitis: review of randomised, double-blind clinical studies conducted in Japan. Clin Drug Investig 2006;26(5):235–46.

72. Bieber T, Vick K, Fölster-Holst R, et al. Efficacy and safety of methylprednisolone aceponate ointment 0.1% compared to tacrolimus 0.03% in children and adolescents with an acute flare of severe atopic dermatitis. Allergy 2007;62(2):184–9.

73. Aoyama H, Tabata N, Tanaka M, et al. Successful treatment of resistant facial lesions of atopic dermatitis with 0.1% FK506 ointment. Br J Dermatol 1995;133(3):494–6.

74. Ruzicka T, Bieber T, Schopf E, et al. A short-term trial of tacrolimus ointment for atopic dermatitis. European Tacrolimus Multicenter Atopic Dermatitis Study Group. N Engl J Med 1997;337(12):816–21.

75. Reitamo S. Tacrolimus: a new topical immunomodulatory therapy for atopic dermatitis. J Allergy Clin Immunol 2001;107(3):445–8.

76. Reitamo S, Rustin M, Ruzicka T, et al. Efficacy and safety of tacrolimus ointment compared with that of hydrocortisone butyrate ointment in adult patients with atopic dermatitis. J Allergy Clin Immunol 2002;109(3):547–55.

77. Fonacier L, Spergel J, Charlesworth EN, et al. Report of the Topical Calcineurin Inhibitor Task Force of the American College of Allergy, Asthma and Immunology and the American Academy of Allergy, Asthma and Immunology. J Allergy Clin Immunol 2005;115(6):1249–53.

78. Reitamo S, Wollenberg A, Schopf E, et al. Safety and efficacy of 1 year of tacrolimus ointment monotherapy in adults with atopic dermatitis. The European Tacrolimus Ointment Study Group. Arch Dermatol 2000;136(8):999–1006.

79. Hanifin JM, Ling MR, Langley R, et al. Tacrolimus ointment for the treatment of atopic dermatitis in adult patients: part I, efficacy. J Am Acad Dermatol 2001;44(Suppl 1):S28–38.

80. Reitamo S, Ortonne JP, Sand C, et al. A multicentre, randomized, double-blind, controlled study of long-term treatment with 0.1% tacrolimus ointment in adults with moderate to severe atopic dermatitis. Br J Dermatol 2005;152(6):1282–9.

81. Boguniewicz M, Fiedler VC, Raimer S, et al. A randomized, vehicle-controlled trial of tacrolimus ointment for treatment of atopic dermatitis in children. Pediatric Tacrolimus Study Group. J Allergy Clin Immunol 1998;102(4 Pt 1):637–44.

82. Schachner LA, Lamerson C, Sheehan MP, et al. Tacrolimus ointment 0.03% is safe and effective for the treatment of mild to moderate atopic dermatitis in pediatric patients: results from a randomized, double-blind, vehicle-controlled study. Pediatrics 2005;116(3):e334–42.

83. Drake L, Prendergast M, Maher R, et al. The impact of tacrolimus ointment on health-related quality of life

of adult and pediatric patients with atopic dermatitis. J Am Acad Dermatol 2001;44(Suppl 1):S65–72.

84. Poole CD, Chambers C, Sidhu MK, et al. Health-related utility among adults with atopic dermatitis treated with 0.1% tacrolimus ointment as maintenance therapy over the long term: findings from the Protopic CONTROL study. Br J Dermatol 2009;161(6):1335–40.

85. Wollenberg A, Reitamo S, Girolomoni G, et al. Proactive treatment of atopic dermatitis in adults with 0.1% tacrolimus ointment. Allergy 2008;63(7):742–50.

86. Papp KA, Breuer K, Meurer M, et al. Long-term treatment of atopic dermatitis with pimecrolimus cream 1% in infants does not interfere with the development of protective antibodies after vaccination. J Am Acad Dermatol 2005;52(2):247–53.

87. Eichenfield LF, Lucky AW, Boguniewicz M, et al. Safety and efficacy of pimecrolimus (ASM 981) cream 1% in the treatment of mild and moderate atopic dermatitis in children and adolescents. J Am Acad Dermatol 2002;46(4):495–504.

88. Wahn U, Bos JD, Goodfield M, et al. Efficacy and safety of pimecrolimus cream in the long-term management of atopic dermatitis in children. Pediatrics 2002;110(1 Pt 1):e2.

89. Murrell DF, Calvieri S, Ortonne JP, et al. A randomized controlled trial of pimecrolimus cream 1% in adolescents and adults with head and neck atopic dermatitis and intolerant of, or dependent on, topical corticosteroids. Br J Dermatol 2007;157(5):954–9.

90. Ling M, Gottlieb A, Pariser D, et al. A randomized study of the safety, absorption and efficacy of pimecrolimus cream 1% applied twice or four times daily in patients with atopic dermatitis. J Dermatolog Treat 2005;16(3):142–8.

91. Ruer-Mulard M, Aberer W, Gunstone A, et al. Twice-daily versus once-daily applications of pimecrolimus cream 1% for the prevention of disease relapse in pediatric patients with atopic dermatitis. Pediatr Dermatol 2009;26(5):551–8.

92. Langley RG, Eichenfield LF, Lucky AW, et al. Sustained efficacy and safety of pimecrolimus cream 1% when used long-term (up to 26 weeks) to treat children with atopic dermatitis. Pediatr Dermatol 2008;25(3):301–7.

93. Papp KA, Werfel T, Fölster-Holst R, et al. Long-term control of atopic dermatitis with pimecrolimus cream 1% in infants and young children: a two-year study. J Am Acad Dermatol 2005;52(2):240–6.

94. Eichenfield LF, Lucky AW, Langley RG, et al. Use of pimecrolimus cream 1% (Elidel) in the treatment of atopic dermatitis in infants and children: the effects of ethnic origin and baseline disease severity on treatment outcome. Int J Dermatol 2005;44(1):70–5.

95. Kaufmann R, Fölster-Holst R, Hoger P, et al. Onset of action of pimecrolimus cream 1% in the treatment of atopic eczema in infants. J Allergy Clin Immunol 2004;114(5):1183–8.

96. Zuberbier T, Heinzerling L, Bieber T, et al. Steroid-sparing effect of pimecrolimus cream 1% in children with severe atopic dermatitis. Dermatology 2007;215(4):325–30.

97. Whalley D, Huels J, McKenna SP, et al. The benefit of pimecrolimus (Elidel, SDZ ASM 981) on parents' quality of life in the treatment of pediatric atopic dermatitis. Pediatrics 2002;110(6):1133–6.

98. Nuovo J, Ellsworth AJ, Larson EB. Treatment of atopic dermatitis with antihistamines: lessons from a single-patient, randomized clinical trial. J Am Board Fam Pract 1992;5(2):137–41.

99. Klein PA, Clark RA. An evidence-based review of the efficacy of antihistamines in relieving pruritus in atopic dermatitis. Arch Dermatol 1999;135(12):1522–5.

100. Kawakami T, Kaminishi K, Soma Y, et al. Oral antihistamine therapy influences plasma tryptase levels in adult atopic dermatitis. J Dermatol Sci 2006;43(2):127–34.

101. Langeland T, Fagertun HE, Larsen S. Therapeutic effect of loratadine on pruritus in patients with atopic dermatitis. A multi-crossover-designed study. Allergy 1994;49(1):22–6.

102. Doherty V, Sylvester DG, Kennedy CT, et al. Treatment of itching in atopic eczema with antihistamines with a low sedative profile. BMJ 1989;298(6666):96.

103. Wahlgren CF, Hagermark O, Bergstrom R. The antipruritic effect of a sedative and a non-sedative antihistamine in atopic dermatitis. Br J Dermatol 1990;122(4):545–51.

104. Berth-Jones J, Graham-Brown RA. Failure of terfenadine in relieving the pruritus of atopic dermatitis. Br J Dermatol 1989;121(5):635–7.

105. Jekler J, Larko O. Combined UVA-UVB versus UVB phototherapy for atopic dermatitis: a paired-comparison study. J Am Acad Dermatol 1990;22(1):49–53.

106. Reynolds NJ, Franklin V, Gray JC, et al. Narrow-band ultraviolet B and broad-band ultraviolet A phototherapy in adult atopic eczema: a randomised controlled trial. Lancet 2001;357(9273):2012–6.

107. Grundmann-Kollmann M, Behrens S, Podda M, et al. Phototherapy for atopic eczema with narrow-band UVB. J Am Acad Dermatol 1999;40(6 part 1):995–7.

108. Krutmann J, Diepgen TL, Luger TA, et al. High-dose UVA1 therapy for atopic dermatitis: results of a multicenter trial. J Am Acad Dermatol 1998;38(4):589–93.

109. Gambichler T, Othlinghaus N, Tomi NS, et al. Medium-dose ultraviolet (UV) A1 vs. narrowband UVB phototherapy in atopic eczema: a randomized crossover study. Br J Dermatol 2009;160(3):652–8.

110. Majoie IM, Oldhoff JM, van Weelden H, et al. Narrowband ultraviolet B and medium-dose ultraviolet A1 are equally effective in the treatment of moderate to severe atopic dermatitis. J Am Acad Dermatol 2009;60(1):77–84.

111. Selvaag E, Caspersen L, Bech-Thomsen N, et al. Optimized UVB treatment of atopic dermatitis using skin reflectance measurements. A controlled, left-right comparison trial. Acta Derm Venereol 2005;85(2):144–6.

112. Valkova S, Velkova A. UVA/UVB phototherapy for atopic dermatitis revisited. J Dermatolog Treat 2004;15(4):239–44.

113. Stern RS, Nichols KT, Vakeva LH. Malignant melanoma in patients treated for psoriasis with methoxsalen (psoralen) and ultraviolet A radiation (PUVA). The PUVA Follow-Up Study. N Engl J Med 1997;336(15):1041–5.

114. Stern RS, Laird N, Melski J, et al. Cutaneous squamous-cell carcinoma in patients treated with PUVA. N Engl J Med 1984;310(18):1156–61.

115. Lindelof B, Sigurgeirsson B, Tegner E, et al. PUVA and cancer: a large-scale epidemiological study. Lancet 1991;338(8759):91–3.

116. Kalliomaki M, Kirjavainen P, Eerola E, et al. Distinct patterns of neonatal gut microflora in infants in whom atopy was and was not developing. J Allergy Clin Immunol 2001;107(1):129–34.

117. Rosenfeldt V, Benfeldt E, Valerius NH, et al. Effect of probiotics on gastrointestinal symptoms and small intestinal permeability in children with atopic dermatitis. J Pediatr 2004;145(5):612–6.

118. Boyle RJ, Bath-Hextall FJ, Leonardi-Bee J, et al. Probiotics for treating eczema. Cochrane Database Syst Rev 2008;4:CD006135.

119. Michail SK, Stolfi A, Johnson T, et al. Efficacy of probiotics in the treatment of pediatric atopic dermatitis: a meta-analysis of randomized controlled trials. Ann Allergy Asthma Immunol 2008;101(5):508–16.

120. Weston S, Halbert A, Richmond P, et al. Effects of probiotics on atopic dermatitis: a randomised controlled trial. Arch Dis Child 2005;90(9):892–7.

121. Fölster-Holst R, Muller F, Schnopp N, et al. Prospective, randomized controlled trial on Lactobacillus rhamnosus in infants with moderate to severe atopic dermatitis. Br J Dermatol 2006;155(6):1256–61.

122. Fried RG. Nonpharmacologic treatments in psychodermatology. Dermatol Clin 2002;20(1):177–85.

123. Brown DG, Bettley FR. Psychiatric treatment of eczema: a controlled trial. Br Med J 1971;2(5764):729–34.

124. Cole WC, Roth HL, Sachs LB. Group psychotherapy as an aid in the medical treatment of eczema. J Am Acad Dermatol 1988;18(2 Pt 1):286–91.

125. Ehlers A, Stangier U, Gieler U. Treatment of atopic dermatitis: a comparison of psychological and dermatological approaches to relapse prevention. J Consult Clin Psychol 1995;63(4):624–35.

126. Horne DJ, White AE, Varigos GA. A preliminary study of psychological therapy in the management of atopic eczema. Br J Med Psychol 1989;62(Pt 3):241–8.

127. King RM, Wilson GV. Use of a diary technique to investigate psychosomatic relations in atopic dermatitis. J Psychosom Res 1991;35(6):697–706.

128. Koblenzer CS. Psychotherapy for intractable inflammatory dermatoses. J Am Acad Dermatol 1995;32(4):609–12.

129. McSkimming J, Gleeson L, Sinclair M. A pilot study of a support group for parents of children with eczema. Australas J Dermatol 1984;25(1):8–11.

130. Linnet J, Jemec GB. Anxiety level and severity of skin condition predicts outcome of psychotherapy in atopic dermatitis patients. Int J Dermatol 2001; 40(10):632–6.

131. Armstrong AW, Kim RH, Idriss NZ, et al. Online video improves clinical outcomes in adults with atopic dermatitis: a randomized controlled trial. J Am Acad Dermatol 2011;64(3):502–7.

132. Shaw M, Morrell DS, Goldsmith LA. A study of targeted enhanced patient care for pediatric atopic dermatitis (STEP PAD). Pediatr Dermatol 2008; 25(1):19–24.

133. Chinn DJ, Poyner T, Sibley G. Randomized controlled trial of a single dermatology nurse consultation in primary care on the quality of life of children with atopic eczema. Br J Dermatol 2002; 146(3):432–9.

134. Grillo M, Gassner L, Marshman G, et al. Pediatric atopic eczema: the impact of an educational intervention. Pediatr Dermatol 2006;23(5):428–36.

135. Staab D, Diepgen TL, Fartasch M, et al. Age related, structured educational programmes for the management of atopic dermatitis in children and adolescents: multicentre, randomised controlled trial. BMJ 2006;332(7547):933–8.

136. Hanifin JM, Reed ML. A population-based survey of eczema prevalence in the United States. Dermatitis 2007;18(2):82–91.

Contact Dermatitis in the United States: Epidemiology, Economic Impact, and Workplace Prevention

Michael W. Cashman, MD[a], Patricia A. Reutemann, MD[a],
Alison Ehrlich, MD, MHS[a,b,*]

KEYWORDS

- Contact dermatitis • Epidemiology • Occupational
- Economic impact • Prevention strategies • Patch testing

Contact dermatitis is defined as either an acute or chronic inflammatory reaction in response to substances that come into contact with the skin. The former is characterized by pruritus, erythema, and vesiculation while the latter involves pruritus, xerosis, lichenification, hyperkeratosis, and fissuring.[1]

Irritant contact dermatitis (ICD) is caused by an external agent acting merely as a chemical or physical irritant, thus eliciting a nonallergic inflammatory host response. The potential to cause irritation and intensity of the reaction depends on certain features of the agent including its concentration, pH, vehicle, and length of exposure. ICD only occurs above a threshold level, which varies from person to person depending on the penetrability and thickness of the stratum corneum.[2] Very strong irritants elicit an acute reaction after first exposure, which occurs within minutes or is delayed up to 8 to 24 hours[3]; however, the majority of ICD cases are attributable to chronic cumulative exposures to milder irritants (water, soap, detergents), environmental factors (low-humidity air, heat, cold) or even repetitive trauma (rubbing, friction, pressure, abrasions). Repetitive exposures create a chronic disturbance of the barrier function allowing even low concentrations of offending agents to penetrate the skin, and subsequently induce a chronic inflammatory response. Irritation is the most common cause of contact dermatitis, and the skin findings vary greatly depending on severity of exposure.[2] **Box 1** lists the most common substances responsible for ICD.

Allergic contact dermatitis (ACD) is caused by an external agent acting as a specific antigen or allergen, producing the classic, delayed, T-cell–mediated (type IV) hypersensitivity response. As an immunologic phenomenon, it tends to involve the surrounding skin and can even spread beyond the initial exposure site. When the allergen elicits an incredible immune response, the skin eruption becomes generalized.[2,3] Systemic ACD (SACD) describes a cutaneous eruption in response to a systemic exposure of a previously sensitized allergen.[1,3] Several routes of exposure have been reported to elicit SACD such as subcutaneous, hematogenous, intravenous, intramuscular, inhalation, and oral ingestion.[4,5] **Table 1** lists the

The authors have nothing to disclose.

[a] School of Medicine and Health Sciences, George Washington University, 2300 I Street, Northwest, Washington, DC 20037, USA

[b] Department of Dermatology, George Washington University Medical Faculty Associates, 2150 Pennsylvania Avenue, Northwest, Suite 6A-402, Washington, DC 20037, USA

* Corresponding author. Department of Dermatology, George Washington University Medical Faculty Associates, 2150 Pennsylvania Avenue, Northwest, Suite 6A-402, Washington, DC 20037.

E-mail address: aehrlich@mfa.gwu.edu

Dermatol Clin 30 (2012) 87–98
doi:10.1016/j.det.2011.08.004

Box 1
The most common irritants

Cleansers

Water/wet work, soaps, detergents, waterless hand cleaners, degreasing agents, bleaches, isopropyl alcohol, benzoyl peroxide

Acids and Bases

Hydrofluoric acid, cement, chromic acid, phosphorus, ethylene oxide, phenol, fluorohydrogenic acid, nonanoic acid, metal salts, inorganic and organic acids

Industrial Solvents

Benzene, toluene, xylene, ethyl benzene, cumene, gasoline, kerosene, Stoddard solvent, hexane, carbon tetrachloride, trichloroethane, tetrachloroethane, trichloroethylene, methylene chloride, ethylene dichloride, methyl alcohol, ethyl alcohol, isopropyl alcohol, glycidyl ethers, ethyl acetate, amyl acetate, butyl acetate, turpentine, ethyl ether, acetone, carbon dioxide, dimethyl sulfoxide, dioxane, styrene, metal working fluids, arsenic, oxalic acid, formic acid, salicylic acid, sodium hypochlorite, alkalis, anhydrides

Chemicals

Sodium, potassium, lithium, phosphorus, phenolic compounds, bromine, iodine, ethylene oxide, aluminum chloride, propylene glycol, sodium lauryl sulfate, butanediol diacrylate, hexanediol diacrylate, tetraethylene glycol diacrylate, anthralin, benzalkonium chloride, 2-chloroethyl sulfide, calcipotriol, 2-chlorovinyl arsine, epichlorhydrine, octyl gallate

Plants

Euphorbiaceae (spurges, crotons, poinsettias, machineel tree). Racunculaceae (buttercup), Cruciferae (black mustard), Urticaceae (nettles), Solanaceae (pepper, capsaicin), Opuntia (prickly pear), furocoumarins

Materials

Fiberglass, wool, rough synthetic clothing, fire-retardant fabrics, noncarbon copy paper

Airborne Irritants

Acids, alkalis, ammonia, anhydrous calcium sulfate, arsenic, calcium silicate, cement, dichlorvos, domestic cleaning products, epoxy resins, formaldehyde, fiberglass, industrial solvents, metallic oxide powders, paper, phenol formaldehyde resins, sawdust, silver, sodium sesquicarbonate, urea-formaldehyde insulating foam, dust foam, wool dust, tear gases

Others

Cosmetics, oils, greases, foods, medications (benzoyl peroxide, tretinoin, diclofenac, podophyllin), animal products

Data from Amado A, Taylor JS, Sood A. Irritant contact dermatitis. In: Wolff K, Goldsmith LA, Katz SI, et al, editors. *Fitzpatrick's dermatology in general medicine.* 7th edition. New York: McGraw-Hill; 2008. Available at: http://www.accessmedicine.com/content.aspx?aID=2950409. Accessed April 15, 2011; and Taylor JS, Sood A, Amado A. Occupational skin diseases due to irritants and allergens. In: Wolff K, Goldsmith LA, Katz SI, et al, editors. *Fitzpatrick's dermatology in general medicine.* 7th edition. New York: McGraw-Hill; 2008. Available at: http://www.accessmedicine.com/content.aspx?aID=3001176. Accessed April 15, 2011.

---

most common allergens responsible for ACD according to patch-test results from the North American Contact Dermatitis Group (NACDG) in 2005 to 2006.

Besides the major division of contact dermatitis as either irritant or allergic, other classifications of contact dermatitis as well as a spectrum of contact responses of the skin exist, and are often underreported to the physician or employer. Subjective irritancy describes idiosyncratic stinging and smarting reactions that occur within seconds to minutes of contact without visible skin changes, and last either momentarily or for several hours.[1,3] Toxic or caustic burns are the most severe form of an acute irritant reaction wherein the skin undergoes necrosis. The most

Table 1	
The most common allergens	
Patch–Test Allergen	Positive Reaction (%)
Nickel sulfate	19.0
Balsam of Peru	11.9
Fragrance mix	11.5
Quaternium-15	10.3
Neomycin	10.0
Bacitracin	9.2
Formaldehyde	9.0
Cobalt chloride	8.4
Methyldibromoglutaronitrile	5.8
p-Phenylenediamine	5.0
Potassium dichromate	4.8
Carba mix	3.9
Thiuram mix	3.9
Diazolidinylurea	3.7
2-Bromo-2-nitropropane-1, 3-diol	3.4
Cinnamic aldehyde	3.1
Imidazolidinylurea	2.9
Propylene glycol	2.9
MCI/MI 100 ppm	2.8
Tixoorto-21-pivalate	2.7

Abbreviation: MCI/MI, methylchloroisothiazolinone/methylisothiazolinone.

Data from Zug KA, Warshae EM, Fowler JF, et al. Patch-test results of the North American Contact Dermatitis Group 2005–2006. Dermatitis 2009;20:149–60.

severe irritants, such as strong acids and bases and oxidizing and reducing agents, create toxic reactions even with a very small amount and brief exposure.[2] Airborne ICD and ACD arise when irritating dusts, volatile chemicals, or allergens suspended in the air become exposed to skin, producing a contact dermatitis. Phototoxic and photoallergic reactions occur when a chemical or drug is absorbed into the skin via oral ingestion, subcutaneous injection, or topical application. The offending agent acts as an irritant or antigen only after exposure to and activation by ultraviolet (UV) light.[6] Finally, occupational contact dermatitis describes any type of contact dermatitis caused by agents present at a place of employment or trade. ACD, ICD, and acute caustic chemical injuries are the most common toxin-related skin problems in the workplace. As such, occupational contact dermatitis (OCD) is the most common occupational skin disease in the United States and in many other countries.[2]

RISK FACTORS

Contact dermatitis is broadly classified into irritant and allergic reactions, thus skin exposure to potential irritants and allergens is a clear prerequisite for its development. However, the multifactorial etiology of contact dermatitis, with numerous extrinsic and intrinsic factors influencing its development, often makes the exact causative agent difficult to determine.[6] Extrinsic factors include occupation, geographic and environmental factors, biochemical properties of allergens and irritants,[6] and cultural factors, while intrinsic factors include age, sex, race, epidermal barrier integrity, atopic constitution, and genetics, all of which contribute to skin reactivity.[7]

Occupation

Occupation is a key factor in the development of contact dermatitis, with 90% to 95% of all occupational skin diseases representing some form of contact dermatitis.[2] OCD was found to be the most common among metalworkers, construction workers, professional hairdressers, waiters, cleaners, health care workers, agricultural workers, chefs, and food workers, with the highest prevalence found among cosmetologists.[7] The most common sources of allergic sensitizations identified were metallic objects followed by drugs, cosmetics, and rubber. As expected, the most common occupations with ACD were hairdressers, construction workers, and metalworkers. In comparison, the most common occupations with ICD were health care workers, agricultural workers, and cleaners, most likely a result of repetitive contact with chemicals and water.[7] Environmental and physical factors decrease the protective barrier of the skin, rendering it much more susceptible to the harmful effects of irritants and allergens. Professions whereby skin is constantly exposed to water lead to maceration of the skin, and repetitive cycles of wetting and drying causes scaling, fissuring, and cracking. These changes weaken the protective seal of the stratum corneum and permit increased cutaneous penetration of molecules.[6] Indeed, "wet work" is the most commonly implicated exogenous factor in OCD, with affected professions including health care professionals, janitors, maids, bartenders, dishwashers, waiters, hair washers, bakers, cooks, and employees in the food service industry.[2,6,7]

Environment

Low-humidity environments decrease ceramide levels in the stratum corneum, producing desiccation and disruption of the epidermal barrier.[2,6] In hot, humid, or occlusive environments, perspiration causes soluble chemicals to dissolve, facilitating easier absorption into the skin. Microtraumatization of the skin also disrupts the protective epidermal barrier, especially in professions where repetitive friction, rubbing, or exposure to harsh, rough materials or fabrics occurs.[6] Professionals who wear protective gloves can create a cycle of occlusion, perspiration, maceration, and subsequent irritation; therefore, its overuse or improper use paradoxically increases the risk of skin dysfunction, penetration by irritants and allergens, and risk of development of contact dermatitis.[2]

Age and Sex

The frequency of positive patch-test results increases with age, reaching a peak between 60 and 69 years. In addition, compared with men (50–59 years), women become sensitized to allergens at a younger age (20–29 years). Age was also found to be associated with specific origins of contact dermatitis, including metals (10–59 years old), cosmetics (20–49 years), household products (30–59 years), and drugs (50–69 years).[7] Regarding ICD, it has been suggested that susceptibility to irritants is enhanced in children, but appears to decline with age.[6] Furthermore, self-reported dermatitis of the hands was most prevalent in young women and decreased with age; however, hand dermatitis in general is significantly more frequent in women than in men.[8] Epidemiologic studies have shown that women carry an increased risk for the development of ICD. In fact, in comparison with men women have reported more intense irritant contact reactions when exposed to alkalis and detergents; however, other studies revealed no gender differences after exposure to certain irritants, thus the intrinsic effect of gender and the risk of ICD is still debatable.[6] Despite this, an increased prevalence of contact dermatitis among women is widely accepted, most likely related to the increased extrinsic differences such as the occupational and domestic exposures between women and men, and less likely due to the intrinsic factors of skin susceptibility between sexes.[8]

Race and Ethnicity

A clinical consensus has established that black skin is less reactive than white skin, which is less reactive than Asian skin; however, one review found that this rarely reached statistical significance.[9] African Americans have greater compaction of the lipid content in their stratum corneum, which most likely confers greater barrier protection from susceptibility to potential allergens and

irritants. Reduced rates of sensitization to weaker allergens such as nickel and neomycin in African Americans compared with Caucasians, as well as an overall reduced rate of ICD in African Americans has been reported. This protection is secondary to increased lipid production rather than a genetic predisposition or immunologic-mediated advantage.[6] In white and black patients patch tested by members of the NACDG, no differences were found in the overall response rate to allergens. However, some differences were found in response to specific allergens, yet it was unclear if these differences were attributable to a genetic basis by race or mere difference in ethnicity of potential exposures between the two groups.[10] One study found a similar incidence rate of allergic reactions between Japanese and Caucasian people, but Japanese people exhibited more severe allergic reactions.[6] Patch testing Japanese and German women with sodium lauryl sulfate revealed no significant differences in skin reaction or barrier function in the measurements of several physiologic parameters after 24 hours; however, Japanese women had significantly more subjective sensory complaints. Although racial differences in the speed of penetration could not be excluded, ethnic differences owing to cultural behaviors could be responsible for these increased feelings of irritation.[11] Furthermore, a comparison of white Europeans patients with Fitzpatrick skin types I to IV with Indian, Pakistani, and Bengali patients with skin type V, who all lived in the same community, resulted in a lower incidence of positive patch-test results among the races of the Indian subcontinent, although no significant difference between the detected responsible allergens was found among these two groups. The decreased incidence of positive reactions is still unclear, but different exposures between these groups as opposed to an innate difference in susceptibility is likely responsible for such findings.[12]

Atopy

Atopic dermatitis (AD) is associated with a higher rate of contact allergy and irritancy, due to disturbed barrier function that heightens the susceptibility to skin irritants and allergens.[13] Numerous studies have repeatedly shown that AD is the single most important risk factor for the development of hand eczema[8]; however, the association between AD and ACD is largely controversial, and the relationship between the two remains unclear.[6,7,13] While a history of atopy increases the risk of developing ACD, there is no evidence suggesting that ACD is more prevalent among atopic patients.[6,7] Furthermore, the rates of positive patch tests in atopics as compared with nonatopics are either similar or not significantly different.[7,13] In fact, no significant difference in patch-test results was elucidated in atopics versus nonatopics among hairdressers, except for increased sensitization to fragrance mix 1 and nickel sulfate within the atopic group.[14] Although atopy may increase the risk of contact dermatitis, patch testing benefits anyone with an unclear etiology of dermatitis regardless of its association with atopic diathesis.

INCIDENCE AND PREVALENCE

Contact dermatitis is a significant public health concern. According to the National Health and Nutritional Examination Survey (NHANES) the prevalence of contact dermatitis in the United States was 136 per 10,000 individuals,[15] determined using data collected over a 1-year period between 1999 and 2006; however, this figure was underreported in comparison with the documented physical examination findings. The National Ambulatory Medical Care Survey conducted in 1995 estimated 8.4 million outpatient visits to American physicians for contact dermatitis, rating it the second most frequent dermatologic diagnosis.[16] The majority of epidemiologic data regarding contact dermatitis has been extrapolated or inferred from government reports on prevalence and incidence, and their impact on occupational skin diseases. Therefore, the remainder of this section focuses on the epidemiology of contact dermatitis in the occupational setting.

While occupational skin diseases encompass a variety of cutaneous pathologies including neoplasms, infections, and injuries, contact dermatitis is by far the most common[2,17–19] work-related skin disorder, accounting for 90% to 95% of all cases.[2,17,20,21] Hands are the most commonly affected area and account for 80% to 90% of cases,[2,6,22–26] while only 10% involve the face.[6] The 2 major subtypes of OCD are irritant and allergic. It is widely quoted in the literature that ICD is responsible for 80% of all OCD cases, with the remaining 20% caused by ACD[2,6,17]; however, a wide variation exists in this distribution.[27] In fact, the NACDG has reported significantly more occupational ACD (60%) then ICD (32%) in the United States.[6]

Specific data on national occupational disease and illness in the United States are available from the United States Bureau of Labor and Statistics (BLS) collected through annual surveys of approximately 160,000 employers selected to represent all private industries nationwide. According to the most recent 2009 survey results, BLS data estimated 25,900 cases of occupational skin diseases or disorders and an incidence rate of 2.9 cases per 10,000 full-time workers. These figures showed a downward trend in comparison with 2008 BLS data, which estimated 35,800 cases and an incidence rate of 3.8 per 10,000 full-time workers.[28] Several studies have examined BLS survey limitations, and the number of actual occupational skin diseases may be on the order of 10 to 50 times higher than figures reported by the BLS, theoretically raising the number of occupational skin disease cases to between 250,000 and 1.25 million.[6,17,29]

The aforementioned BLS figures represent incidence rates and total cases for all occupational skin diseases or disorders and not cases of contact dermatitis specifically. In most countries, the reported incidence rate for OCD varies between 5 and 19 cases per 10,000 full-time workers per year.[6] To determine the OCD incidence rate in the United States based on 2009 BLS data, the extrapolated figures for OCD alone are 23,310 cases (assuming 90% of all occupational skin diseases are due to OCD) and an incidence rate of 2.6 cases per 10,000 full-time workers per year (using the BLS equation to calculate incidence rate). To verify these calculations, the most recent data were obtained by using the searchable BLS databases online. Statistics were pooled from cases coded as (1) dermatitis, (2) ICD, (3) ACD, (4) contact dermatitis and related eczema, (5) dermatitis unspecified, and (6) dermatitis N.E.C. (nowhere else classified), resulting in 6200 total OCD cases and an OCD incidence rate of 0.5 per 10,000 full-time workers.[30] Herein lies a discordance between values reported in the literature and the national statistical data, underscoring the challenge in estimating the incidence rate of OCD, which is especially relevant in the United States.

Many investigators have discussed the possible reasons for such disparate incidence rates including variations in the types of industries in a geographic area, the age and sex distribution of the patients assessed, selection biases inherent among patients referred to tertiary dermatologic centers, the ability of the health care provider to fully assess the worker by patch testing, and the national regulations, reporting, and data collection systems.[27,31,32] For instance, milder cases of OCD are never registered[2,6] or brought to medical attention, and therefore never calculated in the epidemiologic data. In addition, a lack of standardization in case definitions could certainly influence the underestimation of OCD incidence rate.

OCD prevalence provides information on the number of workers affected by contact dermatitis at any one time (eg, point prevalence) or over a defined period of time (eg, period prevalence).[6] In 2005, the ACD prevalence rate was 15% in individuals under the age of 18, and 28% for those over the age of 18. Therefore, the overall period prevalence rate for contact dermatitis estimated 2440 cases per 10,000 individuals per year.[33] OCD prevalence estimates, like OCD incidence rates, vary widely. Such distributions are largely due to differing definitions of contact dermatitis in classifying the allergic type versus the irritant type. Despite these variabilities, a 10% 1-year prevalence and 20% lifetime prevalence are consistently reported estimates in the context of OCD.[2] Investigators who take interest in the accurate determination of OCD prevalence often use hand dermatitis as a clinical surrogate. The first epidemiologic study specifically designed to assess the prevalence of chronic hand dermatitis, as well as its impact on patient-reported outcomes and economic costs in a United States managed care population, projected a 16% prevalence for chronic hand dermatitis nationwide after standardization against the general population with regard to distributions for age, gender, and race.[34]

To collect more precise epidemiologic data for contact dermatitis, many countries have created programs to exercise better surveillance of gathered data to help minimize discrepancies. Such programs include the Health and Occupation Reporting network (THOR) in conjunction with a more specific surveillance scheme called EPI-DERM, both used in the United Kingdom,[35] while the Danish National Board of Industrial Injuries Registry (DNBIIR) is used in Denmark.[36] Data from EPI-DERM gathered between 1993 and 2004 indicated approximately 80% of occupational skin disease cases were caused by contact dermatitis,[35] which closely compares with the estimated 90% in the United States. Slightly lower than the projected prevalence of 16% for hand dermatitis in the United States, the prevalence for hand dermatitis in Europe is between 6.7% and 10.6%.[6,34]

As regards the United States, a sector of the Centers for Disease Control and Prevention (CDC) known as the National Institute of Occupational Health (NIOSH) also publishes historical data on the epidemiology of OCD in addition to the annual data reported by the BLS and other organizations such as NHANES and NACDG. The most recently updated statistics from NIOSH are based on data collected from 1992 to 2001, and provide an overview of the most common occupations and industries with the highest incidence of OCD. Two occupational groups accounted for 56% of all dermatitis cases in 2001: operators, fabricators, and laborers (28.4%), and service workers (27.6%). The specific industries with dermatitis incidence rates higher than the private sector incidence rate of 0.5 per 10,000 full-time workers reported in 2001 included agriculture, forestry, and fishing (1.3 per 10,000 full-time workers), manufacturing (0.7), transportation and public utilities (0.7), and services (0.6). Agriculture had consistently higher incidence rates than other industry sectors during 1992 to 2001 and experienced a 78% rate reduction over this period.[37] A couple of years later, an influential report outlined several key issues, including multiple specialties treating patients, survivor bias, and the plethora of cases never documented, all complicating the epidemiology of OCD and its analysis.[38] These pitfalls are of paramount importance and should be revisited whenever critically evaluating the literature for incidence and prevalence estimates of contact dermatitis.

ECONOMIC IMPACT AND COST TO SOCIETY

Important public health measures of disease involve the total number of cases, the incidence and prevalence, and the economic impact on society. The economic burden of any disease is measured by both its direct and indirect costs. Direct expenses include medical costs, costs associated with disability, workers' compensation, and rehabilitation, while the indirect expenses cover lost workdays (eg, sick leave), loss of productivity, and the possible need for a change in jobs.[38,39] Sources most often report fiscal values in a historical context. The estimated annual cost for contact dermatitis including both direct and indirect expenses in 1984 exceeded $22 million in the United States; however, the actual incidence figures may be 10 to 50 times greater than reported by the BLS. With this in mind, the total annual cost for all occupational skin diseases in 1984 ranged from $222 million to $1 billion, although these estimates did not consider costs of occupational retraining or costs attributable to the effects on quality of life.[17] Furthermore, this historical data only provide an estimated total annual cost for all occupational skin diseases, and not an estimation of costs due to work-related contact dermatitis alone.

Workers' compensation is an additional factor contributing to the direct costs associated with OCD, and is used as a complementary method in the surveillance of skin diseases. Workers' compensation data were first used to analyze injury costs and indemnity duration from OCD in

South Carolina, and examined later by other states for analysis in California, Ohio, and Washington State.[40–43] These investigations significantly contributed to the literature with a fresh perspective, as they validated the effective utility of reviewing workers' compensation data in an effort to identify high-risk industries and their rates of occupational skin disease. Initial analyses seemed very promising for future clinical investigations; however, none examined workers' compensation data for direct costs associated with contact dermatitis and its subsequent economic impact until more recently. A retrospective analysis of workers' compensation claims was performed in Oregon from 1990 to 1997 in order to elucidate the incidence rates, costs, severity, and work-related factors associated with OCD, which revealed a mean total cost of $3552.35 per dermatitis claim, including costs for total temporary disability, medical treatment, partial permanent disability, and vocational rehabilitation.[19] For the 8-year period examined, the total cost of all dermatitis claims amounted to $2,170,489.55, averaging $271,311.94 annually in Oregon.[19] This analysis clearly demonstrates the significant economic burden of OCD, which continues to remain an important problem in need of further attention by employers and researchers alike. The main pitfall with using workers' compensation data to gauge the societal economic burden of OCD in the United States is that no national estimates exist that are based on these claims. Such an estimate would be difficult to obtain because workers' compensation laws, data collection, and reimbursement policies vary by state.[18]

In the United States today, the National Occupational Research Agenda (NORA) partnered with NIOSH estimated an annual cost of at least $1 billion, including workdays and loss of productivity associated with contact dermatitis,[44] implying that their estimate includes both direct and indirect costs. The Lewin Group, Inc also reviewed annual costs associated with OCD, but separately reported direct expenses from indirect expenses, providing more specific information on its economic impact. Direct costs associated with OCD in 2005 were $1.4 billion with $592.6 million for physician and clinic services, and $613 million for treatments and prescription drugs. Indirect costs for the same year were estimated at $499 million, including $268 million due to lost workdays for those affected by the condition, $90 million associated with lost caregiver workdays, and $141 million attributable to restricted activity days.[33] In addition to such insight, the report mentioned their undoubtedly underestimated results. Direct cost calculations excluded

the cost of over-the-counter products used by many patients with contact dermatitis, while indirect costs did not account for patients with mild or moderate disease who did not seek medical attention.[33] Despite this inherent underestimation, these monetary figures likely provide the best approximation of the actual economic burden of OCD in the United States.

BURDEN OF DISEASE ON THE PATIENT

While the societal economic impact of contact dermatitis is largely influenced by its associated costs and expenses, the burden of disease on the individual patient goes far beyond any estimated individual cost. With regard to individual costs, the major influential factor in the burden of OCD on the patient is job interruption. Many patients are unable to afford the loss of income associated with a prolonged 2-week period of lost wages.[2] More severe cases may necessitate job transfer or even lead to frank unemployment, and the notion that a significant proportion of individuals experiences work disruption including loss of employment or job change, often resulting in economic disadvantage, has been reported.[45] Financial stress clearly has a negative impact on an individual with work-related contact dermatitis; however, a change in occupation is indicated only for a minority of affected workers. In fact, in the general population most workers with OCD who change jobs do so for reasons other than dermatitis.[6]

In addition to financial duress, the burden of contact dermatitis on the patient also leads to impaired quality of life (QoL), and QoL outcomes have gained increasing importance over the past decade. Despite its heightened interest, there has been relatively little published with respect to QoL outcomes for contact dermatitis specifically.[45] To address this issue, a dermatology-specific QoL instrument was developed for use in patch-test populations.[46] Approximately 75% of patients reported some impact on self-perception, while 50% experienced interference with activities of daily living and sociality, and only about 25% noted a problem with work or school.[46,47] A QoL questionnaire in another patch-test clinic population investigated QoL outcomes for contact dermatitis, for which 36% of patients reported embarrassment, 35% prevention or interference with work, 32% sleep disturbance, 23% hindrance with housework/shopping/gardening, 20% impedance of social/leisure activities, 15% hindrance with clothes worn, 13% interference with sports activities, and 12% problems with relationships.[45] These results provide evidence that many patients with contact dermatitis suffer from negative QoL outcomes, but more recent attempts to quantify impairment using different quantitative measures have also been reported. Poor QoL scores have been reproduced, averaging 7.8, in responders with more severe cases of OCD on the Dermatology Life Quality Index (DLQI), ranking it just below psoriasis and AD for QoL impairment.[36,39]

Another important aspect to consider when examining the burden of contact dermatitis on a given individual is the psychosocial repercussions associated with the disease. The importance of the hands as tools for communication and expression is manifested by the major psychosocial problems (eg, anxiety, depression, social phobia) suffered by affected individuals.[2] As hands are a means for social communication and expression, it is not surprising that the burden of occupational hand dermatitis negatively influences QoL. In fact, the burden of occupational hand dermatitis may negatively affect sociality or lead to emotional distress in some cases. One study reported 81% of mostly female responders with occupational hand dermatitis, who described some type of emotional or social disturbance—one-half called their condition a handicap with regard to their occupational and leisure activities, one-third required a change of daily activities, and slightly more than one-third reported mood and sleep disturbances and avoided social contact, as people kept their distance from them.[48]

The burden of OCD on the patient should also be assessed in terms of its disease severity, as this varies between individuals. To achieve this, a novel scale known as the Occupational contact Dermatitis Disease severity Index (ODDI) was created, and its validity and reliability tested.[25] Construct validity was verified by comparison with the Global Clinical Dermatology Severity Assessment (GCDSA). Subsequent analysis showed that the ODDI was found to be reliable, with substantial agreement for both intraobserver and interobserver reliability. Internal consistency within the ODDI was nearly perfect (intraclass correlation coefficient ranged from 0.94 to 0.99) and users reported quick and easy use.[25] The ODDI includes an assessment of both visual changes and functional impact, which allows for fluctuations in disease activity and provides a better overall assessment of disease severity than previously published scales.[25] With the ODDI, the burden of work-related contact dermatitis on a given individual will be more accurately determined, more quickly assessed, and generally more useful, especially in the setting of future clinical trials.

PREVENTION STRATEGIES
Avoidance

For specific irritants and allergens present in the workplace, the Occupational Safety and Health Administration (OSHA) mandates all chemical compounds to have a material safety data sheet (MSDS), which was developed after Congress passed the Occupational Safety and Health Act in 1970 and the Hazard Communication Standard in 1986. The MSDS helps identify hazardous ingredients in products used in workplaces.[2] MSDSs typically contain information regarding the physical and chemical characteristics of a substance, health effects, chemical reactivity, chemical and trade names of hazardous ingredients, safe handling precautions, carcinogenicity, emergency and first aid measures, and manufacturer contact information.[15] Despite these regulations, MSDSs are frequently criticized as being ineffective for evaluating potential OCD.[2,15,49] Under current OSHA guidelines, MSDSs can exclude helpful information such as generic names, formulas of hazardous chemicals protecting trade secrets, permissible exposure levels, specific occupations at risk of exposure, and most notably potential skin-sensitizing agents.[49] These sensitizers, otherwise known as contact allergens, are often omitted because the manufacturer deemed them not toxic.[15,50] Sensitizers at a concentration of less than 1% would not be listed on the MSDS in the United States; however, legislation requires sensitizers present at concentrations of more than 0.1% be listed in the European Union.[15] Although the MSDS typically contains the skin irritancy potential for some substances, helping the physician decide whether to use it in a patch test, it is inadequate for the protection and diagnosis of workers with suspected OCD. The manufacturer contact information is a very important component of the MSDS; however, clinicians are often unsuccessful in obtaining any additional information from manufacturers.[50]

For any substance labeled as an allergen identified by patch testing, physician members of the American Contact Dermatitis Society (ACDS) have access to several online databases providing patients with numerous resources of products that are and are not safe to use. The Contact Allergen Management Program (CAMP) is another available service to ACDS members designed to help patients with ACD to find personal care products free of ingredients causing their allergic reactions.[51]

Education

Due to the increasing incidence of OCD, public health interventions and workplace education that focus on prevention are of utmost importance.[52] Concepts for educational interventions have been developed by insurance companies, legislators, and public health institutions.[53] According to the CDC, employers should adhere to a hierarchy of controls to prevent occupational skin disease in workers. Steps include eliminating exposure to harmful chemicals or substituting less hazardous ones, engineering controls to prevent skin contact with such agents, and providing personal protective equipment and educational training programs.[54] Multiple studies have examined the effect of education on the prevalence of OCD in various industries including wet work, food services, cosmetology, health care, and chemical manufacturing. Prevention strategies range from elimination or substitution of harmful exposures, technical control measures, and personal protection to identification of susceptible individuals, education, training, and health surveillance. These educational initiatives stress the proper use of personal protective equipment, awareness of personal and environmental hygiene, and the recognition of early signs and symptoms of OCD. Such efforts have proved to be effective in the primary, secondary, and tertiary prevention of occupational skin diseases in addition to being cost effective.[55] On reviewing the utility and effectiveness of specific prevention programs for hand dermatitis, skin protection, skin care education, rehabilitation, occupational interventions, and coordinated care from allied health professionals have all carried greater importance in comparison with usual care or no intervention at all. Such findings have established moderate evidence in reducing the occurrence of OCD and improving adherence to preventive measures, but only weak evidence in improving clinical and self-reported outcomes.[56] The outcomes of specific instruction courses as tools for preventing occupational skin diseases in Germany were assessed in health care workers, and the investigators reported continual positive outcomes in improved skin health and skin care behaviors 1 year after attending the course.[57]

PATCH TESTING

Many agents can act dually as irritant and allergen, making it very difficult to differentiate between ACD, ICD, and even endogenous eczema clinically or histologically. Not only does patch testing distinguish ACD from ICD, it establishes a causal relationship between ACD and a particular allergen. Therefore, the gold standard for diagnosing ACD is the patch test. Although patch testing is the mainstay for ACD workup, several important factors such as the type of series, test preparation techniques, provider care, patient preparation, time intervals of readings, availability, and cost have all been reported to significantly affect its clinical relevance.[1,58]

According to the principles of evidence-based medicine, patch testing is expected to be cost effective only if there is a strong clinical suspicion for allergy and patients are tested with chemicals relevant to their exposures.[59] Patch testing has a sensitivity and specificity between 70% and 80% when using a standardized general allergen series[60]; however, up to 50% of allergens go undetected unless testing is executed with both standard allergens and allergens present in the culpable environment.[61] Several high-risk occupations have standardized patch-test series commercially available and specifically designed for the most relevant allergens in professions such as hairdressing, metalworking, and dentistry. Testing these additional series significantly increases the probability of detecting allergens relevant to the environmental exposure for each individual.[62] Preemployment patch testing of new trainees in the pharmaceutical and metalworking industries, which are considered high risk for developing contact sensitization, identified certain chemical sensitivities in 7% of subjects.[15] Despite this result, patch tests are not completely reliable, can be costly, require adequate preparation, often result in false positives, and paradoxically cause sensitization in some people. In fact the World Health Organization (WHO) does not recommend testing healthy people, and random or preemptive patch testing is highly discouraged.[15] Therefore it is neither practical nor cost effective to patch-test people unless the clinical suspicion is strong and the most relevant series is chosen.

For highly suspicious cases, patch testing has the greatest QoL benefits and is most cost effective in patients with disease duration of 2 months to 1 year, or with severe, chronic, or recurrent ACD.[63–65] Patch testing is still beneficial in the long-term outcomes of patients even when the results are negative or inconclusive.[66] When this occurs, specialized clinics can significantly aid in the diagnosis of contact dermatitis through advanced and formalized training in patch-test application and interpretation, improved comprehension of when to appropriately test additional series or personal patient products, and through use of prick testing for possible contact urticaria.[62] Increased morbidity, heightened frustration, and higher economic burden on both patient and society have all been reported when this valuable tool goes unused.[67]

List of Acronyms	
ACD	Allergic contact dermatitis
ACDS	American Contact Dermatitis Society
AD	Atopic dermatitis
BLS	United States Bureau of Labor and Statistics
CAMP	Contact Allergen Management Program
CDC	Centers for Disease Control and Prevention
DLQI	Dermatology Life Quality Index
DNBIIR	Danish National Board of Industrial Injuries Registry
EPI-DERM	United Kingdom OCD surveillance; not a true acronym
GCDSA	Global Clinical Dermatology Severity Assessment
ICD	Irritant contact dermatitis
MSDS	Material Safety Data Sheet
NACDG	North American Contact Dermatitis Group
NHANES	National Health and Nutritional Examination Survey
NIOSH	National Institute of Occupational Health
NORA	National Occupational Research Agenda
ODDI	Occupational Contact Dermatitis Disease Severity Index
OSHA	Occupational Safety and Health Administration
QoL	Quality of life
SACD	Systemic allergic contact dermatitis
THOR	The Health and Occupation Reporting Network
WHO	World Health Organization

SUMMARY

Contact dermatitis carries significant public health ramifications. Whether irritant or allergic, contact dermatitis represents a significant cause of morbidity, especially in the workplace. Prevention of OCD can be achieved through patient education, improved health and safety interventions, and increased awareness of potential irritants or allergens. There is a great need for more effective national tracking systems and better work-related education programs, which are worth striving for in the future.

REFERENCES

1. Bourke J, Coulson I, English J. Guidelines for the management of contact dermatitis: an update. Br J Dermatol 2009;160:946–54.
2. Clark SC, Zirwas MJ. Management of occupational dermatitis. Dermatol Clin 2009;27:365–83.
3. Krasteva M, Kehren MT, Ducluzeau M, et al. Contact dermatitis II. Clinical aspects and diagnosis. Eur J Dermatol 1999;9(2):144–60.
4. Nijhawan RI, Molenda M, Zirwas MJ, et al. Systemic contact dermatitis. Dermatol Clin 2009;27(3): 355–64.
5. Thyssen JP, Maibach HI. Drug-elicited systemic allergic (contact) dermatitis–update and possible pathomechanisms. Contact Dermatitis 2008;59(4): 195–202.
6. Belsito DV. Occupational contact dermatitis: etiology, prevalence, and resultant impairment/ disability. J Am Acad Dermatol 2005;53(2):303–13.
7. Bordel-Gómez MT, Miranda-Romero A, Castrodeza-Sanz J. Epidemiology of contact dermatitis: prevalence of sensitization to different allergens and associated factors. Actas Dermosifiliogr 2010; 101(1):59–75.
8. Thyssen JP, Johansen JD, Linneberg A, et al. The epidemiology of hand eczema in the general population-prevalence and main findings. Contact Dermatitis 2010;62:75–87.
9. Modjtahedi SP, Maibach HI. Ethnicity as a possible endogenous factor in irritant contact dermatitis: comparing the irritant response among Caucasians, Blacks, and Asians. Contact Dermatitis 2002;47(5): 272–8.
10. Deleo VA, Taylor SC, Belsito DV, et al. The effect of race and ethnicity on patch test results. J Am Acad Dermatol 2002;46(2 Suppl Understanding): S107–12.
11. Aramaki J, Kawana S, Effendy I, et al. Differences of skin irritation between Japanese and European women. Br J Dermatol 2002;146(6):1052–6.
12. Fairhurst DA, Shah M. Comparison of patch test results among white Europeans and patients from the Indian subcontinent living within the same community. J Eur Acad Dermatol Venereol 2008; 22(10):1227–31.
13. Sharma VK, Asati DP. Pediatric contact dermatitis. Indian J Dermatol Venereol Leprol 2010;76(5):514–20.
14. O'Connell RL, White IR, Mc Fadden JP, et al. Hairdressers with dermatitis should always be patch tested regardless of atopy status. Contact Dermatitis 2010;0:177–01.

15. Hogan DJ, Ledet JJ. Impact of regulation on contact dermatitis. Dermatol Clin 2009;27:385–94.

16. Hogan DJ. Allergic contact dermatitis. Medscape Reference. Available at: http://emedicine.medscape.com/article/1049216-overview Updated June 3, 2010. Accessed April 20, 2011.

17. Lushniak BD. Occupational contact dermatitis. Dermatol Ther 2004;17:272–7.

18. Blanciforti LA. Economic burden of dermatitis in US workers. J Occup Environ Med 2010;52(11):1045–54.

19. McCall BP, Horwitz IB, Feldman SR, et al. Incidence rates, costs, severity, and work-related factors of occupational dermatitis. A workers' compensation analysis of Oregon, 1990-1997. Arch Dermatol 2005;141:713–8.

20. Fregert S. Occupational dermatitis in a 10-year material. Contact Dermatitis 1975;1(2):96–107.

21. Mathias CGT. Occupational dermatoses. J Am Acad Dermatol 1988;19(6):1107–14.

22. Koch P. Occupational contact dermatitis. Recognition and management. Am J Clin Dermatol 2001; 2(6):353–65.

23. Dooms-Goossens A, Drieghe J, Dooms M. The computer and occupational skin disease. Philadelphia: Saunders; 1990.

24. Nethercott JR, Holness DL, Adams RM, et al. Patch testing with a routine screening tray in North America, 1985 through 1989: I-IV. Am J Contact Dermatitis 1991;2:122–34, 198–201, 247–54.

25. Curr N, Dharmage S, Keegel T, et al. The validity and reliability of the occupational contact dermatitis disease severity index. Contact Dermatitis 2008;59: 157–64.

26. Skoet R, Olsen J, Mathiesen B, et al. A survey of occupational hand eczema in Denmark. Contact Dermatitis 2004;51:159–66.

27. Holness DL. Characteristic features of occupational dermatitis: epidemiologic studies of occupational skin disease reported by contact dermatitis clinics. Occup Med 1994;9:45–52.

28. Bureau of Labor Statistics. Occupational injuries and illnesses in the United States. Available at: http://www.bls.gov/iif. Accessed April 20, 2011.

29. National Institute for Occupational Safety and Health (NIOSH). National Occupational Survey—Pilot study for development of an occupational disease surveillance method. Rockville (MD): US Department of Health, Education, and Welfare, HEW Publication (NIOSH); 1975. p. 75–162.

30. Bureau of Labor Statistics—Injuries, illnesses, and fatalities databases. Washington, DC: United States Department of Labor; 2009. Available at: http://www.bls.gov/iif/data.htm. Accessed April 20, 2011.

31. Kucenic MJ, Belsito DV. Occupational allergic contact dermatitis is more prevalent than irritant contact dermatitis: a 5-year study. J Am Acad Dermatol 2002;46:695–9.

32. Andersen KE. Multicentre patch test studies: are they worth the effort? Contact Dermatitis 1998;38: 222–3.

33. The Lewin Group, Inc. The burden of skin diseases 2005. Cleveland (OH): The Society for Investigative Dermatology and the American Academy of Dermatology Association; 2005. p. 37–40.

34. Fowler JF, Duh MS, Chang J, et al. A survey-based assessment of the prevalence and severity of chronic hand dermatitis in a managed care organization. Cutis 2006;77:385–92.

35. Schofield JK, Grindlay D, Williams HC, editors. Skin conditions in the UK: a healthcare needs assessment. 1st edition. Nottingham (UK): Centre of Evidence Based Dermatology; 2009. p. 1–146.

36. Cvetkovski RS, Zachariae R, Jensen H, et al. Quality of life and depression in a population of occupational hand eczema patients. Contact Dermatitis 2006;54:106–11.

37. National Institute for Occupational Safety and Health (NIOSH). Worker health chartbook 2004: skin diseases and disorders. Available at: http://www.cdc.gov/niosh/docs/2004-146/ch2/ch2-11.asp.htm. Accessed April 21, 2011.

38. Lushniak BD. The importance of occupational skin diseases in the United States. Int Arch Occup Environ Health 2003;76:325–30.

39. Fowler J. Chronic hand eczema: a prevalent and challenging skin condition. Cutis 2008;82(4):4–8.

40. Shmunes E, Keil JE. Occupational dermatoses in South Carolina: a descriptive analysis of cost variables. J Am Acad Dermatol 1983;9:861–6.

41. O'Malley MA, Mathias CG. Distribution of lost-work-time claims for skin disease in California agriculture: 1978-1983. Am J Ind Med 1988;14:715–20.

42. Mathias CG, Sinks TH, Seligman PJ, et al. Surveillance of occupational skin disease: a method utilizing workers compensation claims. Am J Ind Med 1990;73:363–70.

43. Kaufman JD, Cohen MA, Sama S, et al. Occupational skin diseases in Washington State, 1989 through 1993: using workers compensation data to identify cutaneous hazards. Am J Public Health 1998;88:1047–51.

44. National Institute for Occupational Safety and Health (NIOSH). Developing dermal policy based on laboratory and field studies: a new National Institute for Occupational Safety and Health (NIOSH) research program in response to the National Occupational Research Agenda (NORA). Available at: http://www.cdc.gov/niosh/norahmgp.html. Accessed April 21, 2011.

45. Holness DL. Results of a quality of life questionnaire in a patch test clinic population. Contact Dermatitis 2001;44:80–4.

46. Anderson RT, Rajagopalan R. Development and validation of a quality of life instrument for cutaneous diseases. J Am Acad Dermatol 1997;37:41–50.

47. Rajagopalan R, Anderson RT. The profile of a patient with contact dermatitis and a suspicion of contact allergy (history, physical characteristics and dermatology-specific quality of life). Am J Contact Dermatitis 1997;8:26–31.

48. Meding B, Swanbeck G. Consequences of having hand eczema. Contact Dermatitis 1990;23:6–14.

49. Bernstein JA. Material safety data sheets: are they reliable in identifying human hazards? J Allergy Clin Immunol 2002 Jul;110(1):35–8.

50. Keegel T, Saunders H, LaMontagne AD, et al. Are material safety data sheets (MSDS) useful in the diagnosis and management of occupational contact dermatitis? Contact Dermatitis 2007;57(5):331–6.

51. Contact Allergen Management Program (CAMP) Database. Bunnell (FL): American Contact Dermatitis Society (ACDS). Available at: http://www.contactderm.org. Accessed May 2, 2011.

52. Weisshaar E, Radulescu M, Soder S, et al. Secondary individual prevention of occupational skin diseases in health care workers, cleaners and kitchen employees: aims, experiences and descriptive results. Int Arch Occup Environ Health 2007; 80(6):477–84.

53. Seyfarth F, Schliemann S, Antonov D, et al. Teaching interventions in contact dermatitis. Dermatitis 2011; 22(1):8–15.

54. Centers for Disease Control and Prevention (CDC). Workplace safety & health topics. Available at: http://cdc.gov/niosh/topics/skin/recommendations.html. Updated August 26, 2010. Accessed April 25, 2011.

55. Brown T. Strategies for prevention: occupational contact dermatitis. Occup Med (Lond) 2004;54(7):450–7.

56. van Gils RF, Boot CR, van Gils PF, et al. Effectiveness of prevention programmes for hand dermatitis: a systematic review of the literature. Contact Dermatitis 2011;64(2):63–72.

57. Apfelbacher CJ, Soder S, Diepgen TL, et al. The impact of measures for secondary individual prevention of work-related skin diseases in health care workers: 1-year follow-up study. Contact Dermatitis 2009;60(3):144–9.

58. Frick-Engfeldt M, Gruvberger B, Isaksson M, et al. Comparison of three different techniques for application of water solutions to Finn Chambers. Contact Dermatitis 2010;63(5):284–8.

59. van der Valk PG, Devos SA, Coenraads PJ. Evidence-based diagnosis in patch testing. Contact Dermatitis 2003;48(3):121–5.

60. Nethercott J. The positive predictive accuracy of patch tests. Immunol Allergy Clin N Am 1989;9: 549–53.

61. Wilkinson JD. Identification of factors involved in contact dermatitis. In: Rycroft JG, Menne T, Frosch PJ, et al, editors. Textbook of contact dermatitis. New York: Springer-Verlag; 1991. p. 662.

62. Goulden V, Wilkinson SM. Evaluation of a contact allergy clinic. Clin Exp Dermatol 2000;25(1):67–70.

63. Rajagopalan R, Anderson RT, Sarma S, et al. An economic evaluation of patch testing in the diagnosis and management of allergic contact dermatitis. Am J Contact Dermatitis 1998;9(3):149–54.

64. Rajagopalan R, Kallal JE, Fowler JF Jr, et al. A retrospective evaluation of patch testing in patients diagnosed with allergic contact dermatitis. Cutis 1996;57(5):360–4.

65. Rajagopalan R, Anderson R. Impact of patch testing on dermatology-specific quality of life in patients with allergic contact dermatitis. Am J Contact Dermatitis 1997;8(4):215–21.

66. Slodownik D, Williams J, Frowen K, et al. The additive value of patch testing with patients' own products at an occupational dermatology clinic. Contact Dermatitis 2009;61(4):231–5.

67. Rietschel RL. Human and economic impact of allergic contact dermatitis and the role of patch testing. J Am Acad Dermatol 1995;33(5 Pt 1): 812–5.

Acne Vulgaris: Pathogenesis, Treatment, and Needs Assessment

Siri Knutsen-Larson, MD[a,1], Annelise L. Dawson, BA[a,1],
Cory A. Dunnick, MD[a,*],
Robert P. Dellavalle, MD, PhD, MSPH[b]

KEYWORDS

- Acne vulgaris • Epidemiology • Treatment

Acne vulgaris is a common skin condition with substantial cutaneous and psychologic disease burden. Studies suggest that the emotional impact of acne is comparable to that experienced by patients with systemic diseases, like diabetes and epilepsy.[1–3] In conjunction with the considerable personal burden experienced by patients with acne, acne vulgaris also accounts for substantial societal and health care burden. Americans use more than 5 million physician visits for acne each year, leading to annual direct costs in excess of $2 billion.[4,5] Acne is the most common diagnosis made by dermatologists and is also commonly made by nondermatologist physicians.[6,7] The pathogenesis and existing treatment strategies for acne are complex.[8] This article discusses the epidemiology, pathogenesis, and treatment of acne vulgaris. The burden of disease in the United States and future directions in the management of acne is also addressed.

EPIDEMIOLOGY

Acne is a highly common skin condition. Still, estimates of acne prevalence vary substantially given the absence of a universally accepted diagnostic or grading schema. Additionally, estimates continue to change as the prevalence of acne decreases secondary to improved treatment modalities.[9] Acne is most common in adolescents, affecting approximately 85% of teenagers.[9,10] Acne prevalence after adolescence decreases with increasing age, but disease burden in younger adults is still quite high.[8] A common misconception by the medical and lay community is that acne is a self-limited teenage disease and, thus, does not warrant attention as a chronic disease. Nevertheless, the chronicity of many cases of acne as well as the well-documented psychologic effects of chronic acne contributes to the burden of the disease.[2,3,11]

The average age of onset of acne is 11 years in girls and 12 years in boys.[12,13] Acne is increasing in children of younger ages, with the appearance of acne in patients as young as 8 or 9 years of age. This trend toward earlier development of acne is thought to be related to the decreasing age-of-onset of puberty that has been observed in the United States.[14] Acne is more common in males in adolescence and early adulthood, which

[a] Department of Dermatology, University of Colorado Denver, PO Box 6511, Mail Stop 8127, Aurora, CO 80045, USA
[b] Dermatology Service, Denver Department of Veterans Affairs Medical Center, University of Colorado School of Medicine, Colorado School of Public Health, 1055 Clermont Street, Mail Code #165, Denver, CO 80220, USA
[1] Both authors contributed equally to this article.
* Corresponding author. Department of Dermatology, University of Colorado Denver School of Medicine, Aurora Court F703, PO Box 6510, Aurora, CO 80045.
E-mail address: cory.dunnick@ucdenver.edu

Dermatol Clin 30 (2012) 99–106
doi:10.1016/j.det.2011.09.001

is a trend that reverses with increasing age.[12,13] It is well known that adult acne is more common in women. Adult acne typically represents chronic acne persisting from adolescence, not new-onset disease.[15,16]

Other factors impacting acne prevalence and severity include ethnicity and genetic propensity. Acne age of onset and disease character vary among patients of different ethnicities. Scarring and pigmentary changes are common in skin of color. Propensity to scar and to develop hyperpigmentation is highest among Hispanic and African American patients, respectively.[12,17] These long-term disease consequences are challenging to treat and contribute to the disease burden. In addition, genetic factors impact the propensity to develop acne. Adolescent and adult acne is more common in children of parents with a history of acne.[12,18,19]

Several modifiable factors alter acne risk. Cigarette smoking, for example, raises acne risk with disease severity worsening in a dose-dependent fashion with increasing number of cigarettes smoked daily.[13] Although evidence regarding the impact of dietary factors on acne is equivocal, studies suggest that dairy intake increases acne risk.[20–22] Finally, traditional opinion in dermatology holds that acne tends to improve during summer months when sun exposure is greater.[23] This finding is supported by an observed seasonal decrease in physician visits for acne during summer months.[24] Nevertheless, no studies exist to support this association and use of UV light to treat acne has been rejected.[23] Undoubtedly, acne is a complex disease process influenced by both genetic and environmental factors.

PATHOGENESIS

The pathogenesis of acne is a result of multifaceted processes within the pilosebaceous unit resulting in bacterial overgrowth and inflammation. This condition typically develops at the time of the pubertal transition when changes in the body's hormonal milieu alter pilosebaceous gland function. Initially, follicular epithelial cells differentiate abnormally and form tighter intracellular adhesions and, therefore, are shed less readily. This process leads to the development of hyperkeratotic plugs, or microcomedones, which enlarge progressively to form noninflammatory, closed or open comedones.[25] Circulating and cutaneously derived androgens, often named the primary inciting factor in the development of acne, induce sebum production, further contributing to the development of comedones.[26] Conditions, such as polycystic ovarian syndrome, congenital adrenal hyperplasia, and various endocrine tumors, result in a higher circulating level of androgens and are associated with the development of acne vulgaris.[27]

The corporal distribution of acne depends on pilosebaceous gland density and morphology and, thus, is common in regions where these structures are largest and most abundant: the face, chest, neck, and back. Noninflammatory acne is characterized by the formation of open or closed comedones. Open comedones, or blackheads, demonstrate darkly colored hyperkeratotic plugs within the follicular opening. This dark coloration is related to the oxidation of melanin and not dirt, as is a common public misconception. Closed comedones, or whiteheads, are white to flesh toned in color and seem not to have a central open pore.[25]

Changes in the skin's natural flora accompany this androgen-related increase in sebum production. *Propionibacterium acnes*, a normal component of the cutaneous flora, inhabits the pilosebaceous unit using lipid-rich sebum as a nutrient source. *P acnes*, therefore, flourishes in the presence of increased sebum production, leading to inflammation via complement activation and the release of metabolic byproducts, proteases, and neutrophil-attracting chemotactic factors.[25,28] Inflammatory acne vulgaris lesions, such as papules, pustules, nodules, or cysts, develop when comedones rupture and contents of the pilosebaceous unit spill into the surrounding dermis.[25,29] In severe cases, adjacent cysts may coalesce to form channels or draining sinuses. Inflammatory acne may produce cutaneous scarring or hyperpigmentation that persists long after acne resolution.[25]

PREVENTION

External factors play an important role in the development of acne lesions. Cigarette smoking and dietary factors increase acne risk and disease severity. In addition, certain skin and hair products and use of occlusive clothing articles contribute to acne development. The removal of any of these factors may lead to an improvement in disease severity.

The link between smoking and acne is well established.[13] Even though smoking avoidance and cessation should be encouraged in all patients, this preventive message is especially important for patients suffering from acne. Practitioners should emphasize not only that smoking increases acne risk but also that a dose-dependent relationship exists between daily cigarette use and acne disease severity.

The controversial relationship between diet and acne has been studied for many years. There is no reputable evidence to support a link between acne and chocolate. Recently, however, studies have suggested an association between milk and acne.[20–22] This finding is based on increased levels of insulinlike growth factor 1 in milk causing an increase in circulating androgens. Associations of omega-3 fatty acids, antioxidants, zinc, vitamin A, and iodine with acne have also been proposed. However, all of these areas require further research.[30] Dietary modification alone is not adequate for acne prevention regardless of the association between diet and acne. Individuals with acne wishing to make dietary changes should focus on the avoidance of dairy products as perhaps the most evidence-based intervention.

Facial and hair products, especially cosmetics and hair products containing oils, may lead to an exacerbation of acne lesions.[17,31] In addition, repeated scrubbing with soaps, detergents, and other agents can cause trauma to underlying comedones, thereby increasing inflammation. Thus, individuals with acne should select oil-free or noncomedogenic products and refrain from aggressively rubbing the face.[32] Other factors also contribute to pore occlusion, including tight clothing and head gear. Hence, these articles should be avoided when possible.

TREATMENT

In the United States, there is an overabundance of treatment recommendations for patients with acne. Unfortunately, few of these recommendations are evidenced based and comparative studies are limited.[33] In fact, in 2009, the Institute of Medicine listed acne as a priority for comparative effectiveness research evaluating treatment regimens.[34] Recently published treatment algorithms include A Global Alliance to Improve Outcomes in Acne, those endorsed by the American Academy of Dermatology, and recommendations from a European expert group on oral antibiotics to treat acne.[32,35,36] These recommendations are based on expert opinion given the limited evidence available. All of the guidelines recommend similar approaches focusing on acne severity and degree of inflammation. In addition, acne treatment recommendations may be based on skin type, clinical classification of acne, and preexisting acne scaring.[37] Treatment options include proper skin care, topical and oral antimicrobials, topical and systemic retinoids, benzoyl peroxide, and oral contraceptives for female patients. These treatments are often used in combination to achieve disease resolution.

A primary initial treatment approach is proper skin care. This care includes eliminating the aforementioned extrinsic factors as well as encouraging proper skin hygiene and adherence to prescribed acne treatment regimens. Although it was previously thought that excessive skin cleansing contributes to the formation of acne, several small studies indicate that facial cleansing, even when performed up to 4 times daily, is not harmful and may, in fact, diminish acne severity.[38–40] Patient education in proper hygiene includes counseling regarding appropriate skin cleanser and moisturizer selection.[41]

If skin care alone does not lead to the resolution of cutaneous lesions, topical and systemic antimicrobials may be used. Topical antibiotics may be used to treat mild to moderate acne. Systemic antibiotics are indicated when acne is moderate to severe or if disease manifestations are producing marked psychosocial stress for patients.[28] The purpose of this treatment modality is to decrease the presence of *P acnes* on the skin surface and within the pilosebaceous unit.[42] Antibiotics confer more than antimicrobial properties. They also produce antiinflammatory effects, inhibit neutrophil chemotaxis, and alter compliment pathways, all of which aid in the treatment of acne.[28] Various classes of antibiotics, such as sulfonamides, macrolides, tetracyclines, and dapsone, may be used to treat acne.[28,42]

Widespread and long-term use of antibiotics has led to the development of *P acnes* resistance and has also been associated with *Staphylococcus* resistance.[28,43,44] Thus, when treating with antimicrobials, the prescribing clinician must consider not only local patterns of resistance but also patient adherence to a regimen that will not promote selection for resistant bacterial strains. It is also important to avoid protracted antibiotic courses. Monotherapy with antimicrobials should be avoided, especially when using macrolides that are most often associated with the development of resistance.[28,44] Instead, successful treatment is often seen when pairing antimicrobials with benzoyl peroxide, hormonal therapies, and retinoid preparations.[28,42]

In women with mild to moderate acne, combined oral contraceptives (COCs) can be used. A recent Cochrane review concluded that this method of treatment reduces acne severity when compared with placebo.[45] Even though androgen levels are often normal in women with acne vulgaris, hormonal therapies combating androgens seem to benefit these patients.[46] Progestins tend to be proandrogenic but most COCs are estrogen dominant. Estrogen containing oral contraceptives increase circulating levels of steroid hormone binding globulin which results in lower circulating levels of testosterone. Different COCs contain varying levels of progestins and the implications of this require further research.[45] In women with mild to moderate acne who do not desire childbearing, COCs are a good treatment recommendation. Oral contraceptives are often paired with other acne therapies.[32]

Topical retinoids represent the most commonly prescribed treatment option because they are effective in both the treatment and prevention of acne.[47] The mechanism of action of retinoids involves preventing the primary acne lesion, which decreases inflammation.[48] This drug class is an excellent choice for both initial and maintenance therapy and assists many patients in achieving adequate disease control. Depending on the case, topical retinoids can be paired with benzoyl peroxide, antimicrobials, or with oral contraceptives.

Finally, oral isotretinoin is an option for severe, refractory acne. The mechanism of action includes decreasing sebaceous gland activity with a resultant decrease in sebum secretion. This action effectively diminishes overgrowth of P acnes, which is a key pathogenic factor. The drug also inhibits keratinocyte hyperplasia and instead promotes normal differentiation.[49] Isotretinoin must be prescribed carefully because it carries several black box warnings, including teratogenicity, possible change in mood status, and hypertriglyceridemia, among others.[49,50] This drug is the only acne treatment option that permanently changes the course of the disorder. However, because of the considerable side effects, it should only be used in those with refractory nodular acne.

Given the increasing trend toward treatment with several agents simultaneously, providers have come to rely on the use of combination agents in the treatment of acne. These agents include pairings of topical antibiotics with benzoyl peroxide, topical antibiotics with retinoids, and others. Use of combined agents has been demonstrated to improve patient adherence to prescribed regimens.[51] Given that poor adherence to complex medication regimens limits treatment efficacy and contributes to the chronicity and burden of acne, providers should aim to simplify treatment regimens and use combined agents when feasible.

ACNE SCARRING

Despite the many treatment options, acne scars still develop in some patients. They result from skin damage during the healing process of acne. Acne scars are divided into 2 groups: more common atrophic scars and hypertrophic scars. Treatments for acne scarring include, but are not limited to, topical treatments, chemical peels, dermabrasion, laser, and dermal grafting. Unfortunately, there are no well-accepted guidelines to optimize acne scar treatment. Additional research is required to determine cost-effectiveness and establish the duration of treatment effects.[52]

BURDEN OF TREATMENT

The annual cost of acne treatment is quite high given the prevalence and chronicity of the disease. Acne represents the most common dermatologic diagnosis in the United States.[6,7] A study based on data from 2004 estimates that the annual direct cost of acne management is more than $2.5 billion. Acne ranks second only to skin ulcers and wounds in annual cost burden for dermatologic illness.[4]

In addition to the high cost burden, the treatment of acne produces heavy physician demands. Acne accounts for more than 5 million physician visits annually, or approximately 8% of all dermatologic health care visits.[5,7,53] Two-thirds of physician visits for acne are made by women, suggesting that women are more likely than men to seek medical care for acne.[53,54] Contrary to the perception of acne as a disease of adolescents only, individuals aged older than 18 years account for more than 60% of acne-related visits. Nevertheless, the health care burden of adolescent acne is substantial, with patients aged 12 to 17 years composing nearly 40% of the visits. Although recent studies have demonstrated an increase in acne prevalence for children aged younger than 12 years, these patients account for the minority of health care visits or less than 2% of all physician visits for acne.[54]

AVAILABLE SERVICES

Acne vulgaris is managed in the outpatient setting by both specialist and generalist physicians. Dermatologists provide approximately two-thirds of all acne care in the United States, followed by pediatricians (16%), general/family practitioners (12%), internists (5%), and obstetricians/gynecologists (1%).[55] Long wait times and poor geographic distribution of the dermatologic workforce are 2 factors thought to promote the use of nondermatologist care in acne treatment.[56,57] Furthermore, several characteristics, including being younger than 18 years of age, Hispanic ethnicity, receipt of care in the West or Midwest, and the use of public medical insurance, are predictive of nondermatologist acne care.[55]

Use of nondermatologist care in acne treatment is relevant because it may not be equivalent to the care provided by dermatologists. Studies report differences in prescribing patterns and varying regimen complexity between dermatologists and general practitioners. In particular, generalists are less likely to prescribe topical retinoids and are more likely to prescribe antibiotic monotherapy, which are trends not in line with the present recommendations.[47,58]

Overall, generalists receive limited training in the treatment of dermatologic disease. US medical schools provide on average only 21 hours of dermatology training before graduation, and dermatologic training in pediatric and internal medicine residencies is limited.[59–61] Dermatologists diagnose acne many times more frequently then do their generalist counterparts and this quantity of experience also contributes to the expertise of dermatologists in treating acne.[7,62] Even so, the role of nondermatologist care of acne should not be undervalued, given the substantial burden of acne. Medical school and residency training programs should place greater emphasis on dermatologic education. Future efforts to develop standardized, evidence-based acne treatment guidelines may assist nondermatologists in providing comparable acne care.

In addition to the acne treatment by physicians, there has also been a growing trend toward the use of physician assistants (PAs) and other midlevel providers in the management of dermatologic disease. In fact, dermatologists are second only to ophthalmologists in their use of PAs. In 1997, 1 in every 32 patients visiting a dermatology clinic was seen by a PA, which is a proportion that is thought to have increased markedly since that time. PAs work under the supervision of a physician; however, more than one-quarter of patients seeing a PA for dermatologic complaints are not directly evaluated by a physician.[63] To the authors' knowledge, no exact figures are available for the use of PAs in the treatment of acne specifically. Nevertheless, anecdotal experience indicates that acne is a condition commonly managed by dermatology PAs and that the use of PAs to evaluate acne may diminish the costs associated with acne management. Further analyses of the efficacy and cost of PA management of acne are warranted.

In addition to the care resources offered through physicians and midlevel providers, many online resources are available to patients suffering from acne. The American Academy of Dermatology (www.aad.org) offers detailed patient information on acne and also hosts a searchable database that aids patients in locating dermatologists in their geographic region. Acne-Net (http://skincarephysicians.com/acnenet/index.html) provides similar patient material online. Social networking and other online media sources host abundant content describing acne management. Although much of this online content is unregulated and should be interpreted carefully, numerous reliable health information sources exist. Physicians should be aware of the many accurate online resources to which they can direct patients as well as the unregulated content their patients may be accessing.

FUTURE DIRECTIONS

Going forward, several priorities should guide acne research and management efforts. First, it is imperative that comparative effectiveness research is emphasized and evidence-based treatment strategies are established for acne. Not only will this enhance patient outcomes but this will also allow for better control of the costs and physician demands associated with acne treatment. The establishment of optimal treatment regimens would be expected to diminish the chronicity and, hence, burden of acne disease. Furthermore, standardized recommendations would help enable nondermatologist physicians to provide appropriate care and assist in meeting the demands of acne management. Likewise, medical school and residency training programs must emphasize dermatology education. Generalists commonly manage dermatologic illness and their ability to effectively do so relies heavily on adequate training.

Efforts to explore alternative care resources should be supported. Already, the use of PAs and other midlevel providers has been established in dermatologic practice. Further analyses of the efficacy and cost-effectiveness of midlevel provider care should be pursued. Additionally, in recent years, the use of the teledermatology and Internet-based dermatologic care in the treatment of acne has been explored. The use of digital images to monitor treatment progress has been proposed and may be reliable with certain assessment measures, such as total inflammatory lesion count.[64] Similarly, online follow-up visits for acne have been demonstrated to produce equivalent patient outcomes.[65] The use of digital and online resources to treat acne may diminish cost burden and assist in making dermatology services available to patients in regions with limited dermatologic resources.

Finally, cellular phone and Internet technology may be used to promote adherence to treatment regimens through the use of patient reminders.

List of Acronyms

COCs	Combined oral contraceptives
IGF-I	Insulin like growth factor I
P Acnes	Propionibacterium Acnes

Adolescents and young adults, the patients most impacted by acne, are simultaneously highly receptive to the use of technology and prone to medication noncompliance. Improved treatment adherence could help to diminish the acne burden of disease. Physicians must proceed creatively yet cautiously as they develop new approaches to manage acne and control disease burden.

SUMMARY

Acne vulgaris is a common dermatologic disease that results in high monetary and physician use demands in the United States. The pathogenesis and treatment of acne is complex and requires ongoing research to establish best-practice guidelines. In the meantime, physicians should emphasize existing evidence-based recommendations, including the use of topical retinoids and avoidance of antibiotic monotherapy, in the treatment of acne. Moreover, clinicians must continue to pursue innovative strategies, such as the use of nonphysician providers, teledermatology, and other technologic resources, as a means by which to enhance acne management and limit the substantial burden of this prevalent disease.

REFERENCES

1. Mallon E, Newton J, Klassen A, et al. The quality of life in acne: a comparison with general medical conditions using generic questionnaires. Br J Dermatol 1999;140:672–6.
2. Dalgard F, Gieler U, Holm JO, et al. Self-esteem and body satisfaction among late adolescents with acne: results from a population survey. J Am Acad Dermatol 2008;59:746–51.
3. Uhlenhake E, Yentzer BA, Feldman SR. Acne vulgaris and depression: a retrospective examination. J Cosmet Dermatol 2010;9:59–63.
4. Bickers DR, Lim HW, Margolis D, et al. The burden of skin diseases: 2004. J Am Acad Dermatol 2006; 55(3):490–500.
5. Fleischer AB Jr, Feldman SR, Rapp SR. Introduction. The magnitude of skin disease in the United States. Dermatol Clin 2000;18(2):xv–xxi.
6. Thompson TT, Feldman SR, Fleischer AB. Only 33% of visits for skin disease in the US in 1995 were to

dermatologists: is decreasing the number of dermatologists the appropriate response? Dermatol Online J 1998;4(1):3.
7. Stern RS. Dermatologists and office-based care of dermatologic care in the 21st century. J Investig Dermatol Symp Proc 2004;9(2):126–30.
8. Collier C, Harper J, Cantree W, et al. The prevalence of acne in adults 20 years and older. J Am Acad Dermatol 2007. Available at: http://www.eblue.org. Accessed January 10, 2011.
9. Stathakis V, Kilkenny M, Marks R. Descriptive epidemiology of acne vulgaris in the community. Australas J Dermatol 1997;38:115–23.
10. Kraning K, Odland G. Prevalence, morbidity and cost of dermatologic diseases. J Invest Dermatol 1979;73:395–401.
11. Gollnick HPM, Finlay AY, Shear N. Can we define acne as a chronic disease? Am J Clin Dermatol 2008;9(5):279–84.
12. Dreno B, Poli F. Epidemiology of acne. Dermatology 2003;206:7–10.
13. Schafer T, Nienhaus A, Vieluf D, et al. Epidemiology of acne in the general population: the risk of smoking. Br J Dermatol 2001;145:100–4.
14. Friedlander SF, Eichenfield LF, Fowler JF, et al. Acne epidemiology and pathophysiology. Semin Cutan Med Surg 2010;29:2–4.
15. Goulden V, Clark S, Cunliffe W. Post adolescent acne: a review of clinical features. Br J Dermatol 1997;136:66–70.
16. Goulden V, Stables I, Cunliffe WJ. Prevalence of facial acne in adults. J Am Acad Dermatol 1999; 41(4):577–80.
17. Taylor SC, Cook-Bolden F, Rahman Z, et al. Acne vulgaris in skin of color. J Am Acad Dermatol 2002;46(Suppl 2):S98–106.
18. Ghodsi SZ, Orawa H, Zouboulis CC. Prevalence, severity, and severity risk factors of acne in high school pupils: a community-based study. J Invest Dermatol 2009;129:2136–41.
19. Goulden V, McGeown CH, Cunliffe WJ. The familial risk of adult acne: a comparison between first-degree relatives of affected and unaffected individuals. Br J Dermatol 1999;141:297–300.
20. Davidovici BB, Wolf R. The role of diet in acne: facts and controversies. Clin Dermatol 2010;28:12–6.
21. Spencer EH, Ferdowsian HR, Barnard ND. Diet and acne: a review of the evidence. Int J Dermatol 2009; 48:339–47.
22. Adebamowo C, Spiegelman D, Berkey CS, et al. Milk consumption and acne in teenaged boys. J Am Acad Dermatol 2008;58:787–93.
23. Gfesser K, Worret WI. Seasonal variations in the severity of acne vulgaris. Int J Dermatol 1996;35: 116–7.
24. Hancox JG, Sheridan SC, Feldman SR, et al. Seasonal variation of dermatologic disease in the

USA: a study of office visits from 1990 to 1998. Int J Dermatol 2004;43:6–11.

25. Brown SK, Shalita A. Acne vulgaris. Lancet 1998;351(9119):1871–6.

26. Chen W, Thibouot D, Zouboulis CC. Cutaneous androgen metabolism: basic research and clinical perspectives. J Invest Dermatol 2002;119(5):992–1007.

27. Imperato-McGinley J, Gautier T, Cai L, et al. The androgen control of sebum production. Studies of subjects with dihydrotestosterone deficiency and complete androgen insensitivity. J Clin Endocrinol Metab 1993;76:524–8.

28. Tan AW, Tan HH. Acne vulgaris: a review of antibiotic therapy. Expert Opin Pharmacother 2005;6(3):409–18.

29. Rubin E. Essential pathology. 3 edition. Baltimore (MD): Lippincott Williams & Wilkins; 2001.

30. Bowe W, Joshi S, Shalita A. Diet and acne. J Am Acad Dermatol 2010;61(1):124–41.

31. Nguyen Q, Kim Y, Schwartz R. Management of acne vulgaris. Am Fam Physician 1994;50(1):89–99.

32. Gollnick H, Cunliffe W, Benson D, et al. Management of acne: a report from a global alliance to improve outcomes in acne. J Am Acad Dermatol 2003;49:S1–37.

33. Williams HC, Dellavalle RP, Garner S. Acne vulgaris. Lancet 2011. [Epub ahead of print].

34. Ratner R, Eden J, Wolman D, et al. Initial national priorities for comparative effectiveness research. Institute of Medicine. Washington, DC: National Academies Pr; 2009.

35. Strauss J, Krowchuk DP, Leyden J. Guidelines of care for acne vulgaris management. J Am Acad Dermatol 2007;6(4):651–63.

36. Dreno B, Bettoli V, Oschendorf F, et al. European expert group on oral antibiotics in acne. European recommendations on the use of oral antibiotics for acne. Eur J Dermatol 2004;14:391–9.

37. Haider A, Shaw J. Treatment of acne vulgaris. JAMA 2004;292(6):726–35.

38. Choi JM, Lew VK, Kimball AB. A single-blinded, randomized, controlled clinical trial evaluating the effect of face washing on acne vulgaris. Pediatr Dermatol 2006;23(5):421–7.

39. Draelos ZD. The effect of daily facial cleanser for normal to oily skin on the skin barrier of subjects with acne. Cutis 2006;78(Suppl 1):34–40.

40. Choi YS, Suh HS, Yoon MY, et al. A study of the efficacy of cleansers for acne vulgaris. J Dermatolog Treat 2010;21:201–5.

41. Goodman G. Cleansing and moisturizing in acne patients. Am J Clin Dermatol 2009;10:S1–6.

42. Leyden J, Rosso JD, Webster G. Clinical considerations in the treatment of acne vulgaris and other inflammatory skin disorders: a status report. Dermatol Clin 2009;27:1–15.

43. Eady EA. Bacterial resistance in acne. Dermatology 1998;196(1):59–66.

44. Eady EA, Gloor M, Leyden JJ. Propionibacterium acnes resistance: a world wide problem. Dermatology 2003;206(1):54–6.

45. Arowojolu A, Gallo M, Lopez L, et al. Combined oral contraceptive pills for the treatment of acne. Cochrane Database Syst Rev 2009. Available at: http://www.ncbi.nlm.nih.gov/pubmed/17253506. Accessed January 15, 2011.

46. Bolognia J, Jorizzo J, Rapini R. Dermatology, vol 1. 2nd edition. Philadelphia: Elsevier; 2003.

47. Yentzer BA, Irby CE, Fleischer AB, et al. Differences in acne treatment prescribing patterns of pediatricians and dermatologists: an analysis of nationally representative data. Pediatr Dermatol 2008;25(6):635–9.

48. James W. Acne. N Engl J Med 2005;352(14):1463–72.

49. Ward A, Brogden R, Heel R, et al. Isotretinoin. A review of its pharmacological properties and therapeutic efficacy in acne and other skin disorders. Drugs 1984;28(1):6–37.

50. Brelsford M, Beute T. Preventing and managing the side effects of isotretinoin. Semin Cutan Med Surg 2008;197(3):197–206.

51. Yentzer BA, Ade RA, Fountain JM, et al. Simplifying regimens promotes greater adherence and outcomes with topical acne medications: a randomized controlled trial. Cutis 2010;86:103–8.

52. Fabbrocini G, Annunziata M, D'arco V, et al. Acne scars: pathogenesis, classification and treatment. Dermatol Res Pract 2010;2010:893080.

53. Stern RS. Medication and medical service utilization for acne 1995-1998. J Am Acad Dermatol 2000;43:1042–8.

54. Yentzer BA, Hick J, Reese EL, et al. Acne vulgaris in the United States: a descriptive epidemiology. Cutis 2010;86:94–9.

55. Armstrong AW, Idriss N, Bergman H. Physician workforce for acne care in the United States, 2003 through 2005. Arch Dermatol 2009;145(10):1195–6.

56. Resneck J Jr. Too few or too many dermatologists? Difficulties in assessing optimal workforce size. Arch Dermatol 2001;137(10):1295–301.

57. Tsang MW, Resneck JS Jr. Even patients with changing moles face long dermatology appointment wait-times: a study of stimulated patient calls to dermatologists. J Am Acad Dermatol 2006;55(1):54–8.

58. Balkrishnan R, Fleischer AB Jr, Paruthi S, et al. Physicians underutilize topical retinoids in the management of acne vulgaris: analysis of U.S. national practice data. J Dermatolog Treat 2003;14:172–6.

59. McCarthy GM, Lamb GC, Russell TJ, et al. Primary care-based dermatology practice: internists need more training. J Gen Intern Med 1991;6:52–6.

60. Ramsay DL, Weary PE. Primary care in dermatology: whose role should it be? J Am Acad Dermatol 1996; 35:1005–8.

61. Prose NS. Dermatology training during the pediatric residency. Clin Pediatr 1988;27:100–3.

62. Fleischer AB, Herbert CR, Feldman SR. Diagnosis of skin disease by non-dermatologists. Am J Manag Care 2000;6:1149–56.

63. Clark AR, Monroe JR, Feldman SR, et al. The emerging role of physician assistants in the delivery of dermatologic health care. Dermatol Clin 2000; 18(2):297–302.

64. Bergman H, Tsai KY, Seo SJ, et al. Remote assessment of acne: the use of acne grading tools to evaluate digital skin images. Telemed J E Health 2009; 15(5):426–30.

65. Watson AJ, Bergman H, Williams CM. A randomized trial to evaluate the efficacy of online follow-up visits in the management of acne. Arch Dermatol 2010; 146(4):406–11.

US Skin Disease Assessment: Ulcer and Wound Care

Alina Markova, BA[a],*, Eliot N. Mostow, MD, MPH[b,c]

KEYWORDS

- Chronic ulcers • Venous leg ulcers • Pressure ulcers
- Diabetic neuropathic foot ulcers

Chronic ulcers are a growing cause of patient morbidity and contribute significantly to the cost of health care in the United States.[1,2] Chronic ulcers or wounds are breaks in the skin of greater than 6 weeks or with frequent recurrence. The most common etiologies of chronic ulcers include venous leg ulcers (VLUs), pressure ulcers (PrUs), diabetic neuropathic foot ulcers (DFUs), and leg ulcers of arterial insufficiency. From the etiologic classification alone, comorbid conditions are identified that have significant impact on patient morbidity and mortality. Beyond that, however, the specific issues surrounding an open skin ulcer create problems related to drainage, odor, and often ambulatory function. Chronic wounds account for an estimated $6 to $15 billion annually in US health care costs. It is difficult to get accurate measurements on this, however, because these patients are often seen in a variety of settings or simply fail to access the health care system.[1,2] A detailed analysis published in 2004 noted that skin ulcer and wound care incurred approximately $9.5 billion in total direct health care costs in the United States (**Table 1**), making this a potential target for significant savings if improvements can be made in prevention and treatment.[3]

VLU

VLUs are the most frequent type of chronic ulcer in the ambulatory care setting. VLUs are classically on the lower leg and often show signs of venous insufficiency including varicose veins and red–brown hemosiderin discoloration in the surrounding skin. By definition, unless considered a mixed-type ulcer, these patients have an adequately functioning lower limb arterial system (ankle–brachial pressure index [ABI] >0.80 and/or presence of palpable distal limb pulse).[4] While it is difficult to get accurate and current estimates of incidence and prevalence, data demonstrate that VLUs affect about 1% of adults and make up 40% to 70% of all chronic leg ulcers.[5,6] Based on data from a 25-year period in Minnesota and 1990 US population data, it was estimated that that 21,000 new patients were diagnosed with a venous ulcer annually.[5] With increasing population and people living longer, that number would be expected to be higher today. The venous leg ulcer overall age- and sex-adjusted incidence is 18.0 cases per 100,000 person–years. The age-adjusted incidence from 1984 to 2001 was higher among women than men (20.4 cases vs 14.6 cases per 100,000 person–years).[5] This incidence increases with age, with VLUs as the most common wounds among ambulatory elderly.[7] Health care costs directly resulting from VLUs have been estimated to range from $150 million to over $1 billion per year in the United States and over $40,000 per patient over a lifetime.[5,8–10]

Prevention and Treatment

Patients with a previous VLU have twenty-fold higher risk of a recurrence.[11] Additional VLU predictors include advanced age, decubitus ulceration, diabetes, rheumatoid arthritis, falls, and

[a] Alpert Medical School of Brown University, 222 Richmond Street, Box G-9286, Providence, RI 02912, USA
[b] Department of Dermatology, Case Western Reserve University School of Medicine, Cleveland, OH 44106, USA
[c] Department of Dermatology, Northeast Ohio Medical University, Rootstown, OH, USA
* Corresponding author. The Warren Alpert Medical School of Brown University, Box G-9286, Providence, RI 02912.
E-mail address: alina_markova@brown.edu

Dermatol Clin 30 (2012) 107–111
doi:10.1016/j.det.2011.08.005
0733-8635/12/$ – see front matter © 2012 Elsevier Inc. All rights reserved.

Table 1
United States annual direct cost of skin ulcers and wounds in 2004

Annual Direct Cost	($ millions)
Hospital inpatient	$7931.9
Office visits	$497.6
Hospital emergency room	$243.3
Prescription drugs	$222.3
Hospital Outpatient Department	$149.9

Data from Bickers DR, Lim HW, Margolis D, et al. The burden of skin diseases: 2004 a joint project of the American Academy of Dermatology Association and the Society for Investigative Dermatology. J Am Acad Dermatol 2006;55(3):490–500.

cataracts. Morbidities associated with lower extremity ulcers include complications of wound infection such as sepsis, gas gangrene, osteomyelitis, necrotizing fasciitis, and death.

VLUs have healing rates of 57% and 75% after 10 weeks and 16 weeks, respectively.[12] Local ulcer care is a tenet of appropriate management in venous ulcers. Standard venous ulcer care consists of compression and simple wound dressing. High-level compression greater than 25 mm Hg[4,13] shows a significant benefit over low compression. Patient compliance with compression treatment is a critical component of successful wound care. Compression treatment prolongs the mean time to ulcer recurrence from 18.7 months in noncompliant patients to 53.0 months in compliant patients. Certain wound dressings are thought to improve the proportion of ulcer healed, as well as the duration of time to heal when compared with the standard protocol. However, a Cochrane review of 42 randomized–controlled trials revealed no benefit of one dressing over another, suggesting that the dressing beneath the compression is less important than the compression for ulcer healing. Ulcer recurrence may sometimes be decreased with superficial vein surgery to correct venous reflux. Unlike the diabetic and arterial foot ulcer, VLU generally does not result in amputation; instead it becomes a chronic, malodorous wound that substantially impairs the patient's quality of life, although comorbid conditions increase the risk of complications from infection that subsequently lead to cellulitis, sepsis, and death. The management team must consider various prognostic factors in treating VLUs and should recognize patients who are candidates for standard therapies and those who qualify for adjuvant interventions to increase the probability of

wound healing and decrease likelihood for ulcer recurrence. Wound size (>10 cm^2) and age (>12 months) have been shown to be of significant prognostic value in selecting a treatment.[14] Health care providers should be encouraged to use adjuvant therapies earlier in the treatment course for those patients with such increased wound size and duration.

Other Considerations

Compression bandaging for VLUs requires additional time and expertise and is sometimes inadequately reimbursed.[15] Less than 20% of VLU patients were reported to receive adequate compression.[1] The current health care model may not incentivize physicians to deliver basic wound care using gold standards of treatment for VLUs, and patients who cannot afford additional dressings and treatments for more aggressive compression are less likely to comply with recommended therapies.

DFU

DFUs result from structural deformities due to diabetic peripheral motor neuropathy that weakens intrinsic muscles of the feet.[13] Coupled with sensory neuropathy, the feet of diabetics are at increased risk for wound development secondary to mechanical stress and tissue breakdown.[13] The prevalence of diabetes and its complications is increasing, with current estimates that 8.3% of the US population is affected. DFUs have an annual incidence rate of 1% to 4% in the United States, and diabetic patients have a 15% to 25% lifetime risk of acquiring these ulcers.[16] Patients with DFUs have a mean age of 69 years, and nearly 60% of patients are men. DFU prevalence was 6.5 cases per 1000 diabetics aged younger than 44 years of age, rising progressively to 10.3 cases per 1000 diabetics over age 75.[17] Average DFU episode duration was 87 plus or minus 83 days.[18] Ulcer progression may lead to osteomyelitis in 15% of DFU patients, and lower limb amputations in 16% of patients, with at least 80% of amputations preceded by an ulcer.[17] DFU patients also experience decreased survival when compared with non-DFU diabetics.[16,17] Furthermore, patients with neuropathic and ischemic DFUs have 45% and 55% 5-year mortality, respectively. Patients with unhealed DFUs experience a significant reduction in quality of life scores, in addition to frustration, anxiety, and limited activities of daily living (ADL). Patients with DFUs average more outpatient visits (35.08 visits verus 13.05), emergency department visits (0.42 visits vs 0.18), hospital admissions, and longer length of stays (6.03 vs 1.46

days) versus non-DFU diabetics annually, thus contributing significantly to health care costs and resource needs.[17] Still, most DFU patients are treated as outpatients. The average DFU ulcer episode cost is estimated at slightly over $13,000 and correlates with ulcer grade severity.[18] A grade 1 DFU episode costs $1,892, while grade 4 or 5 ulcers approach $28,000.[18]

Prevention and Treatment

Tertiary prevention plays a significant role in lower extremity ulcers. Patients with arterial insufficiency may benefit from smoking cessation, effective offloading, and pressure reduction, while diabetics may further benefit from improved glycemic control to reduce ulcer risk.[19] Glycemic control may also reduce the risk for amputations in patients with pre-existing ulcers.[20]

The goal in DFU treatment is complete wound healing. Standard wound care consists of debridement, infection control, offloading through total contact casting (TCC), and dressings to maintain a moist wound bed. Overall DFU healing rates remain low; 24% and 30% of diabetic neuropathic ulcers attain complete healing after 12 weeks and 20 weeks of standard wound care, respectively.[21] The percent reduction in wound area during the first 4 weeks of standard wound care is a major predictor of treatment outcome. Controlled trials did not demonstrate significant benefit of prophylactic antibiosis in DFU patients.[4] Wound Healing Society (WHS) 2008 guidelines urge practitioners to consider the use of topical, device, or systemic advanced-care agents for wounds with less than 50% reduction in area after 4 weeks of standard wound care. Advanced-care therapies include platelet-derived growth factor, other cytokine growth factors, negative pressure wound therapies (NPWTs), electrical stimulation, hyperbaric oxygen therapy (HBOT), and living skin equivalents (LSEs). The cost of care for DFU patients is 5.4 times greater in the year after the first ulcer episode and 2.8 times higher in the second year as compared with diabetics without foot ulcers. Costs associated with the addition of advanced therapy are higher for the first 5 months, equivalent at 5 months, and decreased from months 6 to 12. The higher costs are offset by the avoidance of serious adverse events, resections, and amputations. When compared with standard wound care, the addition of advanced therapies results in 12% lower costs, 24% more ulcer-free days, 67% less time with an infected ulcer, and a 63% lower risk of amputation. Annually, 50,000 patients in the United States require amputations for osteomyelitis, which most commonly began as DFUs.

Other Consideration

The Medicare reimbursement system encourages the use of more expensive therapies over more economical ones. For example, although TCC is a reasonable standard of care for DFU offloading, it is difficult and time-consuming for the provider with a low reimbursement (facility loses $18 per TCC), while LSE is more expensive, with improved reimbursement (facility gains $422 per LSE application).[1] There have been no comparative effectiveness studies comparing these two modalities, however, and the LSE has randomized trial data to support its efficacy.[22]

PRU

PrUs develop due to the compression and localized damage of skin and the underlying tissue between a bony prominence and an external surface.[13] PrU incidence has grown by 63% in recent years.[23] Over 25 million patients are treated annually for PrU. Pressure ulcers are found in 15% of acute-care, 26% of hospitalized, 43% of nursing home, and 39% of spinal cord injury patients, with a predominance in those bed bound.[23] PrUs increase the length of hospitalization by an average of 11 days.[23] The average hospital charge per PrU patient was nearly $50,000 in 2006.[23] Sixty-thousand deaths each year are associated with complications from PrUs.[24] Pressure ulcers are a unique financial burden to hospitals, as Medicaid and Medicare have recently classified hospital-acquired stage 3/4 PrUs as "never events," thus no longer reimbursing cost of care for these ulcers. PrUs do not have a separate diagnostic-related group category; therefore charges are fragmented into different diagnostic categories.[23] As a result, direct cost resulting from PrUs is difficult to assess and is often underestimated.[23] While average hospital charge per pressure ulcer patient was noted to be $48,000 in 2006, a smaller study that accounted for all direct costs related to PrUs reported an average cost of $124,000 to $129,000 per patient hospital stay.[23]

Prevention and Treatment

Pressure ulcers often require long-term hospitalizations and multiple hospital admissions. Prevention consists of skin surveillance and frequent repositioning. Treatment involves debridement, coverage with moisture-retentive dressings, patient nutrition management, and infection control.[25] A dietary consultation my help determine appropriate nutritional interventions.[25,26] Half of stage 2 and 95% of stage 3/4 ulcers do not heal within 8 weeks.

Efforts to follow current prevention and wound-healing guidelines should be emphasized.[24]

CHRONIC ULCERS: THE MANAGEMENT TEAM

The multidisciplinary team consisting of dermatologists, plastic surgeons, vascular surgeons, orthopedic surgeons, endocrinologists, podiatrists, and wound care nurses allows for improved patient care.[27] Orthopedic surgeons often care for patients with Charcot foot deformities, many of whom will later develop neuropathic DFUs. Plastic surgeons play an important role in treating decubitus ulcers with flaps, grafts, and extensive surgical debridement. If an increase in blood flow may improve wound healing, vascular surgery should be considered to assess the potential for surgical intervention. Dermatologists often manage chronic ulcer cases that are not candidates for surgical intervention; in these cases, the goal becomes palliation, but they are often essential to making an accurate diagnosis, especially when the etiology is more complex, such as secondary to malignancies, atypical infections, vasculitis, or pyoderma gangrenosum.

CHRONIC ULCER: GUIDELINES TO CARE

There are many guidelines and standards of care to be considered in the management of chronic wounds. The Tax Relief and Health Care Act of 2006 authorized the establishment of a pay-for-performance program, Physician Quality Reporting Initiative (PQRI). A 2% bonus payment was linked to whether physicians met certain treatment goals in a given time frame. These incentives included performing peripheral neuropathy evaluations in diabetics and prescribing appropriate footwear for, as well as providing compression therapy annually to, patients over age 18 with a diagnosis of venous ulcer. This initiative failed to include important gold standards such as offloading for DFUs as treatment goals, limiting their potential impact on wound care. The National Guideline Clearinghouse (NGC), Wound Healing Society (www.woundheal.org), and the Association for the Advancement of Wound Care have created a few of the multiple treatment guidelines available today. Implementation of these guidelines remains inadequate.[28–34] One study found significant variability among 4 sites with respect to guideline adherence; the site with the highest percentage of implementation also achieved the best wound healing rates (70% vs 24%).[29] The high number of guidelines makes integration into the health care system especially challenging; the unification of available protocols would allow for implementation into today's complex and diverse medical system.

List of Acronyms	
ABI	Ankle-Brachial Pressure Index
ADL	Activities of daily living
DFU	Diabetic foot ulcer
HBOT	Hyperbaric oxygen therapy
LSE	Living skin equivalent
NGC	National Guideline Clearinghouse
NPWT	Negative pressure wound therapies
PQRI	Physician Quality Reporting Initiative
PrU	Pressure ulcer
TCC	Total contact casting
VLU	Venous leg ulcer
WHS	Wound Healing Society

Unfortunately, guideline standardization is limited by lacking comparative effectiveness research and insufficient funding for research in ulcer prevention and treatment.[35] There is a need for a strong central organization to promote the prevention and treatment of lower extremity ulcers, thus allowing for improved quality and effective care for this growing patient population.

REFERENCES

1. Fife CE, Carter MJ, Walker D. Why is it so hard to do the right thing in wound care? Wound Repair Regen 2009;18(2):154–8.
2. Gordois A, Scuffham P, Shearer A, et al. The health care costs of diabetic peripheral neuropathy in the US. Diabetes Care 2003;26(6):1790–5.
3. Bickers DR, Lim HW, Margolis D, et al. The burden of skin diseases: 2004 a joint project of the American Academy of Dermatology Association and the Society for Investigative Dermatology. J Am Acad Dermatol 2006;55(3):490–500.
4. Kantor J, Margolis DJ. Management of leg ulcers. Semin Cutan Med Surg 2003;22(3):212–21.
5. Heit JA, Rooke TW, Silverstein MD, et al. Trends in the incidence of venous stasis syndrome and venous ulcer: a 25-year population-based study. J Vasc Surg 2001;33(5):1022–7.
6. Kantor J, Margolis DJ. A multicentre study of percentage change in venous leg ulcer area as a prognostic index of healing at 24 weeks. Br J Dermatol 2000;142(5):960–4.
7. Margolis DJ, Bilker W, Santanna J, et al. Venous leg ulcer: incidence and prevalence in the elderly. J Am Acad Dermatol 2002;46(3):381–6.

8. Rudolph DM. Pathophysiology and management of venous ulcers. J Wound Ostomy Continence Nurs 1998;25(5):248–55.

9. Gloviczki P, Gloviczki ML. Evidence on efficacy of treatments of venous ulcers and on prevention of ulcer recurrence. Perspect Vasc Surg Endovasc Ther 2009;21(4):259–68.

10. Olin JW, Beusterien KM, Childs MB, et al. Medical costs of treating venous stasis ulcers: evidence from a retrospective cohort study. Vasc Med 1999;4(1):1–7.

11. Takahashi PY, Chandra A, Cha SS, et al. A predictive model for venous ulceration in older adults: results of a retrospective cohort study. Ostomy Wound Manage 2010;56(4):60–6.

12. Marston WA, Carlin RE, Passman MA, et al. Healing rates and cost efficacy of outpatient compression treatment for leg ulcers associated with venous insufficiency. J Vasc Surg 1999;30(3):491–8.

13. Fonder MA, Lazarus GS, Cowan DA, et al. Treating the chronic wound: a practical approach to the care of nonhealing wounds and wound care dressings. J Am Acad Dermatol 2008;58(2):185–206.

14. Margolis DJ, Allen-Taylor L, Hoffstad O, et al. The accuracy of venous leg ulcer prognostic models in a wound care system. Wound Repair Regen 2004; 12(2):163–8.

15. Carter MJ. Cost-effectiveness research in wound care: definitions, approaches, and limitations. Ostomy Wound Manage 2010;56(11):48–59.

16. Snyder RJ, Hanft JR. Diabetic foot ulcers—effects on QOL, costs, and mortality and the role of standard wound care and advanced-care therapies. Ostomy Wound Manage 2009;55(11):28–38.

17. Driver VR, Fabbi M, Lavery LA, et al. The costs of diabetic foot: the economic case for the limb salvage team. J Vasc Surg 2010;52(Suppl 3):17S–22S.

18. Stockl K, Vanderplas A, Tafesse E, et al. Costs of lower-extremity ulcers among patients with diabetes. Diabetes Care 2004;27(9):2129–34.

19. Singh N, Armstrong DG, Lipsky BA. Preventing foot ulcers in patients with diabetes. JAMA 2005;293(2): 217–28.

20. Mehmood K, Akhtar ST, Talib A, et al. Clinical profile and management outcome of diabetic foot ulcers in a tertiary care hospital. J Coll Physicians Surg Pak 2008;18(7):408–12.

21. Margolis DJ, Kantor J, Berlin JA. Healing of diabetic neuropathic foot ulcers receiving standard treatment. A meta-analysis. Diabetes Care 1999;22(5):692–5.

22. Veves A, Falanga V, Armstrong DG, et al. Graftskin, a human skin equivalent, is effective in the management of noninfected neuropathic diabetic foot ulcers: a prospective randomized multicenter clinical trial. Diabetes Care 2001;24(2):290–5.

23. Brem H, Maggi J, Nierman D, et al. High cost of stage IV pressure ulcers. Am J Surg 2010;200(4): 473–7.

24. Brem H, Lyder C. Protocol for the successful treatment of pressure ulcers. Am J Surg 2004;188:9–17.

25. Baranoski S. Raising awareness of pressure ulcer prevention and treatment. Adv Skin Wound Care 2006;19(7):398–405 [quiz: 405–7].

26. Dorner B, Posthauer ME, Thomas D. National Pressure Ulcer Advisory Panel. The role of nutrition in pressure ulcer prevention and treatment: National Pressure Ulcer Advisory Panel white paper. Adv Skin Wound Care 2009;22:212–21.

27. Mostow EN. Wound healing: a multidisciplinary approach for dermatologists. Dermatol Clin 2003; 21(2):371–87.

28. Searle A, Gale L, Campbell R, et al. Reducing the burden of chronic wounds: prevention and management of the diabetic foot in the context of clinical guidelines. J Health Serv Res Policy 2008;13(Suppl 3): 82–91.

29. Jones KR, Fennie K, Lenihan A. Evidence-based management of chronic wounds. Adv Skin Wound Care 2007;20(11):591–600.

30. Van Hecke A, Grypdonck M, Defloor T. Guidelines for the management of venous leg ulcers: a gap analysis. J Eval Clin Pract 2008;14(5): 812–22.

31. Fretheim A, Schunemann HJ, Oxman AD. Improving the use of research evidence in guideline development: 15. Disseminating and implementing guidelines. Health Res Policy Syst 2006;4:27.

32. Oxman AD, Schunemann HJ, Fretheim A. Improving the use of research evidence in guideline development: 14. Reporting guidelines. Health Res Policy Syst 2006;4:26.

33. Warriner RA 3rd, Carter MJ. The current state of evidence-based protocols in wound care. Plast Reconstr Surg 2010;127(Suppl 1):144S–53S.

34. Marshall JL, Mead P, Jones K, et al. The implementation of venous leg ulcer guidelines: process analysis of the intervention used in a multicentre, pragmatic, randomized, controlled trial. J Clin Nurs 2001;10(6):758–66.

35. Passman MA; Writing Group IV of the Pacific Vascular Symposium 6, Elias S, et al. Nonmedical initiatives to decrease venous ulcers prevalence. J Vasc Surg 2010;52(Suppl 5):29S–36S.

Melanoma: Epidemiology, Diagnosis, Treatment, and Outcomes

William Tuong, BA[a], Lily S. Cheng, BS[a],
April W. Armstrong, MD, MPH[b],*

KEYWORDS

- Melanoma • Epidemiology • Cause • Prevention
- Treatment • Prognosis

Melanoma is an aggressive type of skin cancer that carries significant morbidity and mortality. Although increased awareness of melanoma has led to more diligent screening, improved understanding of melanoma tumorigenesis has guided the development of therapeutic options. This article reviews melanoma epidemiology, cause, clinical presentation, diagnosis, prevention, treatment, and prognosis, with particular emphasis on melanoma care in the United States.

EPIDEMIOLOGY
Incidence

Although overall cancer incidence in the United States has annually declined,[1] melanoma incidence has increased rapidly in the past few decades.[2,3] In 1973, the incidence of melanoma in the United States was 6.8 per 100,000 people; from 2003 to 2007, incidence increased to 20.1 per 100,000 people.[4] It was estimated that more than 68,000 Americans (38,870 men and 29,260 women) were diagnosed with melanoma in 2010.[5] This number was up from the 54,200 new cases (29,900 men and 24,300 women) of melanoma expected in 2003.[6]

In 2010, cutaneous melanoma was estimated to be the fifth and seventh most common cancer diagnosed in men and women, respectively.[5] Based on the US Surveillance, Epidemiology, and End Results (SEER) Program cancer incidence rates collected from 2004 to 2006, men have a 2.67% (1 in 37) lifetime risk of developing melanoma, whereas women are less likely to develop the disease in their lifetime (1.79%, 1 in 56).[5] Overall, in both men and women, the lifetime risk of developing melanoma is 1.93%.[4]

Gender differences seem to exist in melanoma incidence. In the United States, melanoma is more prevalent in men compared with women. In 1975, 9.2 per 100,000 men and 7.4 per 100,000 women were diagnosed with melanoma. In 2003 to 2007, incidence increased to 25.6 per 100,000 in men and 16.2 per 100,000 in women.[7] Despite these current gender differences, melanoma incidence may be increasing in younger women because of increased ultraviolet (UV) radiation exposure and use of tanning beds.[8]

The incidence of melanoma also differs between races. Specifically, the incidence of melanoma is significantly lower in nonwhite populations.[9] According to SEER data, 1.1 black people and 27.8 white people per 100,000 individuals were

The authors have nothing to disclose relevant to this article.

[a] Department of Dermatology, University of California Davis School of Medicine, 3301 C Street, Suite 1400, Sacramento, CA 95816, USA

[b] Dermatology Clinical Research Unit, Teledermatology Program, Department of Dermatology, University of California Davis Health System, University of California Davis School of Medicine, 3301 C Street, Suite 1400, Sacramento, CA 95816, USA

* Corresponding author.

E-mail address: aprilarmstrong@post.harvard.edu

Dermatol Clin 30 (2012) 113–124
doi:10.1016/j.det.2011.08.006
0733-8635/12/$ – see front matter Published by Elsevier Inc.

diagnosed with melanoma in 2007.[4] However, African Americans were much more likely to be diagnosed with metastatic melanoma compared with white people, a stage characterized by therapy resistance and higher mortality.[5] This disparity in melanoma stage and poorer prognosis at diagnosis was also described in a recent study comparing Hispanic people with non-Hispanic white people.[10]

Researchers have questioned whether the increase in melanoma incidence is a true epidemic or an artifact of increased surveillance and improved screening programs. However, evidence suggests that the current increase in melanoma incidence may be caused by true increases in disease incidence. First, incidence increased faster in the 1970s,[11] before the start of a nationwide early detection initiative in 1985 that helped increase the awareness of skin cancer among health care providers and the general public.[12] Second, a recent report found the highest incidence of melanoma in individuals of lower socioeconomic status, a population with decreased access to health services and therefore less regular screening.[3] Third, behaviors associated with increased risk for melanoma, like sun exposure and tanning bed use, have increased in the past decade.[13]

Mortality

Despite more vigilant screening and early detection efforts, melanoma mortality has not appreciably declined. From 1975 to 1989, melanoma mortality annually increased by 1.6%, although this trend seems to be stabilizing.[4] From 2003 to 2007, the median age at death for cutaneous melanoma was 68 years.[7] During this period, the mortality was approximately 0.1% for those less than 20 years old, 2.7% for those between 20 and 34 years old, 6.3% for those between 35 and 44 years old, 14.3% for those between 45 and 54 years old, 19.6% for those between 55 and 64 years old, 20.9% for those between 65 and 74 years old, 24.1% for those between 75 and 84 years old, and 11.9% for those 85 years and older.[4] In 2010, approximately 8700 people (5670 men, 3030 women) were estimated to have died of melanoma.[5]

Based on data from 2003 to 2007, the age-adjusted mortality was 2.7 per 100,00 individuals per year. Within the same age group, mortality caused by melanoma was higher in men compared with women. In men, there was a significant 2.3% annual increase in mortality between the years 1975 and 1989, and a 0.2% annual increase from 1989 to 2007. In women, mortality increased

0.8% annually between the years 1975 and 1988; however, between the years 1988 and 2007, mortality decreased annually by −0.6%.[4]

Five-year survival rates have significantly improved annually since the 1970s. From 1975 to 1977, the 5-year survival rate was 78.1% in men and 86.9% in women. The 5-year survival rate from 1999 to 2006 significantly increased to 91.1% in men and 95.1% in women ($P<.05$).[4] Survival was highest in women, individuals less than the age of 45 years at diagnosis, and those diagnosed with localized melanoma.[4,14]

ETIOLOGY
Pathogenesis and Tumor Progression

Primary melanoma is a malignant neoplasm of neural crest–derived melanocytes, specialized pigmented cells predominately found in the basal layer of the epidermis. The normal function of melanocytes is to produce and transfer a dark pigment called melanin to mitotically active keratinocytes, which are also found in the epidermis. The transferred melanin is concentrated in the perinuclear space of keratinocytes and protects the nucleus from UV radiation damage.[15]

The transformation of melanocytes to tumor cells occurs in both genetically normal and predisposed patients. Although melanoma pathogenesis is complex and not completely understood, it likely involves interactions between environmental factors, accumulation of sequential genetic alterations, activation of oncogenes, inactivation of tumor suppressor genes, and impaired DNA repair.[16,17]

Three distinct pathogenic steps have been proposed in melanoma tumor progression. In an early-stage tumor, the melanoma may be confined to the epidermis and displays only radial (or lateral) growth. When melanoma progresses, it can develop into microinvasive melanoma, in which microscopic extensions invade the superficial papillary dermis. More advanced melanomas can progress to the vertical growth phase, which is characterized by invasive growth with discernable involvement deep into the dermis. In this stage of growth, the melanoma has gained the potential to metastasize.[18]

Genetic Mechanisms

Many different genes have been associated with increased risk for melanoma. The more well-characterized mutations involve the highly penetrant gene products of familial melanoma syndromes: p16 (also called cyclin-dependent kinase inhibitor 2A [CDKN2A], or inhibitor of cyclin-dependent kinase 4A, INK4A), alternate reading frame (*ARF*), and cyclin-dependent kinase 4 (*CDK4*). The low-penetrance melanocortin-1 receptor (*MC1R*) gene has also been associated with increased melanoma risk. In addition, a *BRAF* mutation has been ascertained in up to 60% of cutaneous melanomas and is the target of new mutation-specific therapies, like RG7204 (also referred to as PLX4032 and RO5185426), which are undergoing clinical testing.[19,20] The best-characterized mutation involves the p16/ARF locus of chromosome 9p21, and this is discussed in more depth later.[21–23]

p16/ARF
The p16/ARF locus is the best-characterized high-penetrance melanoma gene locus.[21–23] This locus encodes 2 tumor suppressor proteins that are essential in the pathways of cell growth regulation and apoptosis.[24] The first is *p16* and the second is *ARF* (also called *p14*).[16,25]

Germline mutations in 1 or both of these gene products are associated with familial melanoma, and have been ascertained in 25% to 50% of familial melanoma kindreds worldwide and in approximately 10% of patients with multiple primary melanoma.[26] Identifying individual contributions of *p16* and *ARF* to melanoma tumorigenesis is difficult because melanoma pedigrees with *ARF*-only mutations are scarse.[27–29]

The penetrance of these gene mutations has been estimated in recent studies, but the complexities of genetic analyses have provided variable results. The Melanoma Genetics Consortium analyzed data from 385 high-risk families (defined as having at least 3 confirmed melanoma cases in a family) to calculate p16/ARF penetrance.[30] By 50 years of age, p16/ARF penetrance reached 0.13 in Europe, 0.50 in the United States, and 0.32 in Australia. By 80 years of age, penetrance increased to 0.58 in Europe, 0.76 in the United States, and 0.91 in Australia.[30] In population-based studies, penetrance estimates were 14% (95% confidence interval [CI], 8.0%–22%) by age 50 years, 24% (95% CI, 15%–34%) by age 70 years, and 28% (95% CI, 18%–40%) by age 80 years.[31]

Risk Factors

Although genetic research on melanoma tumorigenesis is ongoing, numerous other risk factors for melanoma are well documented. Natural and artificial UV radiation, previous and family history, nevi, and several other factors are discussed later.

Natural UV radiation exposure
The role of solar radiation in the development of melanoma is well documented. Solar radiation has been classified as carcinogenic to humans by the International Agency for Research on Cancer (IARC), an agency of the World Health Organization that classifies carcinogens.[32] Average annual amounts of UV radiation positively correlate with melanoma incidence.[33] In addition, latitudinal and altitudinal gradients are observed in melanoma incidence, with the highest incidence occurring in higher altitudes or lower latitudes where UV intensity is greater.[34,35]

Frequency of sunburn, an indirect measurement of intermittent sun exposure, also confers increased risk for melanoma. Although experts have commonly focused on childhood sunburns as a major risk factor for melanoma development, recent studies have shown that the point in life when UV exposure occurs may not be as important to subsequent cancer risk. A meta-analysis found a positive association of melanoma incidence, with an odds ratio (OR) of 1.91 (95% CI, 1.69–2.17) for those with frequent sunburns compared with those with no or rare sunburns in their lifetime.[36] A more recent meta-analysis of 25 studies showed that sunburns, regardless of age, conferred increased melanoma risk.[37] In addition, a case-control study found a twofold increase in melanoma risk in individuals who had more than 5 sunburns, regardless of their timing in life.[38]

Artificial UV radiation exposure (indoor tanning)
Almost 30 million people in the United States tan indoors, including 2.3 million adolescents.[39] In the Health Information National Trends Study, 18.1% of women and 6.3% of men reported using indoor tanning equipment in the past 12 months.[40] Overall, indoor tanning has become increasingly popular in the past decades despite the accumulation of compelling evidence on the dangers of artificial UV radiation in melanoma development.[39]

Through a landmark meta-analysis, the IARC helped confirm the association between indoor tanning and melanoma. This confirmation also contributed to the designation of UV-emitting tanning devices as a group 1 carcinogen by the World Health Organization. Ever use of indoor tanning equipment was associated with increased risk of melanoma (relative risk 1.15; 95% CI, 1.00–1.31). In addition, first exposure of indoor tanning before 35 years of age was associated with a relative risk of 1.75 (95% CI, 1.35–2.26).[41]

Family and personal history
An association between family history and melanoma risk has been described in numerous studies. Patients who reported at least 1 first-degree relative diagnosed with melanoma had approximately a twofold higher risk of developing

melanoma compared with those without a family history.[42,43] Having a parent who had multiple melanomas confers the highest relative risk of 61.78 (95% CI, 5.82–227.19).[44]

A personal history of either melanoma or non-melanoma skin cancer is also a significant risk factor for developing melanoma. A prospective study found that the 5-year risk of developing a second primary melanoma was 11.4%, with the risk increasing for those with atypical nevi or a family history of melanoma.[45] In addition, 30.9% of individuals developed a third primary melanoma within 5 years.[45] The relative risk for developing melanoma in individuals with a personal history of nonmelanoma skin cancer, like squamous cell carcinoma, basal cell carcinoma, or premalignant actinic keratoses, was between 2.8 and 17.[46–48]

Nevi

The number of nevi is positively correlated with UV exposure and is used as a surrogate measurement of UV-induced cutaneous damage.[49] Studies have shown that approximately 25% of melanoma cases are attributable to the presence of 1 or more atypical nevi (also known as a dysplastic nevi), whereas 27% of melanoma cases are attributable to a high common nevus count (more than 50 common nevi).[50] Patients with greater than 1 atypical nevus have an increased relative risk for melanoma of 3.63 (95% CI, 2.85–4.62).[50] In addition, relative risk increases linearly with total body common nevus count.[50]

Other risk factors

Melanoma risk increases with age and is greater in men.[9] It occurs most commonly in white people,[5] with risk inversely related to degree of pigmentation.[51] Similarly, the redhead phenotype characterized by hair color, fair skin, inability to tan, and propensity to freckle is also associated with increased risk of melanoma.[52]

Certain medical conditions can increase risk for melanoma. Xeroderma pigmentosum is an autosomal recessive disorder that is characterized by exquisite hypersensitivity to sunlight and the inability to repair UV-induced DNA damage. Affected individuals younger than 20 years have a greater than 1000-fold increased risk for melanoma as well as other cutaneous neoplasms.[53]

Psoriasis is a common autoimmune disease that causes inflammation of the skin and joints. Psoralen and ultraviolet A (PUVA) therapy has been a widely and successfully used treatment to induce remission in psoriasis. In 2001, the third report of the PUVA Follow-up Study showed that the incidence of invasive melanoma was threefold

higher in patients receiving at least 250 treatments and at least 15 years from first PUVA therapy compared with cohort patients exposed to lower doses of PUVA.[54]

CLINICAL PRESENTATION
Clinical Morphology

Early clinical recognition of melanoma is essential in the successful treatment of this cancer. Pigmented cutaneous lesions can be initially evaluated using the ABCD acronym (asymmetry, border irregularity, color variegation, and diameter).[55] Recently, it has been recommended that E for evolving lesions be added to this list of parameters.[56] Not all melanomas present with all 5 features; it is the combination of the different ABCDE parameters that makes a cutaneous lesion a suspect for early melanoma.[57]

Asymmetry

Most early malignant melanomas grow at an irregular rate, resulting in asymmetry. This asymmetry differs from benign pigmented lesions, which are typically round and symmetric.

Border irregularity

The uneven growth rate usually causes malignant melanomas to have an irregular border, unlike benign pigmented lesions, which typically present with regular margins.

Color variegation

Macular melanomas are often variegated, containing variable hues of tan, brown, black, red, and white. Benign lesions are generally uniform in color.

Diameter

Most malignant melanomas have diameters of at least 6 mm at the time of diagnosis.

Evolution

Clinicians should note any evolving nevi, particularly focusing on changes to shape, size, symptoms (itching), surface (bleeding, papular or nodular formation), and pigmentation over time.

The ABCDE criteria can be useful in early melanoma detection, but its clinical usefulness is limited in several ways. First, the criteria are commonly applied to radial growth phase melanomas and are not typically helpful in evaluating melanomas with vertical growth involvement. Second, it is difficult to apply these criteria to amelanotic melanomas, like desmoplastic melanomas, because these lesions are characteristically non-pigmented or have minimal residual pigmentation. However, the ABCDE criteria are often used in conjunction with other methods to improve diagnostic accuracy. An increasingly used method is dermoscopy, a noninvasive technique that aids in the visualization of subsurface structures and recognition of early melanoma.[58]

Anatomic Distribution

The anatomic distribution of melanoma lesions seems to differ by sex and age. In men, they are commonly located on the trunk (55%), especially the back (39%).[59] Another study calculated a relative tumor density (RTD) value, the ratio of the observed to the expected numbers of cases by site assuming even distribution of melanoma over all body sites.[60] The RTD was significantly increased in the back (3.4) and the upper arm (1.7) for men less than 50 years of age.[60] Men more than of 50 years of age showed a significantly higher RTD for the ear (8.5), face (6.0), neck (3.4), and the back (2.6).[60]

In women, 42% of melanoma lesions were localized to the lower extremities, with 24% on the lower leg. The second most common site was the trunk (25%), with 17% on the back.[59] For women less than 50 years of age, only the back had a significantly raised RTD of 2.3. For those more than 50 years old, the density was significantly higher in the face (5.8), upper arm (2.2), and leg (1.5).[60]

DIAGNOSIS
Biopsy

Skin biopsy remains the standard of practice for diagnosing cutaneous melanoma. Excisional, incisional, shave, and punch biopsies are common techniques. However, excisional biopsy with a 1 mm to 2 mm margin of adjacent normal-appearing skin is the preferred technique for cutaneous lesions suspicious for melanoma.[61] This method helps to ensure that the entire lesion is removed and provides important prognostic information for staging.[62,63]

Incisional biopsies may be indicated in certain clinical circumstances such as facial or acral involvement, low clinical suspicion, or very large lesion. However, subtotal incisional biopsies for melanoma may be inadequate for accurate staging of melanoma.[64]

Punch biopsies are commonly used to initially assess suspicious cutaneous lesions, and may also be more appropriate when sampling larger lesions. Properly performed punch biopsies that extend to subcutaneous fat can provide accurate T-stage information. However, punch biopsies are limited in diameter and may not encompass the entire lesion, which hampers the assessment of key pathologic findings like overall size and symmetry. Especially in the case of larger lesions, partial sampling with punch biopsies can also lead to misdiagnosis.[63]

Shave biopsy is frequently performed for suspected epidermoid carcinoma as well as melanoma because it is efficient and easy to perform. However, shave biopsy should be deep enough to avoid transecting the base of the melanoma.[62] This method has been criticized for its potential to compromise accurate diagnosis, staging, and thus optimal treatment decision making.[63,65] To explore the appropriateness of shave biopsy in melanoma diagnosis, Zager and colleagues[63] retrospectively analyzed a consecutive series of 600 patients undergoing treatment of cutaneous melanoma. They found that only 3% of patients were determined to have a more serious melanoma on wide local excision after a preliminary diagnosis was made with shave biopsy. Nevertheless, although shave biopsy is simple to perform, efficient, and commonly used clinically, it is sometimes debated whether it is an acceptable method for the diagnosis of melanoma.

Major Clinical Subtypes of Melanoma

Four major subtypes of melanoma have been described: superficial spreading melanoma, nodular melanoma, lentigo maligna melanoma, and acral lentiginous melanoma. The less common melanoma subtypes include nevoid melanoma, desmoplastic melanoma, clear cell sarcoma, and solitary dermal melanoma.

Superficial spreading melanoma

Superficial spreading melanoma is the most common melanoma subtype, accounting for 50% to 80% of all melanoma diagnoses.[62] The name is derived from a prolonged radial (lateral) growth phase before invasive (vertical) growth commences. It most likely occurs on sun-exposed areas, such as the back in men and the lower limbs in women, but can occur in any anatomic location. Although these melanomas can arise from a precursor nevus, most occur de novo.

Clinically, a superficial spreading melanoma appears variegated with a sharply marginated and irregular border. It typically presents with multiple shades of tan, brown, gray, black, violet, pink, and, rarely, blue or focal areas of hypopigmentation.[66] At the time of diagnosis, most superficial spreading melanomas are at least 6 mm in diameter and confined to the radial growth phase, which is associated with a good prognosis.[67] Advanced lesions often have a diameter greater than 25 mm and can have palpable nodular areas extending several millimeters above the skin surface[66,67]; at this stage, lesions are commonly invasive (vertical growth) and are associated with poorer prognosis.[67]

Superficial spreading melanoma is characterized histologically by pagetoid and nested epithelioid cells in the intraepidermal portion. Poor circumscription with variable epidermal thickening is also common. Cytologically, the melanocytes may have 1 or more large nuclei with an abundant cytoplasm that is often amphophilic, eosinophilic, or finely pigmented with melanin granules.[66]

Nodular melanoma

Nodular melanoma comprises 20% to 30% of cases.[62] By definition, the cancer cells in nodular melanoma have an early onset of the vertical growth phase.[68] They are more common in men, and usually found on the trunk in men and legs in women.[67] Clinically, they are thick on palpation and pigmented a dark brown, black, or blue-black color in a uniform manner. Histologically, there is no intraepidermal nested melanocytic proliferation beyond the edges of the dermal component (usually no more than 3 rete lateral to the dermal tumor).[66]

Lentigo maligna melanoma

Lentigo maligna melanoma commonly occurs in older individuals with sun-damaged skin and has a predilection for sun-exposed areas such as the malar region, temple, nose, forehead, neck, and forearms.[67]

Clinically, lentigo maligna melanoma commonly presents as a gradually enlarging tumor that is flat and variably pigmented a tan, brown, and black color. In addition, the tumor is typically asymmetrical with irregular borders. Lentigo maligna begins as a small lesion, but can reach several inches in diameter if neglected.[67] However, transformation is slow and it may take 10 to 50 years before invasive growth becomes apparent.[69] Although the tumor is mostly flat, a slightly raised focus of vertical growth may be palpated or detected with tangential lighting.[66]

Histologically, atypical melanocytes proliferate in a lentiginous manner in sun-damaged skin that exhibits epidermal atrophy, solar elastosis, and dermal thinning. The nuclei commonly appear large and hyperchromatic.[66] Multinucleated giant cells, also known as star-burst giant cells, containing as many as 30 nuclei, may be present in the basal layer of the epidermis.[70] Lesion progression frequently presents with the confluence of melanocytes, nesting, and pagetoid epidermal invasion.[66]

Acral lentiginous melanoma

Acral lentiginous melanoma is the least common subtype, accounting for less than 5% of all melanomas.[67,71] However, this subtype accounts for 70% of melanomas seen in African Americans,[62] and is the predominate form of melanoma in other nonwhite populations.[72] They are distinguished by their involvement of hairless areas like subungual, palmar, and plantar regions.[67,73]

Clinically, an acral lentiginous melanoma usually begins as a variably colored macule that develops irregular borders and variegation in pigment, usually brown or black, as it increases in size with time.[67] The surface may have a papule or nodule that is associated with the vertical growth phase; however, flat lesions may have dermal involvement as well.[67] Histologically, early acral lentiginous melanomas show diffuse lentiginous proliferation of atypical melanocytes along the basal layer.[73] As the lesion progresses, it typically presents with confluent lentiginous and nested growth with some pagetoid epidermal invasion.[74]

Subungual melanoma typically presents as a brown or black longitudinal band that extends from the nail bed epithelium to the proximal nail fold and cuticle. The involvement of the proximal nail fold is known as Hutchinson sign and serves as a clue to distinguish melanoma from other types of lesions such as subungual hematoma.[67] Subungual melanoma may or may not cause nail dystrophy; however, it sometimes presents as a subungual mass with variable degrees of pigmentation, ulceration, and nail plate destruction.[75]

Staging

Staging of melanoma is based on the tumor-node-metastasis (TNM) staging criteria. The TNM categories described by the American Joint Committee on Cancer (AJCC) consider histopathologic factors such as primary tumor thickness, ulceration status, and rate of mitosis. Mitotic rate has recently emerged as an important prognostic factor and is expressed as the number of mitoses per square millimeter of primary tumor. The AJCC no longer recommends using the Clark level as a staging criterion because it is not an independent prognostic factor when mitotic rate is included in the analysis. In addition, as the TNM acronym implies, the number of metastatic nodes and presence of metastases is also important.[61]

Primary tumor

The primary tumor (T) is based on thickness, with T1 being less than 1 mm, T2 from 1.01 to 2.00 mm, T3 from 2.01 to 4.00 mm, and T4 being greater than 4 mm.

Regional lymph nodes

Nodal metastases are rated from N0 meaning no regional lymph node (N) involvement, N1 meaning 1 regional lymph node involvement, N2 meaning 2 to 3 regional lymph node involvement, to N3 meaning 4 or more regional lymph node involvement or matted nodes.

Distant metastasis

The absence of distant metastases (M) is signified by M0 and the presence of distant metastases is signified by M1.

TNM combinations correspond to 1 of 5 stages.[61] An accurate staging system facilitates the grouping of patients based on similar risk in terms of disease progression and natural history. In turn, this helps physicians with treatment decision making for a specific patient population.[62]

> Stage 0: carcinoma in situ (TisN0M0)
> Stage I A/B: includes lesions up to 2 mm with no nodal or distant metastases (T1aN0M0, T1bN0M0, T2aN0M0).
> Stage II A/B/C: includes larger lesions, greater than 2 mm without positive nodes or distant metastases (T2bN0M0, T3aN0M0, T3bN0M0, T4aN0M0, T4bN0M0).
> Stage III: includes lesions of any size with positive lymph nodes (TxN1M0, TxN2M0, TxN3M0).
> Stage IV: includes lesions of any size with distant metastases (TxNxM1).

PREVENTION

Because research suggests that UV light exposure contributes to the development of nonmelanoma skin cancers and possibly melanoma, limiting UV light exposure may prevent the development of skin cancers.[76,77] The United States Preventive Services Task Force currently recommends that primary care physicians counsel patients on sun-protective strategies, including regular application of sunscreen and avoidance of indoor tanning.[78] Although sun protection has been shown to reduce rates of nonmelanoma skin cancers, increasing evidence suggests that regular use of sunscreen may also confer a protective effect on the development of melanoma.[79,80] The American Academy of Dermatology (AAD), American Cancer Society, and American Academy of Family Physicians all recommend sun-protective behaviors.[79,81,82] Avoidance of ultraviolet light exposure may be especially beneficial in individuals with a genetic predisposition to melanoma development.[77]

Various other strategies to prevent melanoma are also being investigated.[83,84] To date, no pharmacotherapy has been definitively shown to prevent the development of melanoma. Medications that have been studied in small, early-stage clinical trials include antilipidemics, nonsteroidal antiinflammatory drugs, immune modifiers, and retinoids.[83] Certain natural products have also been investigated, including resveretrol, lycopene, selenium, green tea, ginseng, and other botanicals.[84] Most of these supplements have not been shown to decrease the risk of melanoma, but case-control studies have found that vitamin D and vitamin E supplementation may be associated with a reduction in the severity of disease.[84,85]

Secondary prevention of melanoma involves the early detection of melanoma. The United States Preventive Services Task Force does not recommend for or against regular screening in the general population because studies have yet to show definitive benefit of screening melanoma in asymptomatic individuals in the general population.[86] However, the AAD recommends that high-risk individuals be examined regularly by a dermatologist. The AAD also recommends monthly self-examinations and annual physician examinations for persons older than 40 years.[12] Skin self-examinations seem to have high specificity (83%–97%) but low sensitivity (25%–93%) in detecting melanoma in high-risk individuals.[87]

TREATMENT

Surgical excision is the corner stone of melanoma treatment. Wide excision is generally recommended, but the recommended surgical margin varies in the literature. A meta-analysis in the Cochrane Library defines a narrow margin as 1 to 2 cm and a wide margin as 3 to 4 cm; they found a statistically insignificant difference in overall survival between narrow and wide margins.[88] The meta-analysis included all participants (all ages, all ethnic groups) with early-stage (stage I and II) invasive melanoma.[88] Current national guidelines from the National Comprehensive Cancer Network recommend surgical excision margins up to 2 cm.[88] For lesions less than 1 mm in thickness (stage T1), a margin of 1 cm is recommended. For lesions 1 to 4 mm in thickness (stage T2 and T3), a margin of 2 cm is recommended. For lesions greater than 4 mm in thickness (stage T4), a 2-cm margin of resection is generally considered adequate, but more research is necessary to determine optimal surgical margins for varying depths of melanoma.[89,90] For melanoma in situ, a surgical margin of 5 mm is deemed adequate.[90,91]

Mohs micrographic surgery has emerged as another surgical option in cases in which tissue preservation is important, such as melanomas of the head and neck.[92] This method makes use of immediate frozen or paraffin sections to ensure that the tumor is adequately excised. Mohs surgery has been used successfully in cases of lentigo maligna in which the borders are often poorly defined.[93] Mohs surgery may also confer an additional treatment advantage in desmoplastic melanoma, which has a high propensity for perineural invasion.[92]

Sentinel lymph node biopsy is important in melanoma staging, and results from sentinel lymph node biopsy can confer important prognostic information.[94] It is usually recommended for melanomas that are more than 1 mm deep.[90] Some studies also suggest that a survival benefit may exist from sentinel lymph node biopsy procedures for lesions less than 1 mm.[95] However, survival benefit for regional lymphadenectomy following positive sentinel lymph node biopsy is equivocal.[96]

Adjuvant systemic therapies have limited success in the treatment of advanced-stage melanoma. Interferon-α is an adjuvant treatment that is approved by the US Food and Drug Administration (FDA) for stage III melanoma.[97] Meta-analysis studies by the National Cancer Institute have found limited efficacy of interferon-α. Specifically, adjuvant treatment with interferon-α increased 5-year survival by only 3%, although this was statistically significant.[98] A study by the European Organization for Research and Treatment of Cancer yielded similar results.[94] The investigators found that, although interferon-α reduced relapse rate, the overall survival rate remained largely unchanged. Interleukin-2 is another immunotherapeutic that has recently been approved by the FDA for the treatment of metastatic melanoma. High-dose recombinant interleukin-2 has been found to induce remission in 6% of cases of metastatic melanoma.[99]

In 2011, the FDA approved ipilimumab for the treatment of advanced-stage melanoma. Ipilimumab is a monoclonal antibody against cytotoxic T-lymphocyte–associated antigen 4 that incites a T-cell–mediated response against the tumor. In clinical trials, ipilimumab was found to improve patient survival by 4 months in patients with stage III and IV melanoma.[100]

Other new drug therapies, including drugs that target biologic receptors, are currently in development.[101] Among these are bevacizumab, an endothelial growth factor antibody, and sorafenib, a BRAF cellular pathway inhibitor. These agents have shown some efficacy in early clinical trials.[94] In particular, BRAF inhibitor therapy has shown an initial response in 70% to 80% of patients, but disease relapsed within a median time of 9 months in all patients. Thus, it seems that overall survival is not significantly altered by BRAF inhibitor treatment, and further studies are necessary to evaluate efficacy.[102]

Radiotherapy plays a limited role in the treatment of melanoma because melanoma is radioresistant compared with other cancers.[103] The response rate is typically dose dependent. However, because very high doses of radiation are needed to eradicate tumors, radiotherapy is less optimal as primary treatment of melanoma because of its associated adverse effects. However, radiotherapy may be used as an adjuvant therapy when adequate surgical margins cannot be achieved, such as with lesions on the head and neck.[103]

PROGNOSIS

Prognosis is usually good for thin melanomas. Stage I melanoma has a 5-year survival of 91% to 95% and a 10-year survival of 83% to 88%. Stage II melanoma has a 5-year survival of 45% to 79% and a 10-year survival of 32% to 64%. Ulceration is a poor prognostic sign and lowers the survival rate by about 5%.[94] Stage III melanoma has a 5-year survival of 30% to 70%, depending on the degree of node spread.[94] Stage IV melanoma has a 5-year survival of 10% to 20%. Palliative radiation therapy can extend survival to about 6 months in patients with stage IV melanoma.[94]

Metastatic melanoma has a well-known predilection for distant spread and has a median survival time of 6 to 9 months.[94] In advanced regional disease, it commonly metastasizes hematogenously to other skin regions, soft tissues, the lung, the liver, and the brain. The brain is the most common site of metastases in stage IV melanoma and is associated with poorer prognosis compared with other visceral sites. A retrospective review of 6953 patients found that the median survival time of patients with brain metastases from malignant melanoma was 3 to 4 months after diagnosis, and the brain metastases eventually contributed to the death of 94.5% of patients in this group.[104] Lungs are the second most common sites of metastatic disease, after lymph node involvement.[105] In patients who have visceral metastatic disease, the liver is the most common site involved.[106]

NEEDS IN MELANOMA DETECTION AND CARE

Melanoma represents a significant public health concern. Despite substantial research, melanoma incidence is rising faster than any other type of cancer and melanoma mortality has not appreciably declined. However, addressing certain unmet needs may help reduce the public health burden of melanoma.

Potential opportunities are available to improve screening of melanoma. As stated earlier, melanoma is one of the few cancers for which the United States Preventive Services Task Force does not recommend regular screening. Under such guidelines, the detection of early lesions relies heavily on self-screening by patients and general practitioners. This self-screening is a practice that can be highly inefficient and risks delaying a melanoma diagnosis until later stages that are associated with poorer prognosis. Considering current melanoma screening guidelines, the need for effective and user-friendly screening tests for patients and general practitioners is urgent.

Addressing disparities in melanoma prevention strategies targeting underserved communities, particularly African American communities, may be of value as well. Although melanoma incidence is low in African Americans, melanoma diagnoses are typically made at more advanced stages and associated with poorer outcomes. As such, there is an important need for melanoma prevention interventions that are culturally relevant, linguistically accessible, and provide information on the melanoma subtypes (eg, acral lentiginous melanoma) most prevalent in the targeted community.

SUMMARY

Melanoma is a skin cancer that arises from the malignant transformation of melanocytes. Although it is typically considered a pigmented lesion, the clinical presentation of melanoma can vary greatly. With increased efforts in screening and detection of early-stage melanoma, researchers and clinicians hope to improve clinical outcomes for patients with melanoma. Novel immunotherapies directed at specific molecular targets in the pathogenesis of melanoma usher in a new era of treatment of advanced melanoma.

ACKNOWLEDGMENTS

We would like to acknowledge Jonathan Faridian for his efforts in gathering literature.

REFERENCES

1. Howe HL, Wingo PA, Thun MJ, et al. Annual report to the nation on the status of cancer (1973 through 1998), featuring cancers with recent increasing trends. J Natl Cancer Inst 2001;93(11):824–42.
2. Erickson C, Driscoll MS. Melanoma epidemic: facts and controversies. Clin Dermatol 2010;28(3):281–6.
3. Linos E, Swetter SM, Cockburn MG, et al. Increasing burden of melanoma in the United States. J Invest Dermatol 2009;129(7):1666–74.
4. Altekruse S, Kosary C, Krapcho M, et al. SEER cancer statistics review, 1975-2007. 2009. Available at: http://seer.cancer.gov/csr/1975_2007. Accessed April 6, 2011.
5. Jemal A, Siegel R, Xu J, et al. Cancer statistics, 2010. CA Cancer J Clin 2010;60(5):277–300.
6. Jemal A, Murray T, Samuels A, et al. Cancer statistics, 2003. CA Cancer J Clin 2003;53(1):5–26.
7. Fast Stats: an interactive tool for access to SEER cancer statistics. Surveillance Research Program,

List of Acronyms	
AAD	American Academy of Dermatology
ABCD	Asymmetry, border irregularity, color variegation, and diameter
ABCDE	Asymmetry, border irregularity, color variegation, diameter, and evolving lesions
AJCC	American Joint Committee on Cancer
ARF	Alternate reading frame
CDKN2A	Cyclin-dependent kinase inhibitor 2A
CI	Confidence interval
cm	Centimeters
DNA	Deoxyribonucleic acid
FDA	Federal Drug Administration
IARC	International Agency for Research on Cancer
INK4A	Inhibitor of cyclin-dependent kinase 4A
MC1R	Melanocortin-1 receptor
mm	Millimeter
OR	Odds ratio
PUVA	Psoralen and ultraviolet A
RR	Relative risk
RTD	Relative tumor density
SEER	Surveillance, Epidemiology, and End Results
TNM	Tumor, node, metastasis
US	United States
UV	Ultraviolet

National Cancer Institute. Available at: http://seer.cancer.gov/faststats. Accessed November 4, 2011.

8. Hausauer AK, Swetter SM, Cockburn MG, et al. Increases in melanoma among adolescent girls and young women in California: trends by socioeconomic status and UV radiation exposure. Arch Dermatol 2011;147(7):783–9.

9. Rigel DS. Epidemiology of melanoma. Semin Cutan Med Surg 2010;29(4):204–9.

10. Merrill RM, Pace ND, Elison AN. Cutaneous malignant melanoma among white Hispanics and non-Hispanics in the United States. Ethn Dis 2010; 20(4):353–8.

11. Jemal A, Devesa SS, Hartge P, et al. Recent trends in cutaneous melanoma incidence among whites in the United States. J Natl Cancer Inst 2001;93(9): 678–83.

12. Koh HK, Norton LA, Geller AC, et al. Evaluation of the American Academy of Dermatology's National Skin Cancer Early Detection and Screening Program. J Am Acad Dermatol 1996; 34(6):971–8.

13. Robinson JK, Rigel DS, Amonette RA. Trends in sun exposure knowledge, attitudes, and behaviors: 1986 to 1996. J Am Acad Dermatol 1997;37(2 Pt 1): 179–86.

14. Geller AC, Annas GD. Epidemiology of melanoma and nonmelanoma skin cancer. Semin Oncol Nurs 2003;19(1):2–11.

15. Montagna W, Carlisle K. The architecture of black and white facial skin. J Am Acad Dermatol 1991; 24(6 Pt 1):929–37.

16. Pho L, Grossman D, Leachman SA. Melanoma genetics: a review of genetic factors and clinical phenotypes in familial melanoma. Curr Opin Oncol 2006;18(2):173–9.

17. Uribe P, Wistuba II, Solar A, et al. Comparative analysis of loss of heterozygosity and microsatellite instability in adult and pediatric melanoma. Am J Dermatopathol 2005;27(4):279–85.

18. Bandarchi B, Ma L, Navab R, et al. From melanocyte to metastatic malignant melanoma. Dermatol Res Pract 2010;2010. pii: 583748.

19. Smalley KS. Understanding melanoma signaling networks as the basis for molecular targeted therapy. J Invest Dermatol 2010;130(1):28–37.

20. Puzanov I, Burnett P, Flaherty KT. Biological challenges of BRAF inhibitor therapy. Mol Oncol 2011; 5(2):116–23.

21. Cannon-Albright LA, Goldgar DE, Meyer LJ, et al. Assignment of a locus for familial melanoma, MLM, to chromosome 9p13-p22. Science 1992; 258(5085):1148–52.

22. Kamb A, Shattuck-Eidens D, Eeles R, et al. Analysis of the p16 gene (CDKN2) as a candidate for the chromosome 9p melanoma susceptibility locus. Nat Genet 1994;8(1):23–6.

23. Hussussian CJ, Struewing JP, Goldstein AM, et al. Germline p16 mutations in familial melanoma. Nat Genet 1994;8(1):15–21.

24. Lin J, Hocker TL, Singh M, et al. Genetics of melanoma predisposition. Br J Dermatol 2008;159(2): 286–91.

25. Quelle DE, Zindy F, Ashmun RA, et al. Alternative reading frames of the INK4a tumor suppressor gene encode two unrelated proteins capable of inducing cell cycle arrest. Cell 1995;83(6):993–1000.

26. Pollock PM, Harper UL, Hansen KS, et al. High frequency of BRAF mutations in nevi. Nat Genet 2003;33(1):19–20.

27. Randerson-Moor JA, Harland M, Williams S, et al. A germline deletion of p14(ARF) but not CDKN2A in a melanoma-neural system tumour syndrome family. Hum Mol Genet 2001;10(1):55–62.

28. Hewitt C, Lee Wu C, Evans G, et al. Germline mutation of ARF in a melanoma kindred. Hum Mol Genet 2002;11(11):1273–9.

29. Rizos H, Puig S, Badenas C, et al. A melanoma-associated germline mutation in exon 1beta inactivates p14ARF. Oncogene 2001;20(39):5543–7.

30. Bishop DT, Demenais F, Goldstein AM, et al. Geographical variation in the penetrance of CDKN2A mutations for melanoma. J Natl Cancer Inst 2002;94(12):894–903.

31. Begg CB, Orlow I, Hummer AJ, et al. Lifetime risk of melanoma in CDKN2A mutation carriers in a population-based sample. J Natl Cancer Inst 2005; 97(20):1507–15.

32. El Ghissassi F, Baan R, Straif K, et al. A review of human carcinogens–part D: radiation. Lancet Oncol 2009;10(8):751–2.

33. Armstrong BK, Kricker A. The epidemiology of UV induced skin cancer. J Photochem Photobiol B 2001;63(1–3):8–18.

34. Berwick M, Halpern A. Melanoma epidemiology. Curr Opin Oncol 1997;9(2):178–82.

35. Lee JA, Strickland D. Malignant melanoma: social status and outdoor work. Br J Cancer 1980;41(5): 757–63.

36. Elwood JM, Jopson J. Melanoma and sun exposure: an overview of published studies. Int J Cancer 1997;73(2):198–203.

37. Dennis LK, Vanbeek MJ, Beane Freeman LE, et al. Sunburns and risk of cutaneous melanoma: does age matter? A comprehensive meta-analysis. Ann Epidemiol 2008;18(8):614–27.

38. Pfahlberg A, Kolmel KF, Gefeller O. Timing of excessive ultraviolet radiation and melanoma: epidemiology does not support the existence of a critical period of high susceptibility to solar ultraviolet radiation-induced melanoma. Br J Dermatol 2001;144(3):471–5.

39. Levine JA, Sorace M, Spencer J, et al. The indoor UV tanning industry: a review of skin cancer risk,

health benefit claims, and regulation. J Am Acad Dermatol 2005;53(6):1038–44.

40. Choi K, Lazovich D, Southwell B, et al. Prevalence and characteristics of indoor tanning use among men and women in the United States. Arch Dermatol 2010;146(12):1356–61.

41. The association of use of sunbeds with cutaneous malignant melanoma and other skin cancers: a systematic review. Int J Cancer 2007;120(5): 1116–22.

42. Cho E, Rosner BA, Feskanich D, et al. Risk factors and individual probabilities of melanoma for whites. J Clin Oncol 2005;23(12):2669–75.

43. Ford D, Bliss JM, Swerdlow AJ, et al. Risk of cutaneous melanoma associated with a family history of the disease. The International Melanoma Analysis Group (IMAGE). Int J Cancer 1995;62(4): 377–81.

44. Hemminki K, Zhang H, Czene K. Familial and attributable risks in cutaneous melanoma: effects of proband and age. J Invest Dermatol 2003; 120(2):217–23.

45. Ferrone CR, Ben Porat L, Panageas KS, et al. Clinicopathological features of and risk factors for multiple primary melanomas. JAMA 2005;294(13): 1647–54.

46. Green AC, O'Rourke MG. Cutaneous malignant melanoma in association with other skin cancers. J Natl Cancer Inst 1985;74(5):977–80.

47. Marghoob AA, Slade J, Salopek TG, et al. Basal cell and squamous cell carcinomas are important risk factors for cutaneous malignant melanoma. Screening implications. Cancer 1995;75(Suppl 2): 707–14.

48. Lindelof B, Sigurgeirsson B, Wallberg P, et al. Occurrence of other malignancies in 1973 patients with basal cell carcinoma. J Am Acad Dermatol 1991;25(2 Pt 1):245–8.

49. MacKie RM, Hauschild A, Eggermont AM. Epidemiology of invasive cutaneous melanoma. Ann Oncol 2009;20(Suppl 6):vi1–7.

50. Olsen CM, Carroll HJ, Whiteman DC. Estimating the attributable fraction for cancer: a meta-analysis of nevi and melanoma. Cancer Prev Res (Phila) 2010;3(2):233–45.

51. Gandini S, Sera F, Cattaruzza MS, et al. Meta-analysis of risk factors for cutaneous melanoma: III. Family history, actinic damage and phenotypic factors. Eur J Cancer 2005;41(14): 2040–59.

52. Lin JY, Fisher DE. Melanocyte biology and skin pigmentation. Nature 2007;445(7130):843–50.

53. Kraemer KH, DiGiovanna JJ. Xeroderma pigmentosum. GeneReviews [internet]. Seattle (WA): University of Washington, Seattle;2003. Available at: http://www.ncbi.nlm.nih.gov/books/NBK1397. Accessed August 19, 2011.

54. Stern RS. The risk of melanoma in association with long-term exposure to PUVA. J Am Acad Dermatol 2001;44(5):755–61.

55. Friedman RJ, Rigel DS, Kopf AW. Early detection of malignant melanoma: the role of physician examination and self-examination of the skin. CA Cancer J Clin 1985;35(3):130–51.

56. Abbasi NR, Shaw HM, Rigel DS, et al. Early diagnosis of cutaneous melanoma: revisiting the ABCD criteria. JAMA 2004;292(22):2771–6.

57. Rigel DS, Russak J, Friedman R. The evolution of melanoma diagnosis: 25 years beyond the ABCDs. CA Cancer J Clin 2010;60(5):301–16.

58. Wang SQ, Hashemi P. Noninvasive imaging technologies in the diagnosis of melanoma. Semin Cutan Med Surg 2010;29(3):174–84.

59. Garbe C, Leiter U. Melanoma epidemiology and trends. Clin Dermatol 2009;27(1):3–9.

60. Elwood JM, Gallagher RP. Body site distribution of cutaneous malignant melanoma in relationship to patterns of sun exposure. Int J Cancer 1998; 78(3):276–80.

61. Balch CM, Gershenwald JE, Soong SJ, et al. Final version of 2009 AJCC melanoma staging and classification. J Clin Oncol 2009;27(36):6199–206.

62. Au A, Ariyan S. Melanoma of the head and neck. J Craniofac Surg 2011;22(2):421–9.

63. Zager JS, Hochwald SN, Marzban SS, et al. Shave biopsy is a safe and accurate method for the initial evaluation of melanoma. J Am Coll Surg 2011; 212(4):454–60.

64. Karimipour DJ, Schwartz JL, Wang TS, et al. Microstaging accuracy after subtotal incisional biopsy of cutaneous melanoma. J Am Acad Dermatol 2005; 52(5):798–802.

65. Ng JC, Swain S, Dowling JP, et al. The impact of partial biopsy on histopathologic diagnosis of cutaneous melanoma: experience of an Australian tertiary referral service. Arch Dermatol 2010; 146(3):234–9.

66. Duncan LM. The classification of cutaneous melanoma. Hematol Oncol Clin North Am 2009;23(3): 501–13, ix.

67. Porras BH, Cockerell CJ. Cutaneous malignant melanoma: classification and clinical diagnosis. Semin Cutan Med Surg 1997;16(2):88–96.

68. Clark WH Jr, Elder DE, Van Horn M. The biologic forms of malignant melanoma. Hum Pathol 1986; 17(5):443–50.

69. Clark WH Jr, Mihm MC Jr. Lentigo maligna and lentigo-maligna melanoma. Am J Pathol 1969; 55(1):39–67.

70. Cohen LM. Lentigo maligna and lentigo maligna melanoma. J Am Acad Dermatol 1995;33(6):923–36 [quiz: 937–40].

71. Markovic SN, Erickson LA, Rao RD, et al. Malignant melanoma in the 21st century, part 1: epidemiology,

risk factors, screening, prevention, and diagnosis. Mayo Clin Proc 2007;82(3):364–80.

72. Bradford PT, Goldstein AM, McMaster ML, et al. Acral lentiginous melanoma: incidence and survival patterns in the United States, 1986-2005. Arch Dermatol 2009;145(4):427–34.

73. Coleman WP 3rd, Loria PR, Reed RJ, et al. Acral lentiginous melanoma. Arch Dermatol 1980;116(7):773–6.

74. Scolyer RA, Long GV, Thompson JF. Evolving concepts in melanoma classification and their relevance to multidisciplinary melanoma patient care. Mol Oncol 2011;5(2):124–36.

75. Buka R, Friedman KA, Phelps RG, et al. Childhood longitudinal melanonychia: case reports and review of the literature. Mt Sinai J Med 2001;68(4–5):331–5.

76. Narayanan DL, Saladi RN, Fox JL. Ultraviolet radiation and skin cancer. Int J Dermatol 2010;49(9):978–86.

77. Bataille V, de Vries E. Melanoma–Part 1: epidemiology, risk factors, and prevention. BMJ 2008;337:a2249.

78. Lin JS, Eder M, Weinmann S. Behavioral counseling to prevent skin cancer: a systematic review for the U.S. Preventive Services Task Force. Ann Intern Med 2011;154(3):190–201.

79. Bordeaux JS, Lu KQ, Cooper KD. Melanoma: prevention and early detection. Semin Oncol 2007;34(6):460–6.

80. Gimotty PA, Glanz K. Sunscreen and melanoma: what is the evidence? J Clin Oncol 2011;29(3):249–50.

81. Austoker J. Melanoma: prevention and early diagnosis. BMJ 1994;308(6945):1682–6.

82. Rager EL, Bridgeford EP, Ollila DW. Cutaneous melanoma: update on prevention, screening, diagnosis, and treatment. Am Fam Physician 2005;72(2):269–76.

83. Francis SO, Mahlberg MJ, Johnson KR, et al. Melanoma chemoprevention. J Am Acad Dermatol 2006;55(5):849–61.

84. Jensen JD, Wing GJ, Dellavalle RP. Nutrition and melanoma prevention. Clin Dermatol 2010;28(6):644–9.

85. Egan KM. Vitamin D and melanoma. Ann Epidemiol 2009;19(7):455–61.

86. Wolff T, Tai E, Miller T. Screening for skin cancer: an update of the evidence for the U.S. Preventive Services Task Force. Ann Intern Med 2009;150(3):194–8.

87. Hamidi R, Peng D, Cockburn M. Efficacy of skin self-examination for the early detection of melanoma. Int J Dermatol 2010;49(2):126–34.

88. Sladden MJ, Balch C, Barzilai DA, et al. Surgical excision margins for primary cutaneous melanoma. Cochrane Database Syst Rev 2009;4:CD004835.

89. Cascinelli N. Margin of resection in the management of primary melanoma. Semin Surg Oncol 1998;14(4):272–5.

90. Cook J. Surgical margins for resection of primary cutaneous melanoma. Clin Dermatol 2004;22(3):228–33.

91. Dawn ME, Dawn AG, Miller SJ. Mohs surgery for the treatment of melanoma in situ: a review. Dermatol Surg 2007;33(4):395–402.

92. Perkins W. Who should have Mohs micrographic surgery? Curr Opin Otolaryngol Head Neck Surg 2010;18(4):283–9.

93. Kwon SY, Miller SJ. Mohs surgery for melanoma in situ. Dermatol Clin 2011;29(2):175–83.

94. Thirlwell C, Nathan P. Melanoma–part 2: management. BMJ 2008;337:a2488.

95. Phan GQ, Messina JL, Sondak VK, et al. Sentinel lymph node biopsy for melanoma: indications and rationale. Cancer Control 2009;16(3):234–9.

96. Morton DL, Thompson JF, Cochran AJ, et al. Sentinel-node biopsy or nodal observation in melanoma. N Engl J Med 2006;355(13):1307–17.

97. Wheatley K, Ives N, Hancock B, et al. Does adjuvant interferon-alpha for high-risk melanoma provide a worthwhile benefit? A meta-analysis of the randomised trials. Cancer Treat Rev 2003;29(4):241–52.

98. Mocellin S, Pasquali S, Rossi CR, et al. Interferon alpha adjuvant therapy in patients with high-risk melanoma: a systematic review and meta-analysis. J Natl Cancer Inst 2010;102(7):493–501.

99. Agarwala S. Improving survival in patients with high-risk and metastatic melanoma: immunotherapy leads the way. Am J Clin Dermatol 2003;4(5):333–46.

100. Hodi FS, O'Day SJ, McDermott DF, et al. Improved survival with ipilimumab in patients with metastatic melanoma. N Engl J Med 2010;363(8):711–23.

101. Gray-Schopfer V, Wellbrock C, Marais R. Melanoma biology and new targeted therapy. Nature 2007;445(7130):851–7.

102. Flaherty KT. Narrative review: BRAF opens the door for therapeutic advances in melanoma. Ann Intern Med 2010;153(9):587–91.

103. Testori A, Rutkowski P, Marsden J, et al. Surgery and radiotherapy in the treatment of cutaneous melanoma. Ann Oncol 2009;20(Suppl 6):vi22–9.

104. Sampson JH, Carter JH Jr, Friedman AH, et al. Demographics, prognosis, and therapy in 702 patients with brain metastases from malignant melanoma. J Neurosurg 1998;88(1):11–20.

105. Patel JK, Didolkar MS, Pickren JW, et al. Metastatic pattern of malignant melanoma. A study of 216 autopsy cases. Am J Surg 1978;135(6):807–10.

106. Patnana M, Bronstein Y, Szklaruk J, et al. Multimethod imaging, staging, and spectrum of manifestations of metastatic melanoma. Clin Radiol 2011;66(3):224–36.

Nonmelanoma Skin Cancer

Randie H. Kim, MD, PhD[a], April W. Armstrong, MD, MPH[b],*

KEYWORDS

- Nonmelanoma skin cancers • Basal cell carcinomas
- Squamous cell carcinomas • UV exposure

Nonmelanoma skin cancers (NMSCs), largely encompassing basal cell carcinomas (BCCs) and squamous cell carcinomas (SCCs), represent the most commonly diagnosed cancer in the United States, with more than 2 million new cases each year.[1] This article focuses on the recent epidemiologic trends as well as health outcomes of NMSCs in the United States. In addition, current national guidelines, available treatments and care pathways, and clinical trials are discussed.

EPIDEMIOLOGY OF NMSCs

UV radiation has been well established to be the greatest risk factor for the development of NMSCs with several supporting evidence. Epidemiologic studies and observations have shown that there is a predisposition of these cancers to develop on sun-exposed areas.[2] Higher incidence of NMSCs is reported in lighter-skinned populations, populations closer to the equator, and occupational populations with greater outdoor exposure.[3,4] There is also a significantly greater risk of cancer in patients with genetic disorders or mutations that lead to greater UV sensitivity.[5,6] Experimental models have shown that UV radiation can induce skin cancers in animals.[7] Despite this knowledge, NMSCs continue to have a high disease burden in the United States.

Population-based studies for NMSCs present an epidemiologic challenge. NMSCs are not reported to cancer registries[8] because of high cure rates and lack of hospitalizations, rendering statistics regarding incidence and disease burden largely incomplete. Much of the information comes from surveys, which are limited by sampling, underreporting, and finite resources, as well as projected data, which are susceptible to mathematical and analytical assumptions. These challenges make current and future population-based studies even more difficult because these reports suggest that the incidence of NMSC continues to trend upwards.

Incidence of NMSCs in the United States

A 1971 to 1972 National Cancer Institute (NCI) survey from 4 geographic regions in the United States estimated the national incidence of NMSCs to be around 300,000 new cases per year, representing about 50% of the incidence in total cancers in the United States.[9] Because of concerns of ozone depletion and the association between UV exposure and skin cancer, the NCI conducted a second survey from 1977 to 1978 that expanded to 8 geographic regions to evaluate dose-response effects between UV exposure and skin cancer incidence.[2] The incidence of NMSCs from this period was estimated to be 233 per 100,000 per year (480,000 persons).

A 1994 update used a data registry from Kaiser-Permanente, a health maintenance organization (HMO) in Portland, OR, USA, to project age-adjusted incidences of BCCs and SCCs using linear and log-linear regression analyses. These analyses showed that national estimates for the incidence of NMSCs ranged from 0.9 to 1.2 million, again nearly totaling the incidence of all other cancers combined.[10]

[a] Department of Dermatology, University of California Health System, 3301 C Street, Suite 1400, Sacramento, CA 95816, USA
[b] Dermatology Clinical Research Unit, Teledermatology Program, Department of Dermatology, University of California Davis Health System, University of California Davis School of Medicine, 3301 C Street, Suite 1400, Sacramento, CA 95816, USA
* Corresponding author.
E-mail addresses: aprilarmstrong@post.harvard.edu; april.armstrong@ucdmc.ucdavis.edu

Dermatol Clin 30 (2012) 125–139
doi:10.1016/j.det.2011.08.008
0733-8635/12/$ – see front matter Published by Elsevier Inc.

The most recent national estimates of NMSC incidence were determined to be 2,152,500 treated persons and 3,507,693 total number of NMSCs in 2006 based on 2 Medicare databases (2006 Total Claims Data Set and the Medicare Limited Data Set Standard Analytic File 5% Sample Physician Supplier Data) as well as the National Ambulatory Medical Care Survey (NAMCS). These databases provided information on skin cancer procedures for Medicare patients and NMSC-related office visits.[11]

Incidence by Skin Cancer Type

BCCs account for approximately 80% of NMSCs,[2,12] although the ratio of BCCs to SCCs declines in regions closer to the equator,[2,12] with increasing age,[13] and with male gender. For BCCs, the male to female ratio is 1.4 to 1.6, whereas for SCCs, this ratio is 2.8.[2,14,15] The overall lifetime risk for developing NMSC is 1 in 5.[16] The lifetime risk for developing BCCs (28%–33%) is higher than for developing SCCs (7%–11%).[10]

Approximately 80% of BCCs are found on the head and neck in the United States, with the trunk as the second most common site[2,13,14,17]; this suggests that chronic sun exposure and intermittent sun exposure from recreational activities increase the risk of developing BCCs. Variations in BCC anatomic distribution can differ by gender,[18] ethnicity,[2] and geographic location.[19]

SCCs have a greater capacity for invasion and metastasis and account for most of NMSC-related mortality.[20] About 70% to 80% of SCCs occur on the head and neck, followed by the upper extremities as the next most common location,[15,21] indicating that SCC distribution is more strongly correlated with sun-exposed skin. In combination with the increased SCC incidence with age and decline in latitude, cumulative UV exposure is a strong risk factor for cancer development. However, SCCs occur with greater frequency in areas of non–sun-exposed skin in nonwhite populations, particularly African Americans.[22–24]

Time Trends: NMSC Incidence is Increasing

Numerous reports indicate that NMSC incidence is rising.[2,11] Two of the eight geographic regions surveyed in 1977 to 1978 were also previously surveyed in 1971 to 1972. During this 6-year period, there was a 15% to 20% increase in the age-adjusted rates of NMSCs.[2] In the 2006 national estimates, the total number of NMSC-related procedures increased 76.9% from 1,158,298 in 1992 to 2,048,517 in 2006.[11]

Other geographic regions have also reported increases in age-adjusted BCC and SCC incidence rates with varying effects by gender and anatomic distribution (**Table 1**). Overall, BCC incidence increased from 0.95% to 5.30% per year, whereas SCC incidence increased from 4.0% to 23.3% per year.[17,21,25–27] Increases in NMSC incidence, however, are not geographically universal[28] and may be due to more aggressive treatment of precancerous actinic keratosis and increased sun-protective behavior in higher risk areas.

These trends have been attributed to greater UV exposure from ozone depletion,[2] greater sun-seeking behavior and exposure,[21,25] and longer lifespans of the general population.[12] It is also recognized that greater public awareness of skin cancer as well as changes in medical practice, such as more routine biopsies of suspicious lesions, could have led to a perceived increase in incidence.[17] Limitations in data collection may overestimate and underestimate NMSC cases, which can lead to inaccurate conclusions of changing patterns.

NMSC Incidence and Geographic Location

Given the correlation between skin cancer and degree of UV radiation, geographic locations with a greater proximity to the equator and a subsequent higher UV-B index have higher rates of NMSCs. Of the 4 locations surveyed from 1971 to 1972, the age-adjusted incidence of NMSCs was highest in Dallas-Fort Worth at 379 per 100,000 persons.[9] Furthermore, patients in Dallas-Fort Worth had more SCCs relative to BCCs, faster rates of incidence at younger ages, and a significantly higher peak in those aged 75 to 84 years, again underscoring the relationship between UV exposure and NMSCs.

The 1977 to 1978 NCI study surveyed 8 regions that ranged from 47.5° latitude to 30.0° latitude. Geographic trends showed that BCC incidence was 2 to 3 times greater in southern latitudes than at sites of northern latitude, while SCC incidence was about 5 times greater in southern regions.[2] Similar to the 1971 to 1972 study, the ratio of BCCs to SCCs decreased with increased UV-B index. Incidence rates also increased more sharply at younger ages in areas of higher UV-B index.

Individual population studies also support the correlation among geographic region, UV exposure, and skin cancer. By the mid-1980s, multiple epidemiologic studies in Hawaiian populations indicated that published rates of NMSCs in Kauai, a latitude of 22° north, were the highest in the country (922 per 100,000 persons).[29] Compared to a population from Rochester, MN, USA,[14] men in Kauai had a BCC incidence rate 0.3-fold greater than men in Rochester, whereas women in Kauai had a rate 2.4-fold greater.[19] Incidence of Bowen disease was 10-fold greater in Kauai compared with the Rochester population.[30]

The relationship between UV dose response and NMSC incidence can be quantified and used to predict rate increases in different geographic locations. Exponential models correlating incidence with UV-B index indicate that a 1% increase in UV-B index could lead to a 2% increase in NMSC incidence.[2] Rates of SCC are subject to even greater increases by a UV gradient,[31] with incidence doubling for every 8° to 10° decline in latitude.[32]

NMSC Incidence and Age

The average age of NMSC diagnosis ranges from 59 to 65 years for men and 60 to 66 years for women, depending on location.[2] In the 1977 to 1978 NCI study, NMSC incidence was 4 to 8 times higher in those aged 55 to 75 years compared to those younger than 20 years. Incidence rates tended to increase significantly around the fifth decade and peak during the seventh and eighth decades.[2,9] Rates of SCCs generally increase rapidly with age compared with BCCs. However, little is known about NMSCs in younger patients, and recent studies have presented conflicting data.

Estimated age-specific and gender-specific incidences of NMSCs in a Minnesota population younger than 40 years indicated that the incidence of both BCCs and SCCs had significantly increased during the study period between 1973 and 2003.[33] Although greater public awareness and surveillance may lead to increases in incidence, the investigators note no association between tumor size and year of diagnosis or age at diagnosis. They hypothesize that increased sun exposure, the use of tanning, and tobacco use may be other contributors to higher rates of NMSC in younger populations.[33]

In contrast, multivariate analysis using national data from the NAMCS during the same study period, 1973 to 2003, revealed no significant increases in NMSC-related outpatient office visits in individuals younger than 40 years, adjusted for gender, race, and geographic location.[34] In this study, the mean age of a patient with an NMSC-related office visit was 64.7 years in 1979 and 69.0 years in 2003. Further epidemiologic studies in younger populations would no doubt be beneficial.

NMSC Incidence and Race/Ethnicity

One of the major limitations of prior estimates is that NMSC incidence generally refers to white populations because of significantly lower rates of incidence in nonwhite individuals. This limitation is illustrated in the 1978 NCI survey in which the annual age-adjusted incidence rate for African Americans was 3.4 per 100,000 persons compared to 232.6 per 100,000 persons for white populations.[2] In Hispanics, NMSC rates were 6 to 8 times less than that of white populations in New Mexico[2] and 11 to 14 times less in southeastern Arizona.[28] Lower skin cancer rates are attributed to increased epidermal melanin production in darker-skinned individuals,[35] which can confer a photoprotection factor of up to 13.4.[36] However, the importance of epidemiologic studies in non-white populations is increasingly being recognized because morbidity and mortality are often greater.

In African Americans, SCCs are more commonly found than BCCs,[22,23,37] particularly in non–sun-exposed areas such as the lower extremities, anogenital area, and feet.[22–24,37,38] Specifically, SCCs can occur 8.5 times more frequently than BCCs,[39] which suggests that UV exposure may not play a significant role in SCC development in African Americans. Rather, risk factors for SCC development in African American populations include chronic scars, burns, chronic leg ulcers, and chronic inflammation.[22,36,37,40] The tendency of these cancers to arise in non–sun-exposed areas and in areas of chronic trauma or inflammation may be reasons for the greater morbidity and mortality in this population because cancers are more aggressive or are diagnosed at later stages.

In contrast, BCCs in darker-skinned individuals tend to have an anatomic distribution similar to lighter-skinned populations.[38,41] Of the BCC cases seen in African Americans in a Howard University Hospital study, 60% of patients were considered to be of fair complexion and 7% of olive complexion. This is compared to the control group in which only 10% of patients were of fair or olive complexion, highlighting the association between UV exposure and BCC cases.[38] In other ethnic groups, comparisons of ethnic Japanese in Kauai standardized to Japanese populations show that rates of BCCs and SCCs were at least 45 times greater in Hawaii[42] but 12-fold[19] and 5-fold[43] lower than Caucasian Kauaiians, respectively. Histologically, pigmented BCCs are more common in darker-skinned populations,[44,45] which make it difficult to differentiate from other lesions. Thus, despite the lower incidences of NMSCs in nonwhite populations, atypical presentations and distributions of NMSCs in these individuals warrant further consideration during differential diagnosis.

Methods and Challenges to Estimate Incidence

Estimating NMSC incidence has evolved over the past 40 years. One of the major challenges of NMSC incidence is how to account for multiple

Table 1
The increase of NMSC incidence over time

Study	Results	BCC/SCC Changes in Incidence	Greatest Changes in Anatomic Distribution	Reference
Survey to identify newly diagnosed pathology-confirmed BCCs and SCCs in New Hampshire between June 1, 1979, and May 31, 1980, and between July 1, 1993, and June 30, 1994	BCC	1.8-fold increase in men (170–310 per 100,000), 1.8-fold increase in women (91–166 per 100,000)	3.1-fold increase on the trunk in men (26.8–83.2 per 100,000), 3.65-fold increase on lower limbs in women (3.7–13.5 per 100,000)	Karagas et al[17]
	SCC	3.3-fold increase in men (29–97 per 100,000), 4.6-fold increase in women (7–32 per 100,000)	7.5-fold increase on the trunk in men (1.6–12 per 100,000), 7.7-fold increase on lower limbs in women (0.7–5.4 per 100,000)	
Pathology-confirmed SCCs from Kaiser Permanente tumor registry in Portland, Oregon-Vancouver, Washington area between 1960 and 1986	SCC	2.6-fold increase in men (41.6–106.1 per 100,000), 3.1-fold increase in women (9.7–29.8 per 100,000)	No statistically significant differences in rates of increase among head and neck, trunk, and extremity SCCs	Glass and Hoover[21]
ICD-coded newly diagnosed BCCs and SCCs from the British Columbia Cancer Registry between 1973 and 1987	BCC	1.6-fold increase in men (70.8–113.7 per 100,000), 1.5-fold increase in women (61.1–90.7 per 100,000)	Substantial increases on head, neck, and trunk in men and women; more modest increases on extremities	Gallagher et al[25]
	SCC	1.6-fold increase in men (18.4–29.3 per 100,000), 1.7-fold increase in women (9.2–15.4 per 100,000)	Greatest increases on head and neck in men and women	

Description	Type	Incidence trend	Anatomic distribution	Reference
Pathology-confirmed invasive SCCs from the Rochester Epidemiology Project databases in Olmsted County, Minnesota, between 1984 and 1992	SCC	1.5-fold increase in men (125.9–191 per 100,000), 2.1-fold increase in women (46.5–99.6 per 100,000)	Distribution remained relatively constant during study period (data not shown)	Gray et al[26]
Survey to identify newly diagnosed primary NMSCs in North Central New Mexico between 1977 and 1978 and 1998 and 1999	BCC	1.5-fold increase in men (618.7–930.3 per 100,000), 1.2-fold increase in women (398.7–485.5 per 100,000)	5.2-fold increase on the upper limbs in men (16.4–85 per 100,000), 3.8-fold increase on lower limbs in women (6.4–24.1 per 100,000)	Athas et al[27]
	SCC	1.9-fold increase in men (187.5–356.2 per 100,000), 2.1-fold increase in women (71.8–150.4 per 100,000)	5.6-fold increase on lower limbs in men (1.1–6.2 per 100,000), 5-fold increase on lower limbs in women (3.5–17.4 per 100,000)	
Pathology-confirmed NMSCs from the Southeastern Arizona Skin Cancer Registry in Cochise, Pima, and Santa Cruz counties between 1985 and 1996	BCC	Slight decline between 1985 and 1993 with a 24% and a 28% increase between 1993 and 1996 for men and women, respectively	No substantial changes in distribution over time	Harris et al[28]
	SCC	0.7-fold decrease in men (383.1–270.6 per 100,000), 0.7-fold decrease in women (154.1–112.1 per 100,000)	No substantial changes in distribution over time	

represent a significant health outcome that provides a better understanding of disease burden. For instance, treatments of NMSCs in the head and neck region have a substantial negative impact on function and cosmesis. Resulting facial disfigurement is associated with higher risks of depression and psychosocial dysfunction.[74] Development of QOL instruments to measure and assess the psychological, social, and emotional impact of NMSCs have since been developed within the past 20 years.

The Facial Skin Cancer Index (FSCI) was the first NMSC-specific QOL instrument for patients with head and neck NMSCs.[75] Development of the FSCI, now Skin Cancer Index (SCI), revealed that issues regarding appearance, scarring, and self-image were unique and specific concerns to NMSC-treated patients not covered by other health-related QOL instruments. Furthermore, emotional states such as anxiety and frustration were greater concerns than physical handicaps.[76] The SCI comprises of 15 items encompassing the 3 domains of emotion, social factors, and appearance.[77]

Using the SCI and other dermatologic QOL instruments, QOL outcomes for NMSC populations have begun to be explored. In a prospective study, patients received the SCI and a general dermatology QOL instrument, the Dermatology Life Quality Index (DLQI), before and 4 months after treatment with Mohs surgery. The SCI was able to capture improvements in total score as well as in each of the 3 subscales. This improvement was in contrast to the DLQI, which did not demonstrate any significant changes, suggesting that the SCI is a sensitive instrument for measuring clinical response and QOL in patients with NMSC.[78] The study noted that predictors of lower QOL included female gender, populations younger than 50 years, and cancers of the lip. Greater improvements in SCI score occurred in younger patients, patients with lower incomes, patients with no prior history of NMSCs, and patients who underwent less reconstructive surgery.

Other studies have reported other predictors of QOL after NMSC treatment. Chren and colleagues[79] used the Skindex, a validated measure of skin-related QOL that reports subscores on symptoms, emotional effects, and effects on functioning, in a prospective study to examine QOL before and after surgical treatment. Better pretreatment QOL scores were related to marital status, postgraduate education, incomes greater than $30,000 a year, fewer comorbidities, and better physical and mental health. Furthermore, patients with BCCs, tumors not on the head and neck, and smaller tumors also reported better pretreatment QOL. However, the strongest predictor of posttreatment QOL was pretreatment QOL. Other posttreatment QOL predictors included better mental health status, fewer comorbidities, and race.[80]

The Skindex was also used to determine if type of surgical treatment (Mohs surgery, excision, and EDC) could predict posttreatment QOL. Patients treated by Mohs surgery or excision, but not EDC, experienced statistically significant improvements in QOL. There were no differences in QOL improvements between Mohs surgery and excision,[81] which may have future implications when considering relative costs. In contrast, a recent report has suggested that type of treatment is not associated with QOL differences,[82] although the investigators note that their cohort was underpowered to answer this question. Regardless, it is clear that QOL, possibly a more meaningful health outcome for patients with NMSC than morbidity and mortality, merits greater examination.

NMSC Expenditures

Although NMSCs are the most common cancer, related costs represent less than 1% of total cancer costs,[83,84] largely because of effective management in the outpatient setting. As NMSC incidence increases, these costs are expected to correspondingly increase. In addition, as a disease more common in the elderly, Medicare costs due to NMSCs are significant. Indeed, NMSCs were determined to be the fifth most costly cancer to Medicare after lung, prostate, colon, and breast, representing about 4.5% of all Medicare expenditure.[85] Furthermore, between 1992 and 1995, NMSC-related costs to Medicare increased by 41%, while payments for treatment of actinic keratosis increased by 91%. Total cost of NMSCs to Medicare have ranged from $285[84] to $426 million per year. National costs were estimated to be $650 million per year.[83]

NMSC expenditure is largely based on treatment setting and treatment modality. 76% of NMSC-related costs were because of outpatient office visits between 1992 and 1995. The average cost for outpatient procedures was $492. For ambulatory surgery visits and inpatient procedures, the average costs were $1043 and $5537, respectively.[83] Expenditure by specialty revealed that the average cost per episode was $957 for surgeons, $877 for multiple specialists, $296 for primary care physicians, and $521 for other physicians.[86] Dermatologists managed about 50% of identified episodes, with the average cost per episode being $604.[86] In another study, dermatologists managed 82% of NMSC episodes in which performed treatments and procedures included biopsies, excisions, destruction, Mohs micrographic surgery, and reconstructive repairs.[87] Based on such cost differentials, the investigators conclude that dermatologists provide convenient, effective, and economical management for NMSCs.

The type of treatment is another major factor in NMSC expenditure. Cook and Zitelli[88] showed that costs for Mohs micrographic surgery ($1243) were comparable to surgical excision with permanent section margin control ($1167) and less expensive than surgical excision with frozen section margin control ($1400) or ambulatory surgical excision ($1973). Although most of their cases were NMSCs, their study also encompassed non-NMSCs, including malignant melanoma. A subsequent study by Bialy and colleagues,[89] had similar conclusions after evaluating cost comparisons between Mohs surgery and surgical excision of facial and auricular NMSCs only. Mohs surgery costs were comparable to surgical excisions with permanent sections ($937 vs $1029) and significantly less expensive than excisions with frozen sections ($937 vs $1399). A study using a computer-simulated probabilistic decision model determined that Mohs surgery was $292 less expensive than traditional surgical excision and offered a 0.056 quality-adjusted life year advantage, which translated to about 3 weeks of optimal QOL.[90]

These results are in contrast to Medicare treatment costs in which Mohs micrographic surgery was significantly more expensive at $899 per patient than either excision at $239 per patient or local destruction at $221 per patient.[84] One reason for this discrepancy is that these Medicare costs do not include associated pathology or subsequent repair. Indeed, Cook and Zitelli[88] noted that procedure and pathology fees for excisions are unbundled, whereas reimbursements for Mohs surgery include both procedure and pathology. Furthermore, the investigators suggest that greater tissue defects by surgical excision leads to more complex reconstructive repair, contributing to overall increased costs.

A more recent study estimated treatment costs based on assigned 2008 relative value unit values and compared costs for a BCC cheek lesion and SCC arm lesion of different sizes by the following treatment modalities: EDC, imiquimod immunotherapy, Mohs micrographic surgery, traditional surgical excision with permanent section, surgical excision with frozen section, and radiation therapy. For all treatment modalities, a BCC cheek lesion was more expensive to treat than an SCC arm lesion. In addition, treatment costs increased with tumor size. EDC was the cheapest procedure

at an average cost of $471 for a BCC cheek lesion and $392 for an SCC cheek lesion. Mohs micrographic surgery costs were $1263 for cheek BCC and $1131 for arm SCC, which were approximately 25% more expensive than surgical excisions with permanent section and immediate repair. Like prior studies, facility-based treatments and hospital-based treatments were significantly more expensive, ranging from $2200 for an arm SCC treated in an ambulatory surgery setting to $3085 for a cheek BCC treated in a hospital setting. Radiation therapy was the most expensive modality at $3460 for a cheek BCC and $3431 for an arm SCC.[91]

TREATMENT GUIDELINES FOR NMSCS IN THE UNITED STATES

In 2010, the National Comprehensive Cancer Network (NCCN) published updated management guidelines for NMSCs.[92] Approach to management begins with a history and physical examination. A complete skin examination is recommended for a lesion suspicious for BCC and a complete skin and regional lymph node examination for a lesion suspicious for SCC. Suspicious lesions should then be biopsied, including the deep dermis if an infiltrating or deeper process is suspected. If palpable lymph nodes or abnormal lymph nodes are found by imaging, then fine-needle aspiration (FNA) should be done. If results are positive, additional imaging can characterize the size, number, and location of additional abnormal lymph nodes. If the FNA result is negative, an open biopsy of lymph nodes is recommended.

Therapy for NMSCs falls into 1 of 3 categories: surgical treatments, radiation therapy, and superficial therapy. Algorithms regarding choice of treatment require clinical assessment of recurrence or metastatic risk. A lesion exhibiting any high-risk behavior is placed in the high-risk treatment pathway. These risk factors include location and size, well-defined versus ill-defined borders, primary versus recurrent disease, immunosuppression status, sites of prior radiotherapy, perineural invasion, histologic differentiation, and histologic subtype. SCCs have additional risk factors that should be evaluated, including sites of chronic inflammation, rapid growth, and neurologic symptoms.

Surgical treatments include EDC, surgical excision with postoperative margin control, surgical excision with intraoperative frozen section assessment, and Mohs surgery. NCCN guidelines state that Mohs surgery is the preferred method of treatment of all high-risk tumors based on reported efficacy[61,93] and the belief that complete tumor removal by intraoperative tissue margin assessment is critical. Intraoperative frozen section is an alternative to Mohs surgery only if all deep and peripheral margins are assessed. For low-risk tumors (<2 cm and well circumscribed), surgical excision with postoperative margin control can be used. The NCCN panel updated clinical margins of SCCs to 4 to 6 mm to include any peripheral rim of erythema. Surgical excision is also indicated for reexcisions of NMSCs of the trunk and extremities after initial excision with positive margins as well as large primary tumors of the trunk and extremities if 10-mm margins can be obtained. However, if closure of defects requires skin graft placement or tissue rearrangement, intraoperative margin assessment is recommended. EDC is effective for low-risk tumors not located in hair-bearing areas because tumors that extend down to follicles may not be completely removed. Furthermore, should the subcutaneous layer be reached during EDC, current guidelines recommend switching to surgical excision because it would be difficult to distinguish subcutaneous fat from tumor with a curette. Biopsy is also recommended to ensure that there are no high-risk features that might require additional therapy.

Radiation can be an effective method of therapy with excellent cosmesis when used properly. The NCCN panel states that radiation therapy is generally used for patients older than 60 years because of concerns over long-term effects of radiation. Indications for radiation therapy include tumors in high-risk locations up to 15 mm in diameter and up to 20 mm in diameter in middle-risk locations. Tumors of the trunk and extremities as well as the genitals, hands, and feet are generally excluded. Radiation therapy is contraindicated in patients with genetic disorders that predispose them to skin cancers. Radiation is delivered as protracted fractionation for improved cosmesis using either orthovoltage x-ray or electron beam.

Superficial therapy encompasses 5-fluorouracil or imiquimod topical therapy, photodynamic therapy (PDT), and cryotherapy. These therapies can be effective for shallow SCCs in situ and low-risk superficial BCCs. They also represent alternatives for patients who wish to avoid radiation therapy or surgery and for those in whom radiation therapy or surgery is contraindicated.

In a Cochrane review evaluating the efficacy of therapies for BCCs, the investigators conclude that few good quality trials exist.[94] Indeed, only 1 randomized trial with long-term follow-up was identified. In this study, the failure rate of surgery with frozen section margin control was significantly lower than that of radiation therapy for primary facial BCCs after 4-year follow-up (relative risk, 0.09; 95% confidence interval, 0.01–0.69). Furthermore, patients reported better cosmesis with surgery than with radiation therapy.[95] More recently, other randomized controlled trials with long-term follow-up have provided more insight and are summarized in **Table 2**. Mohs micrographic surgery was more effective than surgical excision for treating recurrent BCCs but not primary BCCs.[96] Surgery was more effective than PDT with methyl aminolevulinate (MAL)[97] or 5-aminolevulinic acid,[98] although PDT was associated with better cosmesis. There was no difference in 5-year recurrence rates between MAL-PDT and cryotherapy.[99] In addition, a long-term clinical trial comparing the efficacy of imiquimod therapy to that of surgical excision is on the horizon.[100]

Similarly, a recent Cochrane review of therapies for primary SCCs conclude that very few randomized controlled trials comparing different treatments exist.[101] One randomized controlled trial that met inclusion criteria described the use of adjuvant 13-cis-retinoic acid and interferon-α to prevent recurrences or secondary SCCs after initial treatment with surgery and/or radiation. At 2-year follow-up, there were no differences between the treatment and control group.[102] Most trials were excluded from analysis because they were uncontrolled case series, did not include invasive primary SCCs, or only included patients with recurrent or metastatic disease. This highlights the need for long-term prospective trials in evaluating treatment efficacy of primary SCC lesions.

CURRENT NEEDS IN NMSC RESEARCH

NMSCs represent the most common cancer in the United States, accounting for more than 2 million cases per year.[1] Despite the magnitude of health burden on the US population, there remains many questions regarding the epidemiology, health outcomes, and treatments of NMSCs. This article has highlighted these areas of clinical and research need.

Without a national tumor registry, the identification and reporting of NMSC cases have continued to be a challenge in estimating incidence.[46] However, recent methodologies that take advantage of administrative databases and electronic records have provided more convenient ways of identifying cases. In addition, because of NMSC multiplicity, epidemiologic reports may need to represent data both by persons and by number of tumors to more accurately reflect the nature of the disease and the affected population.

Table 2
Randomized controlled trials comparing treatments for BCCs

Study	Intervention	Results	Reference
Prospective randomized controlled trial for the treatment of primary and recurrent facial BCCs (N = 408, primary BCCs, N = 204 recurrent BCCs)	Surgical excision vs MMS	At 5-y follow-up, recurrence of primary BCCs was 4.1% by surgical excision and 2.5% by MMS (log-rank test χ^2, 0.718; P = .397). Recurrence of recurrent BCCs was 12.1% by surgical excision and 2.4% by MMS (log-rank test χ^2, 5.958; P = .015).	Mosterd et al[96]
Prospective randomized multicenter trial for the treatment of primary nodular BCCs (N = 97 patients, N = 105 primary BCCs)	Surgical excision vs MAL-PDT with red light in 2 or 4 treatments at 1-wk intervals	At 3 mo after treatment, recurrence was 14% by MAL-PDT and 4% by surgical excision (P = .09). Estimated sustained lesion complete response rates at 5-y follow-up were 76% by MAL-PDT and 96% by surgical excision (P = .01). Of the persons pn MAL-PDT, 87% reported excellent or good cosmesis vs 54% of those who underwent surgery (P = .007).	Rhodes et al[97]
Prospective randomized controlled trial for the treatment of primary nodular BCCs (N = 149 patients, N = 173 primary BCCs)	Surgical excision vs ALA-PDT at 585–720 nm light source in 2 treatments	The 3-y cumulative incidence of failure was 2.3% by surgical excision and 30.3% for ALA-PDT (P<.001)	Mosterd et al[98]
Prospective randomized multicenter trial for the treatment of primary superficial BCCs (N = 118 patients, N = 219 primary BCCs)	Cryotherapy with double freeze-thaw cycle vs MAL-PDT with red light in 1 treatment	At 5-y follow-up, recurrence was 20% by cryotherapy and 22% by MAL-PDT (P = .86). Of the patients on MAL-PDT, 60% reported excellent cosmesis vs 16% of those on cryotherapy (P = .00078).	Basset-Seguin et al[99]
Prospective randomized multicenter phase 3 trial for the treatment of nodular and superficial primary BCCs	Surgical excision vs 5% imiquimod cream daily for 6 (superficial) or 12 (nodular) wk	Currently ongoing	Ozolins et al[100]

Abbreviations: ALA, 5-aminolevulinic acid; MAL, methyl aminolevulinate; MMS, Mohs micrographic surgery.

Despite inherent limitations, future studies would likely benefit from a standardized and validated approach that would make trend analysis more reliable.

Similarly, true NMSC mortality rates have been limited by inaccurate death certificates.[69] Although mortality seems to be declining, total number of deaths due to NMSC has increased, likely because of greater longevity and population.[70] Such studies suggest that continued monitoring of UV-associated skin cancers and increased surveillance should be directed at skin cancers with greater risk of mortality.

In addition, as incidence increases, greater health burdens are placed on the population. QOL assessments are an important aspect of health outcomes and reveal that NMSCs affect patients' self-image and emotional state, not adequately captured by other health QOL instruments.[76] NMSC-specific QOL studies likely reflect the impact of this disease on the population more accurately and warrant further investigation.[78]

Treatment modality also seems to have effects on all aspects of health outcomes, including rates of recurrence, QOL, and costs. Of particular interest, Mohs micrographic surgery is associated with lower rates of recurrence[50,61] and is at least equal to and perhaps better than traditional excision at improving QOL.[81,82,90] Although conclusions regarding cost comparisons between Mohs

and non-Mohs procedures remain unclear, outpatient treatments are significantly more cost effective than ambulatory surgery settings and inpatient settings.[103] Thus, physicians should consider all aspects of health-related outcomes when determining the appropriate approach for patients with NMSC.

Current US guidelines recommend the use of Mohs micrographic surgery for any high-risk lesion.[92] However, very few long-term randomized controlled trials comparing the efficacies of alternative therapies for primary NMSCs, especially SCCs, exist.[94,101] This is, perhaps, one of the greatest areas of research needs because cost, cosmesis, and efficacy are all considerations when determining the type of treatment, particularly for low-risk tumors. Such studies would undoubtedly be crucial in developing future treatment guidelines.

REFERENCES

1. Jemal A, Siegel R, Xu J, et al. Cancer statistics, 2010. CA Cancer J Clin 2010;60(5):277–300.
2. Scotto J, Fears TR, Fraumeni JF, et al, Fred Hutchinson Cancer Research Center. Incidence of non-melanoma skin cancer in the United States. Bethesda (MD): U.S. Dept. of Health and Human Services, Public Health Service, National Institutes of Health, National Cancer Institute; 1983.
3. Urbach F. Incidence of nonmelanoma skin cancer. Dermatol Clin 1991;9(4):751–5.
4. Gloster HM Jr, Brodland DG. The epidemiology of skin cancer. Dermatol Surg 1996;22(3):217–26.
5. Lynch HT, Fusaro R, Edlund J, et al. Skin cancer developing in xeroderma pigmentosum patient relaxing sunlight avoidance. Lancet 1981;2(8257): 1230.
6. Brash DE, Rudolph JA, Simon JA, et al. A role for sunlight in skin cancer: UV-induced p53 mutations in squamous cell carcinoma. Proc Natl Acad Sci U S A 1991;88(22):10124–8.
7. Fry RJ, Ley RD. Ultraviolet radiation-induced skin cancer. Carcinog Compr Surv 1989;11:321–37.
8. Young JL, Percy CL, Asire AJ, et al. Surveillance, epidemiology, and end results: incidence and mortality data, 1973-77. Bethesda (MD), Washington, DC: U.S. Dept. of Health and Human Services, Public Health Service, National Institutes of Health. For sale by the Supt. of Docs., U.S. G.P.O; 1981.
9. Scotto J, Kopf AW, Urbach F. Non-melanoma skin cancer among Caucasians in four areas of the United States. Cancer 1974;34(4):1333–8.
10. Miller DL, Weinstock MA. Nonmelanoma skin cancer in the United States. Incidence. J Am Acad Dermatol 1994;30(5 Pt 1):774–8.

List of Acronyms	
BCCs	Basal cell carcinomas
CI	Confidence interval
CPT	Current procedural terminology
DLQI	Dermatology Life Quality Index
EDC	Electrodessication and curettage
FNA	Fine needle aspiration
FSCI	Facial Skin Cancer Index
HMO	Health Maintenance Organization
ICD-9-CM	International Classification of Diseases, 9th edition, Clinical Modification
MAL	Methyl aminolevulinate
NAMCS	National Ambulatory Medical Care Survey
NCCN	National Comprehensive Cancer Network
NCI	National Cancer Institute
NMSCs	Non-melanoma skin cancers
PDT	Photodynamic therapy
QOL	Quality of life
RR	Relative risk
SCCs	Squamous cell carcinomas
SCI	Skin Cancer Index
UV	Ultraviolet

11. Rogers HW, Weinstock MA, Harris AR, et al. Incidence estimate of nonmelanoma skin cancer in the United States, 2006. Arch Dermatol 2010; 146(3):283–7.

12. Diepgen TL, Mahler V. The epidemiology of skin cancer. Br J Dermatol 2002;146(Suppl 61):1–6.

13. Serrano H, Scotto J, Shornick G, et al. Incidence of nonmelanoma skin cancer in New Hampshire and Vermont. J Am Acad Dermatol 1991;24(4):574–9.

14. Chuang TY, Popescu A, Su WP, et al. Basal cell carcinoma. A population-based incidence study in Rochester, Minnesota. J Am Acad Dermatol 1990;22(3):413–7.

15. Chuang TY, Popescu NA, Su WP, et al. Squamous cell carcinoma. A population-based incidence study in Rochester, Minn. Arch Dermatol 1990; 126(2):185–8.

16. Rigel DS, Friedman RJ, Kopf AW. Lifetime risk for development of skin cancer in the U.S. population: current estimate is now 1 in 5. J Am Acad Dermatol 1996;35(6):1012–3.

17. Karagas MR, Greenberg ER, Spencer SK, et al. Increase in incidence rates of basal cell and squamous cell skin cancer in New Hampshire, USA. New Hampshire Skin Cancer Study Group. Int J Cancer 1999;81(4):555–9.

18. Pearson G, King LE, Boyd AS. Basal cell carcinoma of the lower extremities. Int J Dermatol 1999;38(11):852–4.

19. Reizner GT, Chuang TY, Elpern DJ, et al. Basal cell carcinoma in Kauai, Hawaii: the highest documented incidence in the United States. J Am Acad Dermatol 1993;29(2 Pt 1):184–9.

20. Weinstock MA, Bogaars HA, Ashley M, et al. Nonmelanoma skin cancer mortality. A population-based study. Arch Dermatol 1991;127(8):1194–7.

21. Glass AG, Hoover RN. The emerging epidemic of melanoma and squamous cell skin cancer. JAMA 1989;262(15):2097–100.

22. Mora RG, Perniciaro C. Cancer of the skin in blacks. I. A review of 163 black patients with cutaneous squamous cell carcinoma. J Am Acad Dermatol 1981;5(5):535–43.

23. Bang KM, Halder RM, White JE, et al. Skin cancer in black Americans: a review of 126 cases. J Natl Med Assoc 1987;79(1):51–8.

24. McCall CO, Chen SC. Squamous cell carcinoma of the legs in African Americans. J Am Acad Dermatol 2002;47(4):524–9.

25. Gallagher RP, Ma B, McLean DI, et al. Trends in basal cell carcinoma, squamous cell carcinoma, and melanoma of the skin from 1973 through 1987. J Am Acad Dermatol 1990;23(3 Pt 1):413–21.

26. Gray DT, Suman VJ, Su WP, et al. Trends in the population-based incidence of squamous cell carcinoma of the skin first diagnosed between 1984 and 1992. Arch Dermatol 1997;133(6):735–40.

27. Athas WF, Hunt WC, Key CR. Changes in nonmelanoma skin cancer incidence between 1977-1978 and 1998-1999 in Northcentral New Mexico. Cancer Epidemiol Biomarkers Prev 2003;12(10): 1105–8.

28. Harris RB, Griffith K, Moon TE. Trends in the incidence of nonmelanoma skin cancers in southeastern Arizona, 1985-1996. J Am Acad Dermatol 2001;45(4):528–36.

29. Stone JL, Elpern DJ, Reizner G, et al. Incidence of non-melanoma skin cancer in Kauai during 1983. Hawaii Med J 1986;45(8):281–2, 285–6.

30. Reizner GT, Chuang TY, Elpern DJ, et al. Bowen's disease (squamous cell carcinoma in situ) in Kauai, Hawaii. A population-based incidence report. J Am Acad Dermatol 1994;31(4):596–600.

31. Qureshi AA, Laden F, Colditz GA, et al. Geographic variation and risk of skin cancer in US women. Differences between melanoma, squamous cell carcinoma, and basal cell carcinoma. Arch Intern Med 2008;168(5):501–7.

32. Giles GG, Marks R, Foley P. Incidence of nonmelanocytic skin cancer treated in Australia. Br Med J (Clin Res Ed) 1988;296(6614):13–7.

33. Christenson LJ, Borrowman TA, Vachon CM, et al. Incidence of basal cell and squamous cell carcinomas in a population younger than 40 years. JAMA 2005;294(6):681–90.

34. Bivens MM, Bhosle M, Balkrishnan R, et al. Nonmelanoma skin cancer: is the incidence really increasing among patients younger than 40? A reexamination using 25 years of U.S. outpatient data. Dermatol Surg 2006;32(12):1473–9.

35. Montagna W, Carlisle K. The architecture of black and white facial skin. J Am Acad Dermatol 1991; 24(6 Pt 1):929–37.

36. Halder RM, Bridgeman-Shah S. Skin cancer in African Americans. Cancer 1995;75(Suppl 2):667–73.

37. Fleming ID, Barnawell JR, Burlison PE, et al. Skin cancer in black patients. Cancer 1975;35(3):600–5.

38. Halder RM, Bang KM. Skin cancer in blacks in the United States. Dermatol Clin 1988;6(3):397–405.

39. Singh B, Bhaya M, Shaha A, et al. Presentation, course, and outcome of head and neck skin cancer in African Americans: a case-control study. Laryngoscope 1998;108(8 Pt 1):1159–63.

40. Harper JG, Pilcher MF, Szlam S, et al. Squamous cell carcinoma in an African American with discoid lupus erythematosus: a case report and review of the literature. South Med J 2010;103(3):256–9.

41. Matsuoka LY, Schauer PK, Sordillo PP. Basal cell carcinoma in black patients. J Am Acad Dermatol 1981;4(6):670–2.

42. Chuang TY, Reizner GT, Elpern DJ, et al. Nonmelanoma skin cancer in Japanese ethnic Hawaiians in Kauai, Hawaii: an incidence report. J Am Acad Dermatol 1995;33(3):422–6.

43. Chuang TY, Reizner GT, Elpern DJ, et al. Squamous cell carcinoma in Kauai, Hawaii. Int J Dermatol 1995;34(6):393–7.

44. Abreo F, Sanusi ID. Basal cell carcinoma in North American blacks. Clinical and histopathologic study of 26 patients. J Am Acad Dermatol 1991; 25(6 Pt 1):1005–11.

45. Bigler C, Feldman J, Hall E, et al. Pigmented basal cell carcinoma in Hispanics. J Am Acad Dermatol 1996;34(5 Pt 1):751–2.

46. Eide MJ, Krajenta R, Johnson D, et al. Identification of patients with nonmelanoma skin cancer using health maintenance organization claims data. Am J Epidemiol 2010;171(1):123–8.

47. Gold HT, Do HT. Evaluation of three algorithms to identify incident breast cancer in Medicare claims data. Health Serv Res 2007;42(5):2056–69.

48. Baldi I, Vicari P, Di Cuonzo D, et al. A high positive predictive value algorithm using hospital administrative data identified incident cancer cases. J Clin Epidemiol 2008;61(4):373–9.

49. Epstein E. Value of follow-up after treatment of basal cell carcinoma. Arch Dermatol 1973;108(6): 798–800.

50. Rowe DE, Carroll RJ, Day CL Jr. Long-term recurrence rates in previously untreated (primary) basal cell carcinoma: implications for patient follow-up. J Dermatol Surg Oncol 1989;15(3):315–28.

51. Paver K, Poyzer K, Burry N, et al. Letter: the incidence of basal cell carcinoma and their metastases in Australia and New Zealand. Australas J Dermatol 1973;14(1):53.

52. Cade S. Malignant disease and its treatment by radium. Baltimore (MD): Williams & Wilkins; 1940.

53. Lo JS, Snow SN, Reizner GT, et al. Metastatic basal cell carcinoma: report of twelve cases with a review of the literature. J Am Acad Dermatol 1991;24(5 Pt 1):715–9.

54. Cotran RS. Metastasizing basal cell carcinomas. Cancer 1961;14:1036–40.

55. Snow SN, Sahl W, Lo JS, et al. Metastatic basal cell carcinoma. Report of five cases. Cancer 1994; 73(2):328–35.

56. Sahl WJ. Basal cell carcinoma: influence of tumor size on mortality and morbidity. Int J Dermatol 1995;34(5):319–21.

57. Katz AD, Urbach F, Lilienfeld AM. The frequency and risk of metastases in squamous-cell carcinoma of the skin. Cancer 1957;10(6):1162–6.

58. Lund HZ. How often does squamous cell carcinoma of the skin metastasize? Arch Dermatol 1965;92(6):635–7.

59. Epstein E, Epstein NN, Bragg K, et al. Metastases from squamous cell carcinomas of the skin. Arch Dermatol 1968;97(3):245–51.

60. Dinehart SM, Pollack SV. Metastases from squamous cell carcinoma of the skin and lip. An analysis of twenty-seven cases. J Am Acad Dermatol 1989; 21(2 Pt 1):241–8.

61. Rowe DE, Carroll RJ, Day CL Jr. Prognostic factors for local recurrence, metastasis, and survival rates in squamous cell carcinoma of the skin, ear, and lip. Implications for treatment modality selection. J Am Acad Dermatol 1992;26(6):976–90.

62. Tavin E, Persky M. Metastatic cutaneous squamous cell carcinoma of the head and neck region. Laryngoscope 1996;106(2 Pt 1):156–8.

63. Weinberg AS, Ogle CA, Shim EK. Metastatic cutaneous squamous cell carcinoma: an update. Dermatol Surg 2007;33(8):885–99.

64. Marcil I, Stern RS. Risk of developing a subsequent nonmelanoma skin cancer in patients with a history of nonmelanoma skin cancer: a critical review of the literature and meta-analysis. Arch Dermatol 2000;136(12):1524–30.

65. Clayman GL, Lee JJ, Holsinger FC, et al. Mortality risk from squamous cell skin cancer. J Clin Oncol 2005;23(4):759–65.

66. Weinstock MA. The epidemic of squamous cell carcinoma. JAMA 1989;262(15):2138–40.

67. Lewis KG, Weinstock MA. Nonmelanoma skin cancer mortality (1988-2000): the Rhode Island follow-back study. Arch Dermatol 2004;140(7):837–42.

68. Dunn JE Jr, Levin EA, Linden G, et al. Skin cancer as a cause of death. Calif Med 1965;102:361–3.

69. Weinstock MA, Bogaars HA, Ashley M, et al. Inaccuracies in certification of nonmelanoma skin cancer deaths. Am J Public Health 1992;82(2): 278–81.

70. Weinstock MA. Nonmelanoma skin cancer mortality in the United States, 1969 through 1988. Arch Dermatol 1993;129(10):1286–90.

71. Lewis KG, Weinstock MA. Trends in nonmelanoma skin cancer mortality rates in the United States, 1969 through 2000. J Invest Dermatol 2007; 127(10):2323–7.

72. Chen J, Ruczinski I, Jorgensen TJ, et al. Nonmelanoma skin cancer and risk for subsequent malignancy. J Natl Cancer Inst 2008;100(17):1215–22.

73. Kahn HS, Tatham LM, Patel AV, et al. Increased cancer mortality following a history of nonmelanoma skin cancer. JAMA 1998;280(10):910–2.

74. Katz MR, Irish JC, Devins GM, et al. Psychosocial adjustment in head and neck cancer: the impact of disfigurement, gender and social support. Head Neck 2003;25(2):103–12.

75. Rhee JS, Matthews BA, Neuburg M, et al. Creation of a quality of life instrument for nonmelanoma skin cancer patients. Laryngoscope 2005;115(7): 1178–85.

76. Matthews BA, Rhee JS, Neuburg M, et al. Development of the facial skin care index: a health-related outcomes index for skin cancer patients. Dermatol Surg 2006;32(7):924–34 [discussion: 934].

77. Rhee JS, Matthews BA, Neuburg M, et al. Validation of a quality-of-life instrument for patients with nonmelanoma skin cancer. Arch Facial Plast Surg 2006;8(5):314–8.

78. Rhee JS, Matthews BA, Neuburg M, et al. The skin cancer index: clinical responsiveness and predictors of quality of life. Laryngoscope 2007;117(3): 399–405.

79. Chren MM, Lasek RJ, Sahay AP, et al. Measurement properties of Skindex-16: a brief quality-of-life measure for patients with skin diseases. J Cutan Med Surg 2001;5(2):105–10.

80. Chen T, Bertenthal D, Sahay A, et al. Predictors of skin-related quality of life after treatment of cutaneous basal cell carcinoma and squamous cell carcinoma. Arch Dermatol 2007;143(11):1386–92.

81. Chren MM, Sahay AP, Bertenthal DS, et al. Quality-of-life outcomes of treatments for cutaneous basal cell carcinoma and squamous cell carcinoma. J Invest Dermatol 2007;127(6):1351–7.

82. Lee KC, Weinstock MA. Prospective quality of life impact of keratinocyte carcinomas: observations from the Veterans Affairs Topical Tretinoin Chemoprevention Trial. J Am Acad Dermatol 2010;63(6): 1107–9.

83. Chen JG, Fleischer AB Jr, Smith ED, et al. Cost of nonmelanoma skin cancer treatment in the United States. Dermatol Surg 2001;27(12):1035–8.

84. Joseph AK, Mark TL, Mueller C. The period prevalence and costs of treating nonmelanoma skin cancers in patients over 65 years of age covered by Medicare. Dermatol Surg 2001;27(11):955–9.

85. Housman TS, Feldman SR, Williford PM, et al. Skin cancer is among the most costly of all cancers to treat for the Medicare population. J Am Acad Dermatol 2003;48(3):425–9.

86. John Chen G, Yelverton CB, Polisetty SS, et al. Treatment patterns and cost of nonmelanoma skin cancer management. Dermatol Surg 2006;32(10):1266–71.

87. Manternach T, Housman TS, Williford PM, et al. Surgical treatment of nonmelanoma skin cancer in the Medicare population. Dermatol Surg 2003; 29(12):1167–9 [discussion: 1169].

88. Cook J, Zitelli JA. Mohs micrographic surgery: a cost analysis. J Am Acad Dermatol 1998; 39(5 Pt 1):698–703.

89. Bialy TL, Whalen J, Veledar E, et al. Mohs micrographic surgery vs traditional surgical excision: a cost comparison analysis. Arch Dermatol 2004; 140(6):736–42.

90. Seidler AM, Bramlette TB, Washington CV, et al. Mohs versus traditional surgical excision for facial and auricular nonmelanoma skin cancer: an analysis of cost-effectiveness. Dermatol Surg 2009; 35(11):1776–87.

91. Rogers HW, Coldiron BM. A relative value unit-based cost comparison of treatment modalities for nonmelanoma skin cancer: effect of the loss of the Mohs multiple surgery reduction exemption. J Am Acad Dermatol 2009;61(1):96–103.

92. Miller SJ, Alam M, Andersen J, et al. Basal cell and squamous cell skin cancers. J Natl Compr Canc Netw 2010;8(8):836–64.

93. Rowe DE, Carroll RJ, Day CL Jr. Mohs surgery is the treatment of choice for recurrent (previously treated) basal cell carcinoma. J Dermatol Surg Oncol 1989;15(4):424–31.

94. Bath-Hextall FJ, Perkins W, Bong J, et al. Interventions for basal cell carcinoma of the skin. Cochrane Database Syst Rev 2007;1:CD003412.

95. Avril MF, Auperin A, Margulis A, et al. Basal cell carcinoma of the face: surgery or radiotherapy? Results of a randomized study. Br J Cancer 1997; 76(1):100–6.

96. Mosterd K, Krekels GA, Nieman FH, et al. Surgical excision versus Mohs' micrographic surgery for primary and recurrent basal-cell carcinoma of the face: a prospective randomised controlled trial with 5-years' follow-up. Lancet Oncol 2008;9(12): 1149–56.

97. Rhodes LE, de Rie MA, Leifsdottir R, et al. Five-year follow-up of a randomized, prospective trial of topical methyl aminolevulinate photodynamic therapy vs surgery for nodular basal cell carcinoma. Arch Dermatol 2007;143(9):1131–6.

98. Mosterd K, Thissen MR, Nelemans P, et al. Fractionated 5-aminolaevulinic acid-photodynamic therapy vs. surgical excision in the treatment of nodular basal cell carcinoma: results of a randomized controlled trial. Br J Dermatol 2008;159(4): 864–70.

99. Basset-Seguin N, Ibbotson SH, Emtestam L, et al. Topical methyl aminolaevulinate photodynamic therapy versus cryotherapy for superficial basal cell carcinoma: a 5 year randomized trial. Eur J Dermatol 2008;18(5):547–53.

100. Ozolins M, Williams HC, Armstrong SJ, et al. The SINS trial: a randomised controlled trial of excisional surgery versus imiquimod 5% cream for nodular and superficial basal cell carcinoma. Trials 2010;11:42.

101. Lansbury L, Leonardi-Bee J, Perkins W, et al. Interventions for non-metastatic squamous cell carcinoma of the skin. Cochrane Database Syst Rev 2010;4:CD007869.

102. Brewster AM, Lee JJ, Clayman GL, et al. Randomized trial of adjuvant 13-cis-retinoic acid and interferon alfa for patients with aggressive skin squamous cell carcinoma. J Clin Oncol 2007; 25(15):1974–8.

103. Mudigonda T, Pearce DJ, Yentzer BA, et al. The economic impact of non-melanoma skin cancer: a review. J Natl Compr Canc Netw 2010;8(8): 888–96.

Infectious Skin Diseases: A Review and Needs Assessment

Annelise L. Dawson, BA[a],
Robert P. Dellavalle, MD, PhD, MSPH[b],
Dirk M. Elston, MD[c,d],*

KEYWORDS

- Infectious skin disease • Cellulitis • Dermatophyte infection
- Superficial fungal infection • Herpes simplex virus infection
- Epidemiology • Treatment

Infectious skin diseases encompass a vast array of conditions that range in severity from benign to life threatening. The clinical presentation of infectious skin diseases varies based on the type of pathogen involved, the skin layers and structures affected, and the underlying medical condition of the patient. Infectious skin diseases represent common diagnoses made by dermatologists, by primary care physicians, and in the emergency room.[1] Between 1980 and 1996, 48 of every 1000 medical visits were attributed to infectious skin disease—a number that is rising, particularly with the appearance of virulent pathogens such as methicillin-resistant *Staphylococcus aureus* (MRSA).[2,3] Effective treatment of infectious skin disease requires timely identification or estimation of the offending pathogen, and selection of a treatment that is effective against the pathogen and is administered via the optimal route and dosing schedule.

BACTERIAL SKIN DISEASES

Bacterial skin and soft-tissue infections (SSTIs) are the most common type of infectious skin disease, and encompass an array of conditions that may be classified by the skin layers and structures they affect.[2] Impetigo is a superficial, crusting epidermal skin infection that presents in bullous and nonbullous forms. Erysipelas is a streptococcal infection of the superficial dermal lymphatics that demonstrates sharply demarcated, raised borders.[3,4] Cellulitis is an infection of the deeper dermis and subcutaneous tissue with poorly demarcated borders; the vast majority of cases are streptococcal in origin. Clinically the distinction between erysipelas and cellulitis is subtle and, given that both are predominantly streptococcal in origin, many experts consider them to be different presentations of the same disease.[5,6] As such, these infection types are often grouped in clinical reporting and epidemiologic analyses. Cutaneous abscesses are collections of pus in the dermis and subcutaneous tissue. Folliculitis describes superficial infection of hair follicles with pus accumulation in the epidermis. Furuncles, or "boils," represent deeper involvement of hair follicles in which the infection extends into the subcutaneous tissue. Carbuncles occur when adjacent

Funding sources: There were no sources of funding for this article.
Disclosures: The authors have no disclosures relevant to this article.

[a] Department of Dermatology, University of Colorado Denver, PO Box 6511, Mail Stop 8127, Aurora, CO 80045, USA
[b] Dermatology Service, Denver Department of Veterans Affairs Medical Center, University of Colorado School of Medicine, Colorado School of Public Health, 1055 Clermont Street, Mail Code #165, Denver, CO 80220, USA
[c] Department of Dermatology, Geisinger Medical Center, Danville, PA, USA
[d] Ackerman Academy of Dermatopathology, 145 East 32nd Street, 10th Floor, New York, NY 10016, USA
* Corresponding author. Ackerman Academy of Dermatopathology, 145 East 32nd Street, 10th Floor, New York, NY 10016.
E-mail address: dmelston@geisinger.edu

Dermatol Clin 30 (2012) 141–151
doi:10.1016/j.det.2011.08.003
0733-8635/12/$ – see front matter © 2012 Published by Elsevier Inc.

furuncles coalesce to form a single inflamed area. Pus-forming infections tend to be staphylococcal in origin, except for periorificial abscesses, which are often anaerobic. Although all of the preceding are common, cellulitis accounts for the majority of serious bacterial SSTIs.[7,8]

Cellulitis

General

Cellulitis represents an acute spreading infection of the dermis and subcutaneous tissue whose clinical appearance was classically described by Celsus in the first century using the terms "calor," "rubor," "tumor," and "dolor," or warmth, erythema, edema, and tenderness, respectively.[9] Certain characteristics, such as pain out of proportion to physical findings, large bullae, crepitus, and anesthesia, suggest more serious infection.[10] Cellulitis is most common in the lower extremities, but has been documented on all parts of the body.[3] Cellulitis results from breaches in skin integrity that allow for the spread of organisms below the skin surface. Cutaneous disruption via skin trauma, ulceration, edema, surgical incision, preexisting fungal and other superficial infection, and dermatitis may predispose to cellulitis.[5,7,11]

In recent years S aureus has become an increasingly important pathogen, and the emergence of community strains of MRSA has created a dilemma for physicians treating invasive bacterial infections.[12–15] Although S aureus is commonly isolated from surface cultures, positive outcomes with β-lactam antibiotics suggest that even in the age of MRSA, the primary pathogens causing cellulitis remain Streptococcus species in Lancefield groups A, C, and G, especially group A β-hemolytic streptococci.[5,16,17] The presence of erysipelas, lymphangitis, and rapid tissue spread suggest streptococcal infection, while purulence or concomitant abscesses and furuncles increase the probability of staphylococcal infection.[9,18]

If staphylococcal infection is suspected, it is difficult to distinguish between methicillin-sensitive S aureus (MSSA) and MRSA based on clinical information alone.[19,20] Certain factors increase the likelihood of MRSA infection, including a history of recurrent infections, young age, participation in athletic sports, and injection drug use.[21] MRSA infection can be further divided into infection with community-acquired MRSA (CA-MRSA) and health care–associated MRSA (HA-MRSA). It may be clinically relevant to differentiate between the two types because HA-MRSA bacterial isolates display broader antibiotic resistance patterns than do CA-MRSA isolates.[22] Nevertheless, the distinction between CA-MRSA and HA-MRSA infection is blurred as patients move between and community and hospital settings.[19,23,24]

Incidence

Recent analyses have yielded incongruous results with regard to the changing incidence of SSTIs over the last 2 decades. One study endorses that the incidence of SSTIs increased from 32 to 48 clinical visits per 1000 persons per year between 1997 and 2005, which is attributed to the growing incidence of cellulitis and abscesses.[7] Other studies endorse that the overall incidence of SSTIs has not increased over a similar time period, but confirm that visits for cellulitis and abscesses specifically have increased significantly.[8,11] Although their conclusions regarding changing incidence differ, when taken together these studies demonstrate the relative commonness of SSTIs and the increasing incidence of cellulitis in particular. In addition, consensus opinion favors the view that emergency room visits for SSTIs have increased in recent years, nearly tripling between 1995 and 2005. This change is attributed to an increase in diagnoses of MRSA-related cellulitis and abscesses.[7,8,13,25]

Treatment

Most cellulitis cases are treated on an outpatient basis with oral antibiotics. Antibiotics are typically selected empirically without diagnostic cultures, given the low yield of cultures for cellulitis.[5,26,27] Aspiration and punch biopsies show varied results, yielding positive cultures in fewer than 40% of cases.[28] In general, pus and tissue samples are most sensitive if collected before initiating antibiotic treatment.[5] Blood cultures should always be obtained if patients demonstrate signs of systemic involvement.[5,9] When systemic disease is suspected, patients are typically treated on an inpatient basis with intravenous (IV) antibiotics.[21] Necrotizing infection requires emergent debridement and treatment with IV antibiotics.[19] Between 1995 and 2005 approximately 14% of emergency room visits for SSTIs resulted in hospitalization.[13] Recently, however, there has been a trend toward at-home administration of IV antibiotics for some patients.[29,30]

The choice of antibiotics for cellulitis can be challenging. A recent Cochrane review cites lack of evidence from randomized controlled trials to guide antibiotic selection.[6] Given the increasing prevalence of MRSA infection, some investigators suggest that providers assume bacterial antibiotic resistance and select empiric antibiotics active against CA-MRSA.[5,25] This practice may produce suboptimal outcomes, however, as sulfa drugs and tetracyclines are not reliable against many pathogen types. Although the prevalence of inducible resistance to clindamycin is increasing, clindamycin remains an acceptable alternative to beta-lactam agents when clinical or epidemiologic factors suggest the possibility of MRSA infection.[9,13,18,22] Linezolid is expensive, but has demonstrated good outcomes in life-threatening MRSA infections.[9,18] Vancomycin achieves low intracellular levels and has demonstrated poorer outcomes in serious infections.[31,32] Fluoroquinolone and macrolide resistance is now widespread.[22] If patients are treated as outpatients, it is advisable to evaluate their response to treatment after 24 to 48 hours.[5]

Cost of treatment

The cost of cellulitis treatment varies widely based on the severity of disease and the treatment mechanism. Data from 2005 to 2006 suggest a mean cost of $6800 for inpatient treatment of SSTI.[33] There are relatively few United States data on the cost of outpatient treatment of cellulitis with oral medications, though data from other countries suggests that outpatient treatment is substantially less expensive. In the Netherlands, for example, outpatient costs account for only 20% of health care costs associated with cellulitis even though they represent 87% of patients treated for cellulitis.[34]

To offset the cost of inpatient care and improve patient comfort, there has been a trend toward home administration of IV antibiotics, which is nearly half as expensive as inpatient management and produces the same patient outcome.[29,30,35] Other analyses have explored the cost effectiveness of cultures, colonization surveillance, decolonization, and duration of antibiotic treatment. Cultures were found not to be cost effective for the majority of patients with uncomplicated infections, although they are recommended when serious pathogens are suspected.[36] Data regarding the cost effectiveness and benefit of MRSA surveillance and decolonization are mixed.[7,10]

Summary and Future Directions

The emergence of new pathogens will continue to affect health care use and the appropriate choice of antibiotics. CA-MRSA is a key example. This pathogen has become the most common cause of skin infections presenting to emergency departments, and its emergence has led to recommendations that first-line antibiotics be chosen for their MRSA coverage. This advice is premature, as most CA-MRSA infections are abscesses and can be treated surgically without the need for antibiotics. Outcomes data suggest that streptococci remain the principal pathogens involved in cellulitis and that β-lactam drugs still play an important role in the treatment of cutaneous infections. Sulfa and tetracycline antibiotics are both unreliable against streptococci. Ongoing monitoring for disease prevalence and antibiogram data are needed to inform future recommendations (**Table 1**).

FUNGAL SKIN DISEASES

Cutaneous fungal infections may be divided into 3 categories: superficial, deep, and systemic infections. Superficial infections are confined to dead keratinous tissue, the epidermis, and hair follicles, and are caused by dermatophytes, nondermatophyte molds, and yeasts (*Candida* and *Malassezia* species).[37–40] Deep infections demonstrate involvement of all skin layers and often extend into the subcutaneous tissue. These infections occur via direct inoculation of the skin, and include infections such as sporotrichosis, mycetoma, and chromomycosis. Systemic infections with cutaneous manifestations are the least common and often occur in immunocompromised hosts. These infections are usually acquired through inhalation of spores with a primary pulmonary focus, even when skin lesions are the presenting finding.

Table 1
Bacterial skin infections: needs and future directions

Surveillance	Treatment	Future Study
• Predominant bacterial species and strains • Antibiotic susceptibility and resistance • Proportions of SSTIs treated in outpatient, inpatient, emergency room, and other health care settings	• Stronger recommendations for antibiotic selection • Emphasize use of incision and drainage for abscesses • Improved management of predisposing conditions	• Cost-of-treatment analyses • Further assessment of the value of colonization monitoring and decolonization efforts • Antibiotic development • Vaccine development

Histoplasmosis, blastomycosis, and coccidioidomycosis may occur in patients with normal immune function, whereas other infections such as cryptococcosis, aspergillosis, fusariosis, and mucormycosis present primarily in immunocompromised hosts.[37]

Superficial Fungal Infections

General

The majority of fungal infections are superficial cutaneous infections, most of which result from dermatophyte infection.[39] Dermatophytes are fungi that digest keratin as a nutrient source. These fungi colonize the highly keratinized stratum corneum, or outermost layer of the skin, as well as other keratinized structures such as the nail plate and hair follicles.[39,41–43] Such fungi rarely invade viable tissue, and thus do not produce deep cutaneous or systemic infections, nor are they lethal.[39,43] Although many infections demonstrate gross changes to the surrounding and underlying tissue suggestive of deeper infection, this usually represents an inflammatory host response to the overlying dermatophyte infection without true invasion.[43]

Dermatophytes are divided into 3 genera: *Trichophyton*, *Microsporum*, and *Epidermophyton*. More than 40 different species of dermatophyte have been implicated in skin disease; however, most infections are caused by just a few species.[39,41,42] *Trichophyton rubrum* is the most common dermatophyte, and it is estimated that 70% of the United States population will experience at least one *T rubrum* infection in their lifetime.[37,44] Other common species in the United States include *Trichophyton tonsurans* and *Trichophyton mentagrophytes*. The distribution of dermatophytes is not static but instead ever-changing, especially in the era of international migration, travel, and commerce.[39,45] Factors such as socioeconomic status, use of occlusive footwear, and urbanization also affect the varying distribution of pathogen types.[45,46]

Tinea pedis, or "athlete's foot," represents a superficial fungal infection of the foot. This common infection occurs in 1 in 5 adults in the United States during their lifetimes. Worldwide incidence has increased in recent decades, especially with the use of occlusive footwear.[38,40] Ninety-five percent of tinea pedis cases are caused by dermatophytes, with most infections caused by *T rubrum* and *Trichophyton interdigitale* (formerly *Trichophyton mentagrophytes* var. *interdigitale*).[39,44,47] Tinea pedis is classified into 3 primary clinical types: interdigital, moccasin, and vesiculobullous. Interdigital infection involves the toe web spaces and often presents with bacterial superinfection. Moccasin-type tinea pedis demonstrates thickening of the plantar and lateral foot with overlying scale. Vesiculobullous-type tinea pedis demonstrates plantar pustules and vesicles, which may become macerated and superinfected with bacteria.[43]

Tinea unguium, or onchomycosis, is an infection of the nail plate or bed. Fungal infection of these structures leads to nail bed deformity (onchodystrophy) with thickening (hyperkeratosis) and discoloration.[48,49] Eighty-two percent of tinea unguium cases are the result of dermatophyte infection, of which *T rubrum* is most common.[39,44,47] *Candida* species and molds may also cause onchomycosis, particularly in tropical climates.[39] Estimates vary regarding the prevalence of onchomycosis; however, most investigators endorse that these infections affect at least 5% of the adult population and increase in prevalence with age.[50,51]

Tinea corporis is a superficial fungal infection of glabrous skin occurring most commonly on the trunk and limbs, whereas tinea facei affects the face. Both types are referred to as "ringworm" given their tendency to produce annular plaques or patches with a red, raised, scaling border. Tinea corporis and facei are most commonly caused by *Trichophyton*, particularly *T rubrum*, and *Microsporum* species.[39,43,48]

Tinea cruris, or "jock itch," describes infection of the groin region that occurs almost exclusively in adult men.[37] It presents as an erythematous patch involving the inner thigh and inguinal folds while sparing the scrotum and penis. Tinea cruris is often associated with tinea pedis, and it is thought that infection occurs through self-inoculation from the foot. Most cases are caused by infection with *T rubrum* or *T mentagrophytes*, and may be secondarily infected with bacteria or yeast species.[37,39,43]

Tinea capitis represents infection of the scalp and hair.[48] Ninety-five percent of cases are caused by superficial infection with *T tonsurans*.[42] Tinea capitis displays wide variation in presentation and is classified into 4 patterns. First, seborrheic-type demonstrates dandruff-like noninflammatory scaling. Next, "black-dot" tinea capitis produces hair breakage, leading to areas of alopecia with dark spots representing underlying hair follicles. Kerion-type tinea capitis involves the formation of a purulent inflammatory nodule. Finally the favus type, the rarest form, describes an inflammatory alopecia with honey-colored crusts.[37,47,52]

Other common superficial fungal infections include candidiasis and tinea versicolor. Candidiasis is most commonly caused by *Candida albicans* and affects the skin, mucus membranes, nails, or gastrointestinal tract.[37,39,47] Candidiasis is more common in women when accounting for vulvovaginal candidiasis, and in immunosuppressed patients.[37,47,53] Tinea versicolor is a harmless skin disease most common in tropical regions, characterized by overgrowth of *Malassezia* species leading to the formation of hypopigmented or hyperpigmented patches with associated fine scale.[37,39,43,47]

Incidence

Fungal skin infections are estimated to affect more than 20% of the world's population.[39,54] In the United States, prevalence is estimated at 10% to 20% of the population.[43,55] Unlike bacterial skin infections, which must be recognized and treated promptly, fungal infections tend to follow a more indolent course and are less commonly life threatening. These infections are often difficult to treat, and persist despite optimal medical management.[56] Furthermore, fungal remnants frequently remain after treatment; this and genetic predisposition result in a high rate of recurrent infection.[54]

Given that cutaneous fungal infections affect up to 1 in 5 individuals in the United States and tend to follow a chronic, treatment-resistant course, it is not surprising that they account for a large number of physician visits each year. It is estimated that superficial cutaneous fungal infections account for more than 4 million outpatient visits annually, one-third of which are for onchomycosis specifically.[38,53] Physician visits for fungal infections comprise 18% of outpatient visits for infectious skin diseases in the United States, or approximately 0.4% of all outpatient visits.[2]

Treatment

The treatment of superficial fungal infections varies based on the type of infection and the suspected pathogen. For some infection types, including tinea corporis, tinea facei, tinea pedis, tinea cruris, tinea versicolor, and candidiasis, treatment with topical agents may be adequate.[43] Nevertheless, many superficial fungal infections respond poorly to topical agents alone. For example, fewer than 20% of cases of tinea unguium respond to topical treatment, owing to poor penetration of the nail bed.[54] For infections such as tinea unguium, tinea capitis, and other refractory or severe cutaneous fungal infections, use of systemic antifungal agents is the standard of care. Griseofulvin, terbinafine, and azoles such as fluconazole, itraconazole, and ketoconazole are the most widely used systemic antifungal therapies for cutaneous fungal infections. Use of some of these agents can be complicated by drug toxicities for which monitoring of hepatic and renal function is necessary. In recent years, several new drugs with more favorable side-effect profiles have been developed.[43,56]

Cost of treatment

Estimates for the annual cost of treatment of cutaneous fungal infections in the United States vary widely. In a study using data from 1990 to 1994, it was estimated that cutaneous fungal infections account for approximately $220 million in office visit and medication expenses annually.[53] In a 2004 study, the economic burden of cutaneous fungal infections was estimated to be much higher at $1.7 billion annually. This value accounted for the cost of physician visits as well as prescription drug costs, which represented 74% of the total.[55] Despite the discrepancy in costs reported by these studies, it is indisputable that cutaneous fungal infections account for substantial annual health care expenditures in the United States.

Summary and Future Directions

The burden of fungal skin disease is high, and recurrence is common. Simple fungal infections serve as important portals of entry for bacterial sepsis in immunosuppressed patients. Given the aging population and increasing prevalence of immunosuppression, these pathogens will continue to represent a public health burden. Research priorities include improved prophylactic regimens, the feasibility of shorter courses of therapy, and the cost effectiveness of care in various populations (**Table 2**).

Table 2
Fungal skin infections: needs and future directions

Surveillance	Treatment	Future Study
• Predominant dermatophyte infection types and species • Fungal infection types in immunocompromised hosts	• Improved prophylactic treatment • Evaluation of efficacy of shorter treatment courses	• Cost-of-treatment analyses • Identify genetic factors that predispose to fungal infection • Development of antifungals with lesser side effects

VIRAL SKIN DISEASES

Viral diseases of the skin represent a final major category of infectious skin disease. While many viral infections are eliminated after initial infection, some of the most common viruses affecting the skin produce chronic or even life-long infection. Human papillomavirus, for example, which causes common and genital warts, can produce chronic infection that is highly recalcitrant to treatment. Herpesviruses, which produce many common cutaneous diseases including oral and genital herpes, establish permanent infection that fluctuates between latent infection and active disease over the lifetime of the host. The persistence of many viral skin diseases therefore contributes to the high prevalence and economic burden of these infections.

Herpes Simplex Virus Infection

General

The viral family Herpesviridae encompasses some of the most widespread human viruses, including herpes simplex viruses 1 and 2 (HSV-1, HSV-2), varicella zoster virus (VZV), Epstein-Barr virus (EBV), and cytomegalovirus (CMV).[57] Herpesviruses are unique in their ability to produce latent, incurable infection. The herpes simplex viruses, HSV-1 and HSV-2, establish initial infection through mucosa or abraded skin.[58] After initial, or "primary," infection, these viruses travel retrograde from of the point of exposure along sensory neuronal axons to nuclei where they multiply and remain latent.[58–60] After a variable period of time viral reactivation can occur, producing recurrence at the site of the primary infection. Disease recurrence may be precipitated by many factors, including emotional stress, fever, localized trauma, ultraviolet light, menstruation, or immunosuppression.[58,61] Often, however, no clear cause is identified. Furthermore, viral reactivation may lead to shedding of viral particles without symptomatic disease. At any given time, approximately 1% to 5% of individuals with HSV infection demonstrate asymptomatic shedding, which contributes to the spread of disease.[62–64]

The herpes simplex viruses cause a variety of clinical manifestations, of which herpes labialis and herpes genitalis are especially widespread. Herpes labialis, the most common form of herpes infection, presents as vesicular or ulcerative lesions of the oral cavity or perioral skin and mucosa.[61] Herpes labialis is typically caused by HSV-1, which is spread through contact with oral secretions. Herpes genitalis describes the appearance of similar lesions involving the genital mucosa. Most cases of herpes genitalis are caused by HSV-2;

however, recent surveys demonstrate increasing overlap in types with up to 30% of herpes genitalis caused by HSV-1.[65]

The clinical presentation of HSV infection is variable and depends on the immune status of the host.[58,59] HSV infections often present with a prodrome of tingling or pain in the region of subsequent disease.[57,61] Most primary HSV-1 infections are asymptomatic, whereas primary HSV-2 infections tend to be severe, with painful vesicle formation and ulceration as well as constitutional symptoms such as fever and lethargy.[57,61,65] HSV-1 recurrences typically present as painful, grouped vesicles on an erythematous base on the vermillion border of the lip, lasting 2 to 3 days. The lesions subsequently develop ulceration with crusting, and ultimately heal in 4 to 5 days.[62] HSV-2 recurrences present with similar skin findings, but tend to be less severe than primary infection and without constitutional symptoms.[61,62] Most diagnoses of HSV infection are made by clinical evaluation alone. Nevertheless, several diagnostic tests are available, including Tsanck smear, viral culture, serologic testing, direct fluorescent antibody studies, and tissue biopsy.[59,64,66]

Herpes simplex virus can produce several other dermatologic disease manifestations, including eczema herpeticum (HSV superinfection of atopic dermatitis), herpetic whitlow (digital HSV infection), and herpes gladiatorum (corporeal HSV infection related to direct skin-to-skin contact occurring in athletic competition).[57] Ophthalmologic manifestations, such as herpes keratitis, may lead to loss of vision with chronic infection. Finally, HSV may cause life-threatening infection including herpes encephalitis and neonatal herpes. Neonatal herpes is most often acquired through vertical transmission from mothers at the time of delivery.[61] Thus, examination for active genital HSV infection should be performed prior to vaginal delivery.

Incidence

The incidence of herpes simplex virus infection is quite high, which may be attributed in part to the fact that once HSV infection is acquired it cannot be cured. Far fewer Americans self-report a history of herpes labialis or genitalis than are actually seropositive for HSV. Serologic analyses demonstrate that 60% to 80% of adults are seropositive for HSV-1 and 20% to 30% of adults are seropositive for HSV-2.[67–71] The prevalence of HSV-2 infection has increased by 30% in recent decades, which some investigators have attributed to changing sexual practices.[70] In general, HSV-2 tends to produce more frequent recurrences than does HSV-1.[72]

Treatment

There is no cure for HSV infection, so treatment is focused on attenuating symptoms, decreasing the frequency of recurrences, and reducing viral shedding.[66] Antivirals have undergone remarkable development over the past 3 decades. Nucleoside reverse transcriptase inhibitors, such as acyclovir, valacyclovir, and famciclovir, are first-line agents in the treatment of primary oral or genital HSV infection.[73,74] For herpes labialis, long-term prophylactic oral acyclovir may reduce the frequency of disease recurrence.[62,75] If prophylactic acyclovir is not used, oral acyclovir may also be initiated at the time of disease recurrence, and has been demonstrated to decrease pain and healing time. The benefits of oral acyclovir are optimized if treatment is initiated early in the prodromal phase.[76] Other oral treatment options for recurrent herpes labialis include famciclovir and valacyclovir.[74,77–79] Several topical agents such as penciclovir are available; however, their effects are modest at best.[80]

The treatment of herpes genitalis is similar to that of herpes labialis. Prophylactic oral acyclovir reduces viral shedding and disease outbreaks.[75] Oral acyclovir, famciclovir, and valacyclovir may also be used in the treatment of genital recurrences.[78,81–84] Intravenous acyclovir is reserved for the treatment of life-threatening HSV infections, including herpes encephalitis, neonatal herpes, and severe infections in immunocompromised patients.[57] Several other antiviral options exist, including penciclovir, docosanol topical, foscarnet, and cidofovir. Foscarnet and cidofovir demonstrate greater toxicity and are used only in the treatment of acyclovir-resistant HSV infections.[74]

Treatment resistance

HSV resistance to standard acyclovir treatment is very low, at less than 1% in immunocompetent hosts, even with a history of antiviral treatment.[85,86] Recent studies indicate, however, that rates of HSV resistance are significantly higher in immunocompromised patients, including patients with AIDS, receiving chemotherapy, and undergoing organ transplantation. In immunocompromised hosts, HSV resistance to acyclovir is reported at 3% to 7% overall and is as high as 11% to 14% in patients undergoing bone marrow transplantation.[86–88] Although the use of prophylactic acyclovir treatment in immunocompromised patients has increased in recent years, surveillance data suggest that rates of resistance have not grown substantially.[87] Nevertheless, the incidence of severe HSV infections has increased given the rise in iatrogenically induced immunosuppression, including through cancer chemotherapy and transplant-related management.[86]

Previously patients found to have acyclovir-resistant HSV infection were treated with foscarnet. Recent monitoring, however, suggests that foscarnet resistance develops rapidly in more than 50% of these patients.[87,89] Cidofovir may be used to treat patients with acyclovir and foscarnet resistance.[89,90] Vidarabine is considered if the aforementioned treatments fail.[90] Resistant herpes infections not only present treatment challenges in immunocompromised patients but also pose serious risks if they produce severe infections such as neonatal herpes or herpes encephalitis in immunocompetent hosts. Thus, the increase in HSV-resistant strains is a major public health issue requiring ongoing surveillance.

Cost of treatment

Although most HSV infections are not life threatening, these life-long diseases produce uncomfortable cutaneous manifestations and carry substantial emotional weight, prompting many patients to seek treatment, which contributes to the economic burden of disease. However, estimates regarding the total cost of HSV treatment are limited. In a 2004 study, the economic burden of cutaneous herpes simplex and herpes zoster infections together was estimated at $1.7 billion annually in the United States.[55] Herpes zoster

Table 3
Viral skin infections: needs and future directions

Surveillance	Treatment	Future Study and Efforts
• HSV infection in immunocompromised hosts • Patterns of HSV resistance • HSV type and subtype distribution	• Randomized controlled trials to evaluate efficacy of existing antivirals • Increased treatment to reduce viral shedding	• Cost-of-treatment analyses • Improve screening tests for use at the time of delivery • Public health messaging to increase HSV awareness • Antivirals effective against dormant infection • Vaccine development

infections account for approximately $1 billion of this expense, suggesting that HSV infections account for $700 million in annual health care costs.[91] Herpes genitalis infections account for more than $200 million of this total,[92] so the annual economic burden of other cutaneous herpes infections, including herpes labialis, may be extrapolated to be nearly $500 million annually. These values represent rough estimates based on separate analyses and so must be interpreted carefully. Nevertheless, it is clear that the economic burden of cutaneous HSV infection is substantial. Further cost analyses are warranted.

Summary and Future Directions

The public health burden of viral skin diseases is significant because of viral dormancy, the high rate of recurrence, and the risk of infection in neonates and immunocompromised hosts. Research priorities include the need for better screening tests at the time of delivery, ongoing surveillance of antiviral resistance, and efforts to improve antiviral capabilities, including the search for agents effective against dormant infection (Table 3).

SUMMARY

Infectious skin diseases represent a primary category of dermatologic illnesses that account for substantial health and economic burden annually. Ongoing surveillance and monitoring of disease agents is important, given their ever-changing susceptibilities and geographic distribution. Furthermore, continuing antimicrobial and vaccine development is a priority, especially with the emergence of new and virulent pathogens.

List of Acronyms	
CA-MRSA	Community-acquired methicillin-resistant *Staphylococcus aureus*
CMV	Cytomegalovirus
EBV	Epstein-Barr virus
HA-MRSA	Health care–associated methicillin-resistant *Staphylococcus aureus*
HSV	Herpes simplex virus
IV	Intravenous
MRSA	Methicillin-resistant *Staphylococcus aureus*
MSSA	Methicillin-sensitive *Staphylococcus aureus*
SSTI	Skin and soft-tissue infection
VZV	Varicella zoster virus

REFERENCES

1. Fleischer AB Jr, Feldman SR, Rapp Introduction SR. The magnitude of skin disease in the United States. Dermatol Clin 2000;18(2):xv–xxi.
2. Armstrong GL, Pinner RW. Outpatient visits for infectious diseases in the United States, 1980 through 1996. Arch Intern Med 1999;159:2531–6.
3. Rogers RL, Perkins J. Skin and soft tissue infections. Prim Care 2006;33:697–710.
4. Bisno AL, Stevens DL. Streptococcal infections in skin and soft tissues. N Engl J Med 1996;334:240–5.
5. Stevens DL, Bisno AL, Chambers HF, et al. Practice guidelines for the management of skin and soft tissue infections. Clin Infect Dis 2005;41:1373–406.
6. Kilburn SA, Featherstone P, Higgins B, et al. Interventions for cellulitis and erysipelas. Cochrane Database Syst Rev 2010;6:CD004299.
7. Hersh AL, Chambers HF, Maselli JH, et al. National trends in ambulatory visits and antibiotic prescribing for skin and soft-tissue infections. Arch Intern Med 2008;168:1585–91.
8. McCaig LF, McDonald LC, Mandal S, et al. *Staphylococcus aureus*-associated skin and soft tissue infections in ambulatory care. Emerg Infect Dis 2006;12:1715–23.
9. Dryden MS. Complicated skin and soft tissue infection. J Antimicrob Chemother 2010;65(Suppl 3):iii35–44.
10. Elston DM. Cutaneous manifestations of infectious disease. Med Clin North Am 2009;93:1283–90.
11. Pallin DJ, Espinola JA, Leung DY, et al. Epidemiology of dermatitis and skin infections in United States physicians' offices, 1993-2005. Clin Infect Dis 2009;49:901–7.
12. Gabillot-Carre M, Roujeau JC. Acute bacterial skin infections and cellulitis. Curr Opin Infect Dis 2007;20:118–23.
13. Moran GJ, Krishnadasan A, Gorwitz RJ, et al. Methicillin-resistant *S. aureus* infections among patients in the emergency department. N Engl J Med 2006;355:666–74.
14. Moran GJ, Amii RN, Abrahamian FM, et al. Methicillin-resistant *Staphylococcus aureus* in community-acquired skin infections. Emerg Infect Dis 2005;11:928–30.
15. Moet GJ, Jones RN, Biedenbach DJ, et al. Contemporary causes of skin and soft tissue infections in North America, Latin America, and Europe: report from the SENTRY Antimicrobial Surveillance Program (1998-2004). Diagn Microbiol Infect Dis 2007;57:7–13.
16. Bernard P, Bedane C, Mounier M, et al. Streptococcal cause of erysipelas and cellulitis in adults.

A microbiologic study using a direct immunofluorescence technique. Arch Dermatol 1989;125:779–82.

17. Fridkin SK, Hageman JC, Morrison M, et al. Methicillin-resistant *Staphylococcus aureus* disease in three communities. N Engl J Med 2005;352(14):1436–44.

18. Stevens DL, Eron LL. Cellulitis and soft-tissue infections. Ann Intern Med 2009;150(1):ITC1.

19. Miller LG, Perdreau-Remington F, Bayer AS, et al. Clinical and epidemiologic characteristics cannot distinguish community-associated methicillin-resistant *Staphylococcus aureus* infection from methicillin-susceptible *S. aureus* infection: a prospective investigation. Clin Infect Dis 2007;44:471–82.

20. Bar-Meir M, Tan TQ. *Staphylococcus aureus* skin and soft tissue infectious: can we anticipate a culture result? Clin Pediatr 2010;49(5):432–8.

21. Neapolitano LM. Early appropriate parenteral antimicrobial treatment of complicated skin and soft tissue infections caused by MRSA. Surg Infect 2008; 9(Suppl 1):S17–27.

22. Naimi TS, LeDell KH, Como-Sabetti K, et al. Comparison of community- and health care-associated methicillin-resistant *Staphylococcus aureus* infection. JAMA 2003;290:2976–84.

23. Otter JA, French GL. Nosocomial transmission of community-associated methicillin-resistant *Staphylococcus aureus*: an emerging threat. Lancet Infect Dis 2006;6:753–5.

24. King MD, Humphrey BJ, Wang YF, et al. Emergence of community-acquired methicillin-resistant *Staphylococcus aureus* USA 300 clone as the predominant cause of skin and soft tissue infections. Ann Intern Med 2006;144:309–17.

25. Pallin DJ, Egan DJ, Pelletier AJ, et al. Increased US emergency department visits for skin and soft tissue infections, and changes in antibiotic choices, during the emergence of community-associated methicillin-resistant *Staphylococcus aureus*. Ann Emerg Med 2008;51:291–8.

26. Eron LJ, Lipsky BA. Use of cultures in cellulitis: when, how, and why? [editorial]. Eur J Clin Microbiol Infect Dis 2006;25:615–7.

27. Gould IM, Mackenzie FM, Shepherd L. Use of the bacteriology laboratory to decrease general practitioners' antibiotic prescribing. Eur J Gen Pract 2007;13:13–5.

28. Zahar JR, Goveia J, Lesprit P, et al. Severe soft tissue infections of the extremities in patients admitted to an intensive care unit. Clin Microbiol Infect 2005;11:79–82.

29. Steinmetz D, Berkovits E, Edelstein H, et al. Home intravenous antibiotic therapy programme, 1999. J Infect 2001;42(3):176–80.

30. Corwin P, Toop L, McGeoch G, et al. Randomized controlled trial of intravenous antibiotic treatment for cellulitis at home compared with hospital. BMJ 2005;330:129–34.

31. Weigelt J, Itani K, Stevens D, et al. Linezolid versus vancomycin in treatment of complicated skin and soft tissue infections. Antimicrob Agents Chemother 2005;49(6):2260–6.

32. Sharpe JN, Shively EH, Polk HC Jr. Clinical and economic outcomes of oral linezolid versus intravenous vancomycin in the treatment of MRSA-complicated, lower-extremity skin and soft-tissue infections caused by methicillin-resistant *Staphylococcus aureus*. Am J Surg 2005;189(4):425–8.

33. Menzin J, Maton JP, Meyers JL, et al. Inpatient treatment patterns, outcomes, and costs of skin and skin structure infections because of *Staphylococcus aureus*. Am J Infect Control 2010;38:44–9.

34. Goettsch WG, Bouwes Bavinck JN, Herings RMC. Burden of illness of bacterial cellulitis and erysipelas of the leg in the Netherlands. J Eur Acad Dermatol Venereol 2006;20:834–9.

35. Marton JP, Jackel JL, Carson RT, et al. Costs of skin and skin structure infections due to *Staphylococcus aureus*: an analysis of managed care claims. Curr Med Res Opin 2008;24(10):2821–8.

36. Perl B, Gottehrer NP, Raveh D, et al. Cost-effectiveness of blood cultures for adult patients with cellulitis. Clin Infect Dis 1999;29:1483–8.

37. Wolff K, Johnson RA. Fitzpatrick's color atlas & synopsis of clinical dermatology. 6th edition. New York: McGraw-Hill; 2009. p. 693–759.

38. Panackal AA, Halpern EF, Watson AJ. Cutaneous fungal infections in the United States: Analysis of the National Ambulatory Medical Care Survey (NAMCS) and National Hospital Ambulatory Medical Care Survey (NHAMCS), 1995-2004. Int J Dermatol 2009;48:704–12.

39. Havlickova B, Czaika VA, Friedrich M. Epidemiological trends in skin mycoses worldwide. Mycoses 2008;51(Suppl 4):2–15.

40. Nelson MM, Martin AG, Hefferman MP. Superficial fungal infections: dermatophytosis, onychomycosis, tinea nigra, piedra. In: Fitzpatrick TB, editor. 6th edition, Dermatology in General Medicine, vol. 2. New York: McGraw-Hill; 2003. p. 1989–2005.

41. Aly R. Ecology and epidemiology of dermatophyte infections. J Am Acad Dermatol 1994;31:S21–5.

42. Foster KW, Ghannoum MA, Elewski BE. Epidemiologic surveillance of cutaneous fungal infection in the United States from 1999 to 2002. J Am Acad Dermatol 2004;50:748–52.

43. Vander Straten MR, Hossain MA, Ghannoum MA. Cutaneous infections: dermatophytosis, onchomycosis, and tinea versicolor. Infect Dis Clin North Am 2003;17:87–112.

44. Kemna ME, Elewski BE. A US epidemiologic survey of superficial fungal diseases. J Am Acad Dermatol 1996;35:539–42.

45. Ameen M. Epidemiology of superficial fungal infections. Clin Dermatol 2010;28:197–201.

46. Macura AB. Dermatophyte infections. Int J Dermatol 1993;32:313–23.

47. Keller RA, Henderson DB. Superficial fungal infections. In: Fitzpatrick JE, Morelli JG, editors. Dermatology secrets plus. 4th edition. Philadelphia: Elsevier; 2011. p. 216–23.

48. High WA. Fungal Infections. In: Elston DE, editor. Infectious diseases of the skin. Washington: Manson; 2009. p. 34–59.

49. Elewski BE. Onchomycosis: treatment, quality of life, and economic issues. Am J Clin Dermatol 2000;1(1):19–26.

50. Ghannoum M, Hajjeh R, Scher R, et al. A large-scale North American study of fungal isolates from nails: the frequency of onychomycosis, fungal distribution, and antifungal susceptibility patterns. J Am Acad Dermatol 2000;43:641–8.

51. Elewski B. Prevalence of onychomycosis in patients attending a dermatology clinic in northeastern Ohio for other conditions. Arch Dermatol 1999;133:1172–3.

52. Sobera JO, Elewski BE. Fungal infections. In: Bolognia JL, Jorizzo JL, Rapini RP, et al, editors. Dermatology. New York: Mosby; 2008. p. 1135–63.

53. Smith ES, Fleischer AB, Feldman SR, et al. Characteristics of office-based physician visits for cutaneous fungal infections: an analysis of 1990 to 1994 National Ambulatory Medical Care Survey Data. Cutis 2002;69:191–202.

54. Zuber T, Baddam K. Superficial fungal infection of the skin: where and how it appears help determine therapy. Postgrad Med 2001;109:117–32.

55. Bickers DR, Lim HW, Margolis D, et al. The burden of skin diseases: 2004. A joint project of the American Academy of Dermatology Association and the Society for Investigative Dermatology. J Am Acad Dermatol 2006;55(3):490–500.

56. Zhang AY, Camp WL, Elewski BE. Advances in topical and systemic antifungals. Dermatol Clin 2007;25:165–83.

57. Lin P, Torres G, Tyring SK. Changing paradigms in dermatology: antivirals in dermatology. Clin Dermatol 2003;21:426–46.

58. Whitley RJ, Rolzman B. Herpes simplex virus infections. Lancet 2001;357:1513–8.

59. Fatahzadeh M, Schwartz RA. Herpes simplex virus infections: epidemiology, pathogenesis, symptomatology, diagnosis, and management. J Am Acad Dermatol 2007;57(5):737–63.

60. Miller CS, Danaher RJ, Jacob RJ. Molecular aspects of herpes simplex virus I latency, reactivation, and recurrence. Crit Rev Oral Biol Med 1998;9(4):541–62.

61. Trizna Z. Viral diseases of the skin: diagnosis and antiviral treatment. Paediatr Drugs 2002;4(1):9–19.

62. Vander Straten M, Carrasco D, Lee P, et al. A review of antiviral therapy for herpes labialis. Arch Dermatol 2001;137:1232–5.

63. Wald A, Zeh J, Selke S, et al. Reactivation of genital herpes simplex virus type 2 in asymptomatic seropositive persons. N Engl J Med 2000;342(12): 844–50.

64. Tateishi K, Toh Y, Minagawa H, et al. Detection of herpes simplex virus (HSV) in the saliva from 1000 oral surgery outpatients by the polymerase chain reaction (PCR) and virus isolation. J Oral Pathol Med 1994;23:80–4.

65. Brown TJ, Yen-Moore A, Tyring SK. An overview of sexually transmitted diseases. Part I. J Am Acad Dermatol 1999;41:511–29.

66. Chakrabarty A, Beutner K. Therapy of other viral infections: herpes to hepatitis. Dermatol Ther 2004; 17:465–90.

67. Cernik C, Gallina K, Brodell RT. The treatment of herpes simplex infections, an evidence-based review. Arch Intern Med 2008;168:1137–44.

68. Mertz GJ. Epidemiology of genital herpes infections. Infect Dis Clin North Am 1993;7:825–39.

69. Siegel D, Golden E, Washington AE, et al. Prevalence and correlates of herpes simplex infections. The population-based AIDS in Multiethnic Neighborhoods Study. JAMA 1992;268(13):1702–8.

70. Fleming DT, McQuillan GM, Johnson RE, et al. Herpes simplex virus type 2 in the United States 1976 to 1994. N Engl J Med 1997;337(16):1105–11.

71. Xu F, Sternberg MR, Kottiri BJ, et al. Trends in herpes simplex virus type 1 and type 2 seroprevalence in the United States. JAMA 2006;296:964–73.

72. Viera MH, Amini S, Huo R, et al. Herpes simplex virus and human papillomavirus genital infections: new and investigational therapeutic options. Int J Dermatol 2010;49:733–49.

73. Centers for Disease Control and Prevention. Sexually transmitted diseases treatment guidelines 2002. MMWR Recomm Rep 2002;51:1–78.

74. Brady RC, Bernstein DI. Treatment of herpes simplex virus infections. Antiviral Res 2004;61:73–81.

75. Evans TY, Tyring SK. Advances in antiviral therapy in dermatology. Dermatol Clin 1998;16:409–20.

76. Spruance SL, Stewart JCB, Rowe NH, et al. Treatment of recurrent herpes simplex labialis with oral acyclovir. J Infect Dis 1990;161:185–90.

77. Spruance SL, Jones TM, Blatter MM, et al. High-dose, short-duration, early valacyclovir therapy for episodic treatment of cold sores: results of two randomized, placebo-controlled, multicenter studies. Antimicrob Agents Chemother 2003;47:1072–80.

78. Mubareka S, Leung V, Aoki FY, et al. Famciclovir: a focus on efficacy and safety. Expert Opin Drug Saf 2010;9(4):643–58.

79. Vigil KJ, Chemaly RF. Valcyclovir: approved and off-label uses for the treatment of herpes virus infections in immunocompetent and immunocompromised individuals. Expert Opin Pharmacother 2010;11(11): 1901–13.

80. Spruance SL, Rea TL, Thoming C, et al. Penciclovir cream for the treatment of herpes simplex labialis. A randomized, multicenter, double-blind, placebo-controlled trial. JAMA 1997;277:1374–9.

81. Wald A, Carrell D, Remington M, et al. Two-day regimen of acyclovir for treatment of recurrent genital herpes simplex virus type 2 infection. Clin Infect Dis 2002;34:944–8.

82. Sacks SL, Aoki FY, Diaz-Mitoma F, et al. Patient-initiated, twice-daily oral famciclovir for early recurrent genital herpes. A randomized, double-blind multicenter trial. JAMA 1996;276:44–9.

83. Tyring SK, Douglas JM, Corey L, et al. A randomized, placebo-controlled comparison of oral valacyclovir and acyclovir in immunocompetent patients with recurrent genital herpes infections. Arch Dermatol 1998;143:185–91.

84. Spruance SL, Tyring SK, DeGregorio B, et al. A large-scale, placebo-controlled, dose-ranging trial of peroral valaciclovir for episodic treatment of recurrent herpes genitalis. Arch Intern Med 1996; 156:1729–35.

85. Bacon TH, Boon RJ, Schultz M, et al. Surveillance for antiviral-agent-resistant herpes simplex virus in the general population with recurrent herpes labialis. Antimicrob Agents Chemother 2002;46(9):3042–4.

86. Ziyaeyan M, Alborzi A, Japoni A, et al. Frequency of acyclovir-resistant herpes simplex viruses isolated from the general immunocompetent population and patients with acquired immunodeficiency syndrome. Int J Dermatol 2007;46:1263–6.

87. Danve-Szatanek C, Aymard M, Thouvenot D, et al. Surveillance network for herpes simplex virus resistance to antiviral drugs: 3-year follow-up. J Clin Microbiol 2004;42(1):242–9.

88. Stranska R, Schuurman R, Nienhuis E, et al. A survey of acyclovir-resistant herpes simplex virus in the Netherlands: prevalence and characterization. J Clin Virol 2005;32:7–18.

89. Chen Y, Scieux C, Garrait V, et al. Resistant herpes simplex virus type 1 infection: an emerging concern after allogenic stem cell transplantation. Clin Infect Dis 2000;31(4):927–35.

90. Chilukuri S, Rosen T. Management of acyclovir-resistant herpes simplex virus. Dermatol Clin 2003;21:311–20.

91. White RR, Lenhart G, Singhal PK, et al. Incremental 1-year medical resource utilization and costs for patients with herpes zoster from a set of US health plans. Pharmacoeconomics 2009;27(9):781–92.

92. Tao G, Kassler WJ, Rein DB. Medical care expenditures for genital herpes in the United States. Sex Transm Dis 2000;27(1):32–8.

Needs Assessment for General Dermatologic Surgery

Jonathan M. Olson, MD[a], Murad Alam, MD, MSCI[b,c,d,*],
Maryam M. Asgari, MD, MPH[e,f]

KEYWORDS

- Skin cancer • Actinic keratoses • Melanoma
- Surgical excision

Key Points

- There are several effective treatment modalities for actinic keratoses, including cryotherapy and photodynamic therapy; and for small, low-risk, nonmelanoma skin cancers, including electrodesiccation and curettage, and excision
- For invasive skin cancers and other higher-risk skin cancers, surgical excision is the most effective treatment
- Surgical excision with appropriate margins remains the treatment of choice for melanoma
- Most important recommendation: Large, randomized controlled trials with long duration of follow-up are needed to better delineate the comparative effectiveness of different nonexcisional methods for the treatment of nonmelanoma skin cance

---

Dermatologic surgery includes Mohs surgery, excisional surgery of benign and malignant lesions, other destructive modalities to treat benign and malignant lesions, cutaneous procedures with lasers and energy devices, cosmetic fillers and injectables, and major cosmetic procedures such as liposuction and surgical skin lifts. The cumulative breadth and depth of dermatologic surgery comprises an increasing and integral part of the practice of dermatology. However, there is little evidence to support many aspects of current practice. This article discusses the evidence for general dermatologic surgical procedures, excluding Mohs (discussed in an article elsewhere in this issue) and cosmetic or laser procedures (also discussed in another article in this issue by Asgari and colleagues; and Alam and colleagues elsewhere in this issue).

The authors outline current data and key issues pertaining to cryosurgery, electrodesiccation and curettage, and excisional surgery for malignant and premalignant lesions. Indications, techniques,

---

[a] Division of Dermatology, Department of Medicine, University of Washington School of Medicine, 1959 NE Pacific Street, Room BB-1353, Box 356524, Seattle, WA 98195, USA
[b] Department of Dermatology, Northwestern University Feinberg School of Medicine, 676 North Saint Clair Street, Suite 1600, Chicago, IL 60611, USA
[c] Department of Otolaryngology-Head and Neck Surgery, Northwestern University Feinberg School of Medicine, 676 North Saint Clair Street, Suite 1325, Chicago, IL 60611, USA
[d] Department of Surgery, Northwestern University Feinberg School of Medicine, 251 East Huron Street, Chicago, IL 60611, USA
[e] Division of Research, Kaiser Permanente Northern California, 2000 Broadway, Oakland, CA 94612, USA
[f] Department of Dermatology, University of California at San Francisco, 1701 Divisadero Street, 3rd Floor, San Francisco, CA 94115, USA
* Corresponding author. Department of Dermatology, Northwestern University Feinberg School of Medicine, 676 North Saint Clair Street, Suite 1600, Chicago, IL 60611.
E-mail address: m-alam@northwestern.edu

Dermatol Clin 30 (2012) 153–166
doi:10.1016/j.det.2011.08.011
0733-8635/12/$ – see front matter © 2012 Elsevier Inc. All rights reserved

and effectiveness and outcomes are discussed, and ill-defined areas for future research are highlighted.

CRYOSURGERY
Background

Cryosurgery was introduced at the turn of twentieth century, but was not popularized for the treatment of skin cancers until the 1960s and has been in widespread use since.[1] Liquid nitrogen exists at a temperature of −195°C, and is sufficient to induce tissue temperatures in the −50°C to −60°C range, which are adequate for tissue destruction.[2]

Technique

Cryotherapy is rapid, simple, well tolerated, and effective, though there are few randomized controlled trials documenting its effectiveness, and variation in technique makes generalization of results difficult. Techniques include intralesional, direct-contact, and open-spray techniques, all with or without the use of a thermocouple to directly monitor temperature. Most current use entails use of the open-spray technique with the so-called cryo-gun, which simultaneously permits storage of cryogen and a constant rate of spray discharge. There is no consensus on the number of freeze-thaw cycles, the amount of surrounding tissue that should be frozen, or the appropriate thaw time. In general, malignant lesions require a more prolonged freeze, which is associated with deeper penetration and a higher volume of tissue destruction. Much of the current data is from large case series,[1,3] short of the gold standard of randomized, prospective trials. Several comparative trials, discussed below, have methodological shortcomings, using substandard freezing times or too few cycles of cryotherapy, with predictably poor results. Still needed are large, well-designed, prospective, randomized studies.

Indications

Cryosurgery is recommended for treatment of actinic keratoses (AK) and nonmelanoma skin cancer (NMSC) in recommendations from the British Association of Dermatologists (BAD),[2] American Academy of Dermatologists (AAD),[4] and National Comprehensive Cancer Network (NCCN).[5] A 2011 review found better cosmesis and lower recurrence rates with surgical excision, as well as a preference among both patients and providers for surgical excision over cryotherapy in treatment of NMSC.[6] Because of the uncertainty in appropriate technique and general lack of high-quality data, NCCN guidelines recommend that in patients with low-risk shallow cancers, such as squamous cell carcinoma (SCC) in situ (SCC-IS) or low-risk superficial basal carcinoma, vigorous cryotherapy may be considered.[5] In clinical practice in the United States, cryotherapy is used mostly for the treatment of AK and benign lesions (eg, verruca vulgaris).

Actinic Keratoses

Cryosurgery is very effective in the treatment of AK, with a cure rate of nearly 99% in a large retrospective series.[7] In direct comparison trials, cryotherapy has been shown to be both equivalent to[8] and inferior to[9] photodynamic therapy in the treatment of AK. However, the trial that showed equivalence used 2 cycles of cryotherapy[8] whereas the second trial used a single cycle of cryotherapy with only 20 seconds of thaw time,[9] highlighting the problem of variability in technique. Given the high prevalence of AK and the number and location of typical lesions, cryotherapy remains a recommended standard treatment by both the AAD[10] and the BAD.[11] In the United States, it is the first-line treatment for AK.

Basal Cell Carcinoma and Squamous Cell Carcinoma

At present, there are insufficient data to permit routine recommendation of cryotherapy for treatment of nonmelanoma skin cancer, notwithstanding the relatively impressive cure rates reported in large series. The BAD guidelines recommend cryotherapy for treatment of low-risk basal cell carcinoma (BCC)[2] and "caution" in using cryotherapy for SCC.[12] This sentiment is echoed in the NCCN guidelines, which state "since cure rates can be lower, superficial therapies should be reserved for those patients where surgery or radiation is contraindicated or impractical."[5]

A 1990 article by Graham and Clark[3] compared the results of more than 20 years of data from both their clinic and that of Zacarian,[1] with a combined 6800 patients and 9267 skin cancers, 8124 of which were BCC (87%), with the remainder including SCC, SCC-IS, lentigo maligna, keratoacanthoma (KA), and Kaposi sarcoma. Both open-spray and direct-probe techniques with a single freeze-thaw cycle were used for most lesions, and a double cycle was used for those tumors deemed more resistant because of location, size, depth, or history of recurrence. A thermocouple was used, with at least 60 seconds of measured thaw time. Documented 5-year cure rates were 97% for BCC, 97% for SCC, and 97% for all other lesions treated. Cure rates were nearly identical in the series from Zacarian, using a double freeze-thaw cycle.[1,3] A more recent series from 2004, also using a double freeze-thaw cycle and the open-spray technique, included 30 years of treatment and 4406 new and recurrent BCC and SCC, with an overall cure rate of 98.6%.[13] A randomized trial of cryotherapy versus photodynamic therapy for SCC-IS noted a relatively poor response rate at 1 year of 67%, but closer inspection reveals that a single cycle of cryotherapy, maintained for "a minimum of 20 seconds," is likely far below the required time for adequate treatment.[14] Part of the problem with using cryotherapy for malignant lesions is the uncertainty regarding the duration of the freeze-thaw cycle and the lack of routine availability of thermocouples to monitor temperature. As a consequence, recurrence rates in clinical practice are unacceptably high, and cryotherapy is not routinely used for treatment of nonmelanoma skin cancer in the United States. An ancillary process is the peripheral damage to normal tissue induced by a prolonged freeze-thaw cycle, and the attendant posttreatment tissue necrosis, pain, delayed healing, loss of function, and scarring.

A single randomized trial has been done comparing curettage plus cryotherapy (n = 51) with surgical excision (n = 49) in the treatment of BCC. The investigators found a trend toward higher recurrence rates with cryosurgery, though not statistically significant, and concluded that "owing to the trend toward lower recurrence rates, better cosmetic results, and reduced wound healing time, we believe that SE [surgical excision] should be preferred to C&C [curettage and cryotherapy] in the treatment of primary, nonaggressive BCC of the head and neck."[15]

ELECTROSURGERY
Background

Combined curettage and electrosurgery is often referred to as electrodesiccation and curettage (ED&C). Curettes are typically semisharp rather than surgically honed, to allow separation and sparing of normal tissue from less cohesive tumor tissue by feel. In ED&C, electrofulguration (ie, electrical current arcs without direct tissue contact) or electrodesiccation (ie, probe tip contacts tissue) are typically performed, causing only superficial tissue destruction.[16] Electrocautery, which causes deeper destruction and potentially more extensive scarring, has fallen out of favor largely because of functional and cosmetic concerns associated with

deep scars, including the risk of persistent pain as well as sensory and muscle restriction.

Curettage alone without electrodesiccation leaves positive tumor margins in up to 30% of cases,[17,18] 47% on the head and neck in one series.[19] The high rate of residual tumor compared with the relatively lower rate of clinical recurrence is not entirely understood, and is not readily explained by the possible antitumor effect of inflammation or the healing process.[17,18] In part, the low recurrence rate may be artifactual because the follow-up periods for most studies are brief, and tumors may have recurred after these periods.

Indications and Advantages

ED&C is rapid, well tolerated, simple, safe, effective, and economic.[16] Disadvantages include prolonged healing time, sometimes larger scars, and lack of histologic confirmation of surgical margins. Guidelines are discussed here.

Technique

Technique varies, though most investigators describe curettage followed by electrodesiccation (or electrofulguration), with the cycle repeated 1 to 3 times.[2,12,16,20] A retrospective study from 2006 using curettage alone in treatment of BCC reported 5-year cure rates of 96%.[21] Another study advocating curettage only reported better cosmetic outcome without electrodesiccation, though the cure rate was a lower 90% and objective measurement of cosmesis was lacking.[22] A 1983 study compared 1 versus 3 rounds of ED&C in BCC, with all lesions excised via Mohs surgery to examine margins. After one round of treatment 45% had residual tumor present, compared with 37% of those treated with 3 rounds. No statistical analysis was performed, and clinical follow-up and cure rates were not assessed.[20]

Basal Cell Carcinoma

ED&C is included in the 1992 AAD guidelines for treatment of BCC.[4] The NCCN guidelines regarding BCC state that ED&C is deemed effective for low-risk tumors with several qualifications: (1) not on hair-bearing sites, because of possible extension down follicular units; (2) if the subcutis is reached, excision should be performed, because the ability to detect normal versus tumor tissue by feel is lost; and (3) if ED&C is done without a prior biopsy based on low-risk appearance, biopsy should be taken at the time of curettage.[5] The BAD guidelines conclude that "curettage and cautery is a good treatment for low-risk BCC."[2]

A 1987 review found a recurrence rate of 7.7% for BCC treated with ED&C, compared with 10% for surgical excision and 7.5% for cryosurgery.[23] A prospective study of recurrence rates for more than 600 NMSC with greater than 6 years of follow-up, published in 2011, found recurrence rates of 1.6% for ED&C and 4.2% for excision.[24] A 1991 series of 2314 primary BCC treated by ED&C found 5-year recurrence rates of 3.3% on low-risk sites (neck, trunk, extremities), 5.3% on middle-risk sites (scalp, forehead, preauricular and postauricular, malar area), and 4.5% on high-risk sites (nose, paranasal, nasal-labial groove, ear, chin, and mandibular, perioral, and periocular areas).[25] It is significant that re-currence rates for various modalities are not often directly comparable because treatments are seldom assigned randomly, and even in prospective cohort studies, more aggressive lesions are more frequently treated with modalities that permit histologic margin assessment, such as surgical excision or Mohs surgery.

Squamous Cell Carcinoma

Most guidelines recommend that ED&C for SCC be limited to small, low-risk lesions—well-defined primary tumors 1 cm or less in diameter on the neck, trunk, arms, legs, or sun-exposed sites.[12,16,26] ED&C is not considered appropriate for recurrent SCC or high-risk lesions, as defined by Rowe and colleagues[27] (discussed later). A 2007 review by Neville and colleagues[28] con-cluded that "curettage and electrodesiccation is not suitable for treating recurrent tumors, lesions larger than 2 cm in diameter, tumors extending into the fat, tumors at sites of high risk for recur-rence, or lesions with ill-defined borders." A 2007 review found cumulative 5-year cure rates of 92% for SCC treated by ED&C. The investigators noted a recurrence rate of 4.5% to 17.6% in high-risk locations (nose, paranasal region, naso-labial fold, ear, chin, and mandible, perioral, and periocular areas), compared with a 3.3% recur-rence rate on the trunk and extremities.[28] A small (n = 14) retrospective study of ED&C versus exci-sion from 2010 found no statistically significant difference in cure rates, but again there is the issue of selection bias, with more aggressive lesions likely treated with excision.[29] A recently published prospective cohort study found that of 127 NMSCs treated with ED&C, only 2 recurred over a mean 6.6-year follow-up period.[24] However, the tumors that were treated with ED&C in this study tended to be BCCs on the trunk and extrem-ities, and it is difficult to draw any conclusions regarding suitability of SCC treatment with ED&C.

This low recurrence rate for select superficial BCCs treated with ED&C is promising. No randomized controlled trials have been done comparing ED&C with other modalities in the treatment of BCCs or SCC.

Current guidelines recommend against the rou-tine use of ED&C for treatment of NMSC on the head and face.[26] The evidence supporting these assertions comes from retrospective reviews only, and virtually every author cited herein recommends against use of ED&C for SCC with any of the high-risk criteria defined by Rowe and colleagues[27] (dis-cussed later). In a retrospective review of NMSC treated with either excision or ED&C (72% BCCs, 28% SCCs), 64% were on the head and neck, and recurrence rates for the two modalities were not statistically significant.[30] A retrospective review of 281 SCC treated with ED&C reported a 98% cure rate at 4 years, which included 29 SCCs on the lower lip treated with ED&C, with a cure rate of 89.6%. As already noted, the highest recurrence rates, up to 17.6%, were seen on the face.[28]

At present, there are insufficient data to recom-mend the use of ED&C for routine treatment of SCC on the head and neck. Use of ED&C for SCC on the head and neck remains extremely controversial, and is considered by many practitioners to be insufficient management for this potentially metastatic tumor. For SCC in situ in particular, borders are usually ill defined, and a focal ED&C is very likely to leave a "halo" of malignant cells that can then grow laterally and even invasively. For most SCCs, excluding those at very low risk, excision modalities are preferred because of their ability to verify clear margins.

Lentigo Maligna and Lentigo Maligna Melanoma

Dysplastic melanocytes are known to extend down hair follicles, and may extend well beyond the visible clinical margin of a lentigo maligna.[16] Two retro-spective studies evaluated ED&C in the treatment of lentigo maligna and lentigo maligna melanoma, and both showed inferior cure rates compared with excision, with the investigators recommending against the use of ED&C.[31,32] In the United States, best practice and medicolegal considerations generally preclude the removal of any melanoma, in situ or invasive, by nonexcisional modalities be-cause nonexcisional treatments cannot establish histologic tumor depth or margin negativity.

PHOTODYNAMIC THERAPY
Background

Photodynamic therapy (PDT) uses a photosensi-tizer that is activated by light of a specific wavelength, causing direct cell damage and apoptosis in the target tissue.[33] The use of photosensitizers evolved from eosin red dye in the early twentieth century to hematoporphyrin derivative–based PDT, which uses the porphyrin precursors 5-aminolevulinic acid (5-ALA, or ALA) and its methyl ester form, methylaminolevulinate (MAL). Both agents, applied topically, have good tissue penetration and preferential uptake in altered cells, and are converted to photosensitizing protoporphyrin IX in target tissue.[33,34] ALA is now also available in a liposomal form with enhanced penetration[35] and as a patch,[35,36] both of which show promise in early trials.

ALA, MAL, and other porphyrins maximally absorb light in the Soret band, approximately 405 to 430 nm (the blue spectrum of visible light), with smaller peaks, called Q bands, from 500 to 635 nm (the red spectrum).[34] As wavelength increases, so does depth of penetration—blue light penetrates only to the level of the epidermis, red light at 630 nm penetrates up to 5 mm, or to the level of the reticular and deep dermis, and wavelengths of 700 to 800 nm may penetrate as deep as 1 to 2 cm.[33] Because of these absorption peaks, most studies have used blue and red light sources (white and green exist but are inferior[33,37]), and while blue light is commonly used for intraepidermal processes, only red-light PDT is recommended for nonmelanoma skin cancer.[33] Increased depth of penetration can also be associated with increased pain, the most frequent side effect of PDT treatment, which can be dose and treatment limiting. ALA was associated with significantly more pain when directly compared with MAL in one study.[38] However, differences in the quantity of photosensitizer applied, the surface area of skin treated, the preexisting health and integrity of the treated skin, individual patient variation, the type of light source, and the duration of light exposure are more likely to affect pain than the type of photosensitizer used. For instance, it has been shown that use of daylight is as effective and less painful for activating MAL than the conventional red light associated with standard PDT.[39]

Indications

In the United States, the only use of both ALA-PDT and MAL-PDT approved by the Food and Drug Administration is in treatment of AK. In Canada, PDT is approved for the treatment of AK and BCC, and in 18 European countries, New Zealand, and Australia it is approved for the treatment of AK, BCC, and cutaneous SCC-IS or Bowen disease.[40] Since 2009, the ALA patch has been approved with red light for the treatment of AK in Europe as well.[33] PDT is recommended as treatment for AK and selected lower-risk NMSC in guidelines from the BAD,[41] the NCCN,[5] and the International Society for Photodynamic Therapy.[42] No randomized trials have directly compared PDT with surgical excision for NMSC.

Actinic Keratoses

Both ALA-PDT and MAL-PDT have proven efficacy in treating AK in multiple prospective, randomized, controlled, multicenter trials.[33,41,42] In prospective randomized trials, MAL-PDT showed both equivalent[8] and superior response to cryosurgery,[9] and has been evaluated in a prospective, double-blind, placebo-controlled trial, with 89% remission in the treatment group compared with 38% for placebo.[43] A prospective, randomized, double-blind trial also showed efficacy in treatment and prevention of AK in transplant patients.[44] PDT also has a cosmetic advantage over cryotherapy in the treatment of AK when compared in an intraindividual, right-left manner.[45] Specifically, PDT is less likely to cause focal hypopigmentation than cryotherapy. PDT also has the theoretical advantage of providing a field effect for widespread AK prophylaxis in patients with very extensive actinic damage; in the United States, cryotherapy is used for more focal treatment of AK. Of course, patients with focally restricted AK may better tolerate cryotherapy.

Basal Cell Carcinoma

PDT is effective in treating superficial BCC, though studies reveal much less effectiveness for destruction of other BCC subtypes. The range of reported recurrence rates for superficial BCC is broad, 0% to 31%.[46] The combined clearance rates in 12 case series was 87% for superficial BCC and 53% for nodular BCC.[33] A prospective, open, uncontrolled multicenter trial of patients with superficial and nodular BCC showed 92% clearance for superficial BCC and 87% clearance for nodular BCC at 3 months, clearly an insufficient follow-up period. At 2 years, still an insufficient follow-up period, overall recurrence rate was elevated to 18%.[47] PDT is much less effective than excisional modalities for BCC, and vastly less effective than Mohs surgery, which has a 5-year recurrence rate of 1% for BCC.[48] The use of PDT in treatment of BCC is likely to obtain a field effect (eg, reduction in size and quantity, but not overall cure) in patients who have numerous superficial BCCs, or in patients who cannot tolerate surgery.

Squamous Cell Carcinoma in Situ (Bowen Disease)

There are very limited data regarding the utility of PDT for treatment of SCC. In 2003 a randomized, phase 3 trial compared ALA-PDT with 5-fluoro-uracil cream, with 82% and 42% clearance at 1 year, respectively.[49] A multicenter randomized, placebo-controlled trial from 2006 compared MAL-PDT with cryotherapy and 5-fluorouracil cream, with statistically significant response rates of 80%, 69%, and 67%, for PDT, topical 5-fluorouracil, and cryotherapy, respectively, but the differences were not statistically significant.[14] Overall, the limited size and number of comparative studies, the unacceptably brief follow-up periods, and the theoretical risks associated with a nonexcisional modality for SCC strongly militate against routine use of PDT for the treatment of SCC. It has been suggested that cosmetic outcome is excellent when SCC is treated with PDT, but this is not a convincing argument in the absence of long-term efficacy data.

Acne

PDT is postulated to work in part because *Proprionibacterium acnes* produces endogenous coproporphyrin III,[33] in addition to purely anti-inflammatory effects.[50-52] There is evidence that PDT is effective in the treatment of inflammatory acne, including a prospective, randomized, blinded, placebo-controlled trial with MAL-PDT[50] and a randomized, controlled, investigator-blinded trial with MAL-PDT.[51] Both showed significant improvement in acne lesions with severe side effects, including pain, erythema, edema, exfoliation, vesiculation, pustular eruptions, and hyperpigmentation.[33] Until recently PDT did not appear to be a viable choice in routine treatment of acne, largely because of side effects.[50-52] More recently, it has been shown that a series of 3 treatments with long-incubation PDT activated by red light can induce a prolonged remission in nodulocystic acne approaching the effectiveness of isotretinoin.[53,54] This treatment is associated with substantial recovery time, posttreatment erosions, and severe edema, and patients have to be appropriately counseled. However, it may be a useful alternative for patients with nodulocystic acne who are unable to tolerate or unwilling to consider isotretinoin.

Other Indications

Psoriasis is unlikely to respond to PDT. The results of a small 2006 prospective randomized, double-blind phase 2/3 intrapatient comparison study[55] and a 2005 randomized intrapatient study both found unsatisfactory treatment results with ALA-PDT, plus a high number of dose-limiting side effects. There is a single small study that indicates ALA-PDT may be useful in preventing progression of morphea,[56] and a study of 12 patients showing some benefit in vulvar lichen sclerosis.[57] It was well tolerated in both series, with side effects limited to mild pruritus and discomfort.

EXCISIONS
Atypical Nevi

An atypical or dysplastic nevus (also known as Clark nevus or nevus with architectural disorder) is a clinically abnormal mole that is a risk factor for melanoma and may individually evolve into melanoma. For an individual atypical nevus, the risk of progression to melanoma is estimated to be 1 in 10,000, and overall risk of developing melanoma increases with the number of atypical nevi.[58,59] Estimates of increased melanoma risk range from 2 to 12-fold compared with controls, rising as the number of clinically atypical nevi increases, though no firm relationship or cutoff has been established.[60] There is no standard definition of clinical atypia or of which nevi merit excision, though there is literature support for use of the "ABCDE" system, the so-called ugly duckling sign, the Glasgow 7-point checklist, and use of dermoscopy, including the Menzies method.[61] Excisional biopsy of a clinically atypical nevus often involves complete removal with 2- to 3-mm margins of clinically normal-appearing skin.[60] National Institutes of Health consensus criteria were established in 1992, with suggested reexcision margins of 2 to 5 mm for histologically atypical nevi,[62] but do not include specific indications for reexcision. Recommendations are also hampered by the lack of a precise histologic definition of atypia,[60] as well as variation among pathologists in defining and grading atypia.[63] Some pathologists do not acknowledge the existence of atypical nevi as a precursor lesion for melanoma, and prefer to classify all pigmented lesions as either melanoma or not melanoma. Further, clinical atypia and histologic atypia do not always correlate in type and degree, and the term "atypical" or "dysplastic" is routinely used to describe either clinically or histologically abnormal variants. Histologic appearance is generally considered more convincing. Various systems are used by pathologists to subclassify nevi in either 3 tiers, as mild, moderate, and severe atypia,[61] or a 2-tiered system of low-grade and high-grade atypia.[65] It is unclear whether routine reexcision of histologically moderately dysplastic nevi is warranted, despite widespread practice.[66] Although a recent study found that recurrence rates for atypical nevi (including moderate atypia) with a positive margin were extremely low, with only 3.6% recurrence after 2 years compared with a 3.3% recurrence rate in benign dermal nevi with positive margins,[67] short duration of follow-up and the dearth of similar studies makes this finding of dubious validity. In practice, moderately and severely atypical or dysplastic nevi are routinely reexcised, with severely atypical nevi often surgically treated in a manner similar to melanoma in situ. A further complicating feature resulting in this conservative management is variation among pathologists regarding grading of the degree of atypia, and the boundary between severe atypia and melanoma.

Melanoma

Surgical treatment of melanoma has undergone substantial evolution since Sampson Handley recommended 5-cm surgical margins in 1907 based on a single autopsy.[68,69] That standard stood for much of the twentieth century, and current recommendations retain modest ambiguity: the 2001 guidelines from the AAD recommend 5-mm margins for melanoma in situ, 1-cm margins for invasive melanoma up to 2 mm thick, and 2-cm margins for invasive melanoma greater than 2 mm in thickness[70]; the more current NCCN guidelines differ slightly, recommending 1 to 2-cm margins for tumors between 1 and 2 mm thick,[71] with the same recommendations from the BAD.[72,73]

There is evidence that wider excision affects locoregional recurrence without affecting overall mortality. Two prospective, randomized controlled trials from Sweden, in 2000 and 2003, compared 2-cm and 5-cm margins for melanoma less than 2 mm thick, and found no difference in local recurrence and melanoma-specific survival.[74,75] A 2002 meta-analysis found that margins greater than 1 cm had no impact on disease-free or overall survival for melanomas less than 2 mm thick,[76] and a 2003 meta-analysis found that overall survival, disease-free survival, and recurrence rates were not improved with margins greater than 2 cm.[71] A prospective trial of melanoma greater than 2 mm thick found a higher recurrence rate with 1-cm margins than with 3-cm margins, though there was no impact on overall survival.[77] A Cochrane review from 2009 noted "current randomised [sic] trial evidence is insufficient to address optimal excision margins for primary cutaneous melanoma."[78]

Surgical guidelines regarding depth are less clear. Current recommendations include excision to subcutaneous fat for melanoma in situ, to fascia for all other melanomas.[70,72,79] No prospective trials have assessed this issue, and a 2010 survey study by DeFazio and colleagues noted the lack of scientific support for current recommendations, with significant differences among practitioners in depth of excision for various forms of melanoma.[80] In routine clinical practice, it is not uncommon for conservative management to entail, when feasible, excision to fascia for severely atypical nevus and melanoma in situ.

Debulking and Additional Margin Assessment

Debulking of the complete extent of melanoma and melanoma in situ is frequently performed to assess the lesion depth, and hence determine the appropriate margin. Some lesions initially diagnosed as melanoma in situ may turn out to display invasive foci, thus mandating more extensive surgical treatment, with wider margins and deeper extirpation. Similarly, after melanomas are removed by Mohs surgery, an additional rim of tissue may be excised and sent for permanent section verification of margins.[81]

In theory, cytoreductive surgery, or debulking of primary tumors could potentiate the effect of systemic treatment, with some evidence in dogs[82] and metastatic renal cell carcinoma in humans.[83] To date, there is no evidence that cytoreductive surgery is palliative or curative in metastatic melanoma, and may subject patients to needless morbidity.

Nonmelanoma Skin Cancer

Current NCCN guidelines regard surgical excision as first-line treatment for NMSC.[5] Two extensive reviews found that surgical excision had the lowest recurrence rate among standard treatments for nonmelanoma skin cancers. In 1992 Rowe and colleagues[27] examined all literature from 1940 to 1990 for SCC, and in 2007 Neville and colleagues[28] examined PubMed from inception until 2006 for both SCC and BCC.

Basal Cell Carcinoma

NCCN guidelines recommend 4-mm margins for low-risk BCC and Mohs surgery for high-risk BCC, defined as lesions greater than 20 mm on the trunk and extremities, greater than 10 mm on the face, poorly defined borders, recurrence, systemic immunosuppression, or occurrence at a site of radiation,[5] with this echoed by the BAD.[2] In two prospective trials from the 1960s, recurrence rates were greater than 30% when the margin was positive. When margins were more than 0.5 mm clear microscopically, recurrence dropped to 1.2%; with recurrence of intermediate margins (0–0.5 mm) 12%.[84] Very similar numbers were reported in a recent study.[85] A prospective study in 1987 examined BCC with skin marking followed by Mohs removal. When tumor diameter was less than 2 cm, a 4-mm margin led to complete histologic clearance in 95% of cases.[86] Tumors larger than 2 cm had a statistically significantly higher and unpredictable rate of subclinical extension, with lower clearance rate.[86] A prospective trial in 2003 excised lesions suspicious for either BCC or SCC without a prior biopsy. Analysis of 1-, 2-, 3-, and 4-mm surgical margins showed that a 4-mm margin would provide at least 0.5 mm of microscopically clear margins in 96% of cases.[87] Of significance, from the standpoint of tissue sparing at functionally and cosmetically sensitive sites, a difference of several millimeters in margin (multiplied by 2 for diameter) may often result in qualitatively different healing or repair, with consequent differences in final structure and function.

Squamous Cell Carcinoma

The BAD recommends 4-mm margins for low-risk SCC, 6-mm margins for larger tumors, and Mohs surgery for "high-risk" tumors.[12] The NCCN guidelines are similar, though 4- to 6-mm margins are recommended for lower-risk primary cutaneous SCC.[5] The question of surgical margins has not been well studied in SCC, with no prospective, randomized trials to the authors' knowledge.

The review by Rowe and colleagues[27] established risk factors for increased risk of recurrence in SCC, including (1) diameter greater than 2 cm, (2) depth greater than 4 mm, (3) Clark levels IV and V, (4) poor histologic differentiation, (5) high-risk sites (ear, lip, within scars, non–sun-exposed skin, local recurrence), (6) histologic evidence of perineural involvement, and (7) immunosuppression. Surgical margins in the reviewed studies were variable. For studies with follow-up of 5 years or longer, surgical excision had a recurrence rate of 8.1% compared with 3.0% for Mohs surgery, followed by ED&C at 3.7% and radiation monotherapy at 10.0%.[27] These rates are not strictly comparable because selection bias likely resulted in higher-risk lesions receiving excisions with microscopically controlled margins, or Mohs surgery.

Most recent literature relies heavily on the 1992 work of Brodland and Zitelli,[88] who used Mohs surgery to establish surgical margins for SCC based on microscopic examination, not on clinical

recurrence or outcome. These investigators found that a 4-mm margin completely removed well-defined tumors less than 2 cm in size 95% of the time. For larger tumors, those extending into subcutaneous tissue, and those in high-risk locations (ear, lip, scalp, eyelids, and nose), 6 mm was required for 95% likelihood of clearance.

Keratoacanthoma

Margin recommendations are 4 to 6 mm, the same as those established for standard SCC.[5,12] There are no prospective controlled trials examining surgical margins in the treatment of keratoacanthoma.

Some controversy remains as to whether KA is a benign neoplasm or a subset of SCC, though molecular evidence favors the squamous cell lineage.[89] In controlled experiments pathologists have not been able to easily distinguish KA from SCC using a small set of criteria.[90] Lesions that clinically or histologically appear to be KA that exhibit aggressive growth or resistance to conservative therapies must be reclassified as SCC. Some investigators advocate surgical management before other modalities (5-fluorouracil, imiquimod, oral isotretinoin, intralesional methotrexate, intralesional interferon-2α),[91] though there is no clear standard.

Rare Tumors

Numerous rare and uncommon tumors beyond those discussed here are routinely treated with wide local excision, but space precludes discussing each of them in turn. Of note, Mohs surgery may be appropriate as an excisional modality for each of these, but this treatment is discussed in the article by Asgari and colleagues elsewhere in this issue on Mohs surgery in order to avoid redundancy.

Dermatofibrosarcoma protuberans
Dermatofibrosarcoma protuberans (DFSP) is an uncommon, low-grade, but locally aggressive sarcoma with extensive subclinical extension and frequent local recurrences. Published recurrence rates with surgical excision are 23% with 4-cm margins and 60% with standard surgical excision (2–4 mm).[92] A 2007 meta-analysis found that 4-cm margins were theoretically required for 95% likelihood of clearance of even small to moderate-sized DFSP.[93] A 2009 retrospective comparison of Mohs and wide surgical excision (4 cm) showed more frequent positive margins with wide excision, but no significant difference in recurrence rates; however, the duration of follow-up was likely insufficient to capture

recurrences associated with positive margins in this indolent, slow-growing tumor.[94]

Merkel cell carcinoma

Merkel cell carcinoma (MCC) is a rare but increasingly frequent and very aggressive malignancy, with a high rate of local recurrence, and likelihood of distant metastasis and mortality. With regard to surgical excision, NCCN guidelines for MCC suggest the following: If surgical excision without intraoperative margin assessment is used, a 1- to 2-cm margin should be removed, deep to investing fascia of the muscle or pericranium.[95] Adjuvant management, including referral to a tumor board, lymph node management, and radiation treatment, may be routinely required. Local recurrence exceeds 25% to 30%, regional disease is found in 50% to 60% of patients, and distant metastases occur in 35% of cases.[96]

Atypical fibroxanthoma

Atypical fibroxanthoma (AFX) is a fibrohistiocytic tumor of intermediate malignant potential, with excellent prognosis in general, but rare reports of metastasis and death.[97] A retrospective comparison found no recurrences in 59 cases treated with Mohs surgery, whereas the recurrence rate in the wide local excision group was 8.7% (2 of 23).[98] Margin analysis showed that 2 cm was required for 95% clearance. There are no randomized controlled trials comparing treatment modalities or surgical margins in AFX, and no standardized treatment guidelines.

OTHER TOPICS
Buffering Anesthesia

Although acidity of local anesthetics has not been definitively established as a cause of increased pain with injection, there is credible evidence that buffering with sodium bicarbonate to achieve a more basic solution can decrease pain. A review from 2003 included 63 publications, 22 of which were prospective randomized trials, and found unequivocal evidence that buffering decreased pain with local anesthesia while not affecting onset, duration, or quality of the block. There was some degradation in stability of the anesthetic solutions, particularly solutions that also contained epinephrine. Slower speed of injection and smaller-gauge needle were also favorably associated with decreased pain.[99]

Dissenting literature does exist. A 2010 prospective, randomized, double-blind study of inferior alveolar nerve blocks found that a sodium bicarbonate buffer did not increase the anesthetic success, result in less pain with injection, or provide faster onset of anesthesia.[100] Use of anesthesia in nerve blocks may not be strictly comparable with its use for intradermal infiltration.

Suture Material, Needle Type, and Suturing Technique

A thorough discussion of suture choice is beyond the scope of this article. There are a few prospective trials on which to base recommendations, with choices largely a function of surgeon preference and habit. In dermatologic surgery, a 3/8 reverse cutting needle, in which the convex surface is sharpened, is most commonly used for optimal handling and minimal tissue damage with needle passage. A standard cutting needle, whose concave surface is sharpened, in theory can lead to suture pull-through. Braided or multifilament sutures may be easier to handle than monofilament because they have less "memory," but monofilaments may pass through tissue more smoothly with less snagging and may be associated with lower rates of infection.[101] It is not clear that suture choice directly affects cosmesis, despite case series extolling the virtues of various materials. Readers are referred to a thorough review of suture materials from 2009 for further detail.[101]

Surgical technique is also a very broad subject, with few prospective trials to guide decision making. Of the myriad suture techniques available—simple interrupted, running, running locked, mattress (horizontal, vertical, running), running subcuticular, purse-string, and so forth—the best choice is highly subjective and a matter of surgeon preference and skill. The specific choice of suture technique is likely largely guided by the surgeon's level of expertise with specific techniques, and the surgeon's assessment regarding which techniques from his or her repertoire is best suited for a particular patient or surgical defect.[102] Understanding of anatomy, gentle tissue handling, good eversion of skin edges, and avoiding compromise of blood supply have been mentioned as necessary accompaniments of good suture technique, but none of these factors have been well studied regarding their impact on the function or appearance of closures. Prospective comparative studies enlisting multiple surgeons with equivalent expertise and randomizing patients to different suturing techniques are largely lacking.

Surgical Dressings: Occlusion and Antibiotics

Postoperative wound care is a vital part of the healing process, and there has been a substantial paradigm shift over the last half of the prior century, with the understanding that keeping a wound occluded and moist promotes healing. However, choice of the most appropriate agent from the bewildering variety of topical preparations and dressings is unclear. It is also unclear at present that antibiotic-containing topical preparations offer any advantage in prevention of infection over nonmedicated preparations in clean surgical wounds. A review of surgical wound care found that antibiotic ointments can accelerate wound healing in comparison with vehicle controls. However, the incidence of allergic contact dermatitis, particularly from neomycin, was as high as 34%, and the development of resistance and/or selection of gram-negative organisms is a valid concern. For routine postoperative wound care, plain petrolatum is an effective, low-cost, less antigenic/allergenic choice.[103] More studies are needed to accurately assess optimization of risk with topical antibiotic use, as well as cost and effectiveness of dressing materials.

Optimization of Scarring

Prevention and treatment of postsurgical scarring is a controversial subject, with few good-quality data. In addition to the proven effect of moist wound healing, silicone gel sheeting and an onion extract–based topical gel (Mederma; Merz Pharmaceuticals, Frankfurt am Main, Germany) have been touted for both prevention of postsurgical scarring and treatment of existing scars. A 2006 Cochrane review of silicone gel sheeting found weak evidence of benefit and concluded that trials "are of poor quality and highly susceptible to bias" and "a great deal of uncertainty prevails."[104] A 2006 prospective, double-blind, placebo-controlled trial found that onion extract–based topical gel was no better than plain petrolatum at improving cosmesis or adverse symptoms associated with scars.[105] However, the study was small (n = 24) with limited follow-up (up to 12 weeks in person, 11 months by phone), limiting the applicability of results. Modalities purported to improve scars may seem more successful in clinical practice than in experimental paradigms because scars improve spontaneously over time, with tissue remodeling resulting in flattening, erythema reduction, and contraction over a period of months to years.

SUMMARY

Lower-risk NMSCs at sites off the face can be treated effectively with a range of modalities, including electrodesiccation and surgical excision. AK can be treated effectively with cryotherapy and photodynamic therapy. Virtually all melanomas are treated with excisional modalities. Lower-risk cutaneous SCCs are more likely than BCCs to require treatment with excisional modalities, with SCC of the head and neck rarely treated with

any modality except some form of surgical excision. Several uncommon and rare NMSCs may be appropriately treated with surgical excision (Mohs surgery is discussed in an article by Asgari and colleagues elsewhere in this issue).

Of significance, it is difficult to compare cure and recurrence rates associated with different surgical and procedural modalities for treatment of NMSC. Physicians do not randomly assign patients to disparate treatments (indeed, in the United States patients and Institutional Review Boards may consider such selection unethical and impermissible), and more definitive excisional modalities that permit histologic margin verification are likely used for higher-risk lesions, which are more likely to recur.

Anesthetic selection, suturing technique, intraoperative tissue handling, and wound dressings have been poorly studied. There is little indication as to which techniques are better for optimizing functional and cosmetic outcomes and for minimizing the risks of hypertrophic scar and other adverse events, such as infection. Comparative studies are difficult to perform because of differences in surgeons' technique preferences and their varying levels of expertise with different techniques; further, patients may decline being randomly assigned to particular study arms, and may instead exhort the operating surgeon to use the "best" available technique.

List of Acronyms	
5-ALA or ALA	5-aminolevulinic acid
AAD	American Academy of Dermatologists
AFX	Atypical fibroxanthoma
AK	Actinic keratoses
BAD	British Association of Dermatologists
BCC	Basal cell carcinoma
DFSP	Dermatofibrosarcoma protuberans
ED&C	Electrodesiccation and curettage
KA	Keratoacanthoma
MAL	Methylaminolevulinate
MCC	Merkel cell carcinoma
NCCN	National Comprehensive Cancer Network
NMSC	Nonmelanoma skin cancer
PDT	Photodynamic therapy
SCC	Squamous cell carcinoma
SCC-IS	In situ SCC

REFERENCES

1. Zacarian SA. Cryosurgery of cutaneous carcinomas. An 18-year study of 3,022 patients with 4,228 carcinomas. J Am Acad Dermatol 1983; 9(6):947–56.
2. Telfer NR, Colver GB, Morton CA. Dermatologists BAo. Guidelines for the management of basal cell carcinoma. Br J Dermatol 2008;159(1):35–48.
3. Graham GF, Clark LC. Statistical analysis in cryosurgery of skin cancer. Clin Dermatol 1990;8(1): 101–7.
4. Drake LA, Ceilley RI, Cornelison RL, et al. Guidelines of care for basal cell carcinoma. The American Academy of Dermatology Committee on Guidelines of Care. J Am Acad Dermatol 1992; 26(1):117–20.
5. Miller S, Alam M, Anderson J, et al. Basal and squamous cell skin cancers, Version 1.2011. 2011. Available at: http://www.nccn.org/professionals/physician_gls/f_guidelines.asp. Accessed June 6, 2011.
6. Galiczynski EM, Vidimos AT. Nonsurgical treatment of nonmelanoma skin cancer. Dermatol Clin 2011; 29(2):297–309, x.
7. Lubritz RR, Smolewski SA. Cryosurgery cure rate of actinic keratoses. J Am Acad Dermatol 1982;7(5): 631–2.
8. Szeimies RM, Karrer S, Radakovic-Fijan S, et al. Photodynamic therapy using topical methyl 5-aminolevulinate compared with cryotherapy for actinic keratosis: a prospective, randomized study. J Am Acad Dermatol 2002;47(2):258–62.
9. Freeman M, Vinciullo C, Francis D, et al. A comparison of photodynamic therapy using topical methyl aminolevulinate (Metvix) with single cycle cryotherapy in patients with actinic keratosis: a prospective, randomized study. J Dermatolog Treat 2003;14(2):99–106.
10. Drake LA, Ceilley RI, Cornelison RL, et al. Guidelines of care for actinic keratoses. Committee on Guidelines of Care. J Am Acad Dermatol 1995; 32(1):95–8.
11. de Berker D, McGregor JM, Hughes BR. Subcommittee BAoDTGaA. Guidelines for the management of actinic keratoses. Br J Dermatol 2007;156(2): 222–30.
12. Motley R, Kersey P, Lawrence C. Dermatologists BAo, Surgeons BAoP. Multiprofessional guidelines for the management of the patient with primary cutaneous squamous cell carcinoma. Br J Plast Surg 2003;56(2):85–91.
13. Kuflik EG. Cryosurgery for skin cancer: 30-year experience and cure rates. Dermatol Surg 2004; 30(2 Pt 2):297–300.
14. Morton C, Horn M, Leman J, et al. Comparison of topical methyl aminolevulinate photodynamic therapy with cryotherapy or fluorouracil for treatment of squamous cell carcinoma in situ: results of a multicenter randomized trial. Arch Dermatol 2006;142(6): 729–35.
15. Kuijpers DI, Thissen MR, Berretty PJ, et al. Surgical excision versus curettage plus cryosurgery in the treatment of basal cell carcinoma. Dermatol Surg 2007;33(5):579–87.
16. Sheridan AT, Dawber RP. Curettage, electrosurgery and skin cancer. Australas J Dermatol 2000;41(1): 19–30.
17. Nouri K, Spencer JM, Taylor JR, et al. Does wound healing contribute to the eradication of basal cell carcinoma following curettage and electrodesiccation? Dermatol Surg 1999;25(3):183–7 [discussion: 187–8].
18. Spencer JM, Tannenbaum A, Sloan L, et al. Does inflammation contribute to the eradication of basal cell carcinoma following curettage and electrodesiccation? Dermatol Surg 1997;23(8):625–30 [discussion: 630–1].
19. Suhge d'Aubermont PC, Bennett RG. Failure of curettage and electrodesiccation for removal of basal cell carcinoma. Arch Dermatol 1984;120 (11):1456–60.
20. Edens BL, Bartlow GA, Haghighi P, et al. Effectiveness of curettage and electrodesiccation in the removal of basal cell carcinoma. J Am Acad Dermatol 1983;9(3):383–8.
21. Barlow JO, Zalla MJ, Kyle A, et al. Treatment of basal cell carcinoma with curettage alone. J Am Acad Dermatol 2006;54(6):1039–45.
22. Reymann F. 15 years' experience with treatment of basal cell carcinomas of the skin with curettage. Acta Derm Venereol Suppl (Stockh) 1985;120:56–9.
23. Rowe DE, Carroll RJ, Day CL. Long-term recurrence rates in previously untreated (primary) basal cell carcinoma: implications for patient follow-up. J Dermatol Surg Oncol 1989;15(3):315–28.
24. Chren MM, Torres JS, Stuart SE, et al. Recurrence after treatment of nonmelanoma skin cancer: a prospective cohort study. Arch Dermatol 2011; 147(5):540–6.
25. Silverman MK, Kopf AW, Grin CM, et al. Recurrence rates of treated basal cell carcinomas. Part 2: curettage-electrodesiccation. J Dermatol Surg Oncol 1991;17(9):720–6.
26. Alam M, Ratner D. Cutaneous squamous-cell carcinoma. N Engl J Med 2001;344(13):975–83.
27. Rowe DE, Carroll RJ, Day CL. Prognostic factors for local recurrence, metastasis, and survival rates in squamous cell carcinoma of the skin, ear, and lip. Implications for treatment modality selection. J Am Acad Dermatol 1992;26(6):976–90.
28. Neville JA, Welch E, Leffell DJ. Management of nonmelanoma skin cancer in 2007. Nat Clin Pract Oncol 2007;4(8):462–9.

29. Reschly MJ, Shenefelt PD. Controversies in skin surgery: electrodesiccation and curettage versus excision for low-risk, small, well-differentiated squamous cell carcinomas. J Drugs Dermatol 2010;9(7):773–6.

30. Werlinger KD, Upton G, Moore AY. Recurrence rates of primary nonmelanoma skin cancers treated by surgical excision compared to electrodesiccation-curettage in a private dermatological practice. Dermatol Surg 2002;28(12): 1138–42 [discussion: 1142].

31. Pitman GH, Kopf AW, Bart RS, et al. Treatment of lentigo maligna and lentigo maligna melanoma. J Dermatol Surg Oncol 1979;5(9):727–37.

32. Coleman WP, Davis RS, Reed RJ, et al. Treatment of lentigo maligna and lentigo maligna melanoma. J Dermatol Surg Oncol 1980;6(6):476–9.

33. Babilas P, Schreml S, Landthaler M, et al. Photodynamic therapy in dermatology: state-of-the-art. Photodermatol Photoimmunol Photomed 2010; 26(3):118–32.

34. Alexiades-Armenakas M. Laser-mediated photodynamic therapy. Clin Dermatol 2006;24(1):16–25.

35. Christiansen K, Bjerring P, Troilius A. 5-ALA for photodynamic photorejuvenation—optimization of treatment regime based on normal-skin fluorescence measurements. Lasers Surg Med 2007; 39(4):302–10.

36. Szeimies RM, Stockfleth E, Popp G, et al. Long-term follow-up of photodynamic therapy with a self-adhesive 5-aminolaevulinic acid patch: 12 months data. Br J Dermatol 2010;162(2):410–4.

37. Morton CA, Whitehurst C, Moore JV, et al. Comparison of red and green light in the treatment of Bowen's disease by photodynamic therapy. Br J Dermatol 2000;143(4):767–72.

38. Moloney FJ, Collins P. Randomized, double-blind, prospective study to compare topical 5-aminolaevulinic acid methylester with topical 5-aminolaevulinic acid photodynamic therapy for extensive scalp actinic keratosis. Br J Dermatol 2007; 157(1):87–91.

39. Wiegell SR, Haedersdal M, Philipsen PA, et al. Continuous activation of PpIX by daylight is as effective as and less painful than conventional photodynamic therapy for actinic keratoses; a randomized, controlled, single-blinded study. Br J Dermatol 2008;158(4):740–6.

40. Ortiz-Policarpio B, Lui H. Methyl aminolevulinate-PDT for actinic keratoses and superficial nonmelanoma skin cancers. Skin Therapy Lett 2009;14 (6):1–3.

41. Morton CA, McKenna KE, Rhodes LE, et al. Guidelines for topical photodynamic therapy: update. Br J Dermatol 2008;159(6):1245–66.

42. Braathen LR, Szeimies RM, Basset-Seguin N, et al. Guidelines on the use of photodynamic therapy for nonmelanoma skin cancer: an international consensus. International Society for Photodynamic Therapy in Dermatology, 2005. J Am Acad Dermatol 2007;56(1):125–43.

43. Pariser DM, Lowe NJ, Stewart DM, et al. Photodynamic therapy with topical methyl aminolevulinate for actinic keratosis: results of a prospective randomized multicenter trial. J Am Acad Dermatol 2003;48(2):227–32.

44. Dragieva G, Prinz BM, Hafner J, et al. A randomized controlled clinical trial of topical photodynamic therapy with methyl aminolaevulinate in the treatment of actinic keratoses in transplant recipients. Br J Dermatol 2004;151(1):196–200.

45. Morton C, Campbell S, Gupta G, et al. Intraindividual, right-left comparison of topical methyl aminolaevulinate-photodynamic therapy and cryotherapy in subjects with actinic keratoses: a multicentre, randomized controlled study. Br J Dermatol 2006;155(5):1029–36.

46. Marmur ES, Schmults CD, Goldberg DJ. A review of laser and photodynamic therapy for the treatment of nonmelanoma skin cancer. Dermatol Surg 2004;30(2 Pt 2):264–71.

47. Horn M, Wolf P, Wulf HC, et al. Topical methyl aminolaevulinate photodynamic therapy in patients with basal cell carcinoma prone to complications and poor cosmetic outcome with conventional treatment. Br J Dermatol 2003;149(6):1242–9.

48. Thissen MR, Neumann MH, Schouten LJ. A systematic review of treatment modalities for primary basal cell carcinomas. Arch Dermatol 1999;135(10): 1177–83.

49. Salim A, Leman JA, McColl JH, et al. Randomized comparison of photodynamic therapy with topical 5-fluorouracil in Bowen's disease. Br J Dermatol 2003;148(3):539–43.

50. Hörfelt C, Funk J, Frohm-Nilsson M, et al. Topical methyl aminolaevulinate photodynamic therapy for treatment of facial acne vulgaris: results of a randomized, controlled study. Br J Dermatol 2006;155(3):608–13.

51. Wiegell SR, Wulf HC. Photodynamic therapy of acne vulgaris using methyl aminolaevulinate: a blinded, randomized, controlled trial. Br J Dermatol 2006;154(5):969–76.

52. Hongcharu W, Taylor CR, Chang Y, et al. Topical ALA-photodynamic therapy for the treatment of acne vulgaris. J Invest Dermatol 2000;115(2):183–92.

53. Sakamoto FH, Lopes JD, Anderson RR. Photodynamic therapy for acne vulgaris: a critical review from basics to clinical practice: part I. Acne vulgaris: when and why consider photodynamic therapy? J Am Acad Dermatol 2010;63(2):183–93 [quiz: 193–4].

54. Sakamoto FH, Torezan L, Anderson RR. Photodynamic therapy for acne vulgaris: a critical review

from basics to clinical practice: part II. Understanding parameters for acne treatment with photodynamic therapy. J Am Acad Dermatol 2010;63(2): 195–211 [quiz: 211–2].

55. Schleyer V, Radakovic-Fijan S, Karrer S, et al. Disappointing results and low tolerability of photodynamic therapy with topical 5-aminolaevulinic acid in psoriasis. A randomized, double-blind phase I/II study. J Eur Acad Dermatol Venereol 2006;20(7):823–8.

56. Karrer S, Abels C, Landthaler M, et al. Topical photodynamic therapy for localized scleroderma. Acta Derm Venereol 2000;80(1):26–7.

57. Hillemanns P, Untch M, Pröve F, et al. Photodynamic therapy of vulvar lichen sclerosis with 5-aminolevulinic acid. Obstet Gynecol 1999;93(1):71–4.

58. Holly EA, Kelly JW, Shpall SN, et al. Number of melanocytic nevi as a major risk factor for malignant melanoma. J Am Acad Dermatol 1987;17(3):459–68.

59. Bauer J, Garbe C. Acquired melanocytic nevi as risk factor for melanoma development. A comprehensive review of epidemiological data. Pigment Cell Res 2003;16(3):297–306.

60. Friedman RJ, Farber MJ, Warycha MA, et al. The "dysplastic" nevus. Clin Dermatol 2009;27(1): 103–15.

61. Tran KT, Wright NA, Cockerell CJ. Biopsy of the pigmented lesion—when and how. J Am Acad Dermatol 2008;59(5):852–71.

62. NIH Consensus conference. Diagnosis and treatment of early melanoma. JAMA 1992;268(10):1314–9.

63. Shapiro M, Chren MM, Levy RM, et al. Variability in nomenclature used for nevi with architectural disorder and cytologic atypia (microscopically dysplastic nevi) by dermatologists and dermatopathologists. J Cutan Pathol 2004;31(8):523–30.

64. Shea CR, Vollmer RT, Prieto VG. Correlating architectural disorder and cytologic atypia in Clark (dysplastic) melanocytic nevi. Hum Pathol 1999; 30(5):500–5.

65. Pozo L, Naase M, Cerio R, et al. Critical analysis of histologic criteria for grading atypical (dysplastic) melanocytic nevi. Am J Clin Pathol 2001;115(2): 194–204.

66. Fung MA. Terminology and management of dysplastic nevi: responses from 145 dermatologists. Arch Dermatol 2003;139(10):1374–5.

67. Goodson AG, Florell SR, Boucher KM, et al. Low rates of clinical recurrence after biopsy of benign to moderately dysplastic melanocytic nevi. J Am Acad Dermatol 2010;62(4):591–6.

68. Handley W. The pathology of melanocytic growths in relation to their operative treatment [lecture I]. Lancet 1907;1:927–33.

69. Handley W. The pathology of melanocytic growths in relation to their operative treatment [lecture II]. Lancet 1907;1:996–1003.

70. Sober AJ, Chuang TY, Duvic M, et al. Guidelines of care for primary cutaneous melanoma. J Am Acad Dermatol 2001;45(4):579–86.

71. Haigh PI, DiFronzo LA, McCready DR. Optimal excision margins for primary cutaneous melanoma: a systematic review and meta-analysis. Can J Surg 2003;46(6):419–26.

72. Miller S, Alam M, Anderson J, et al. Melanoma. 2011. Available at: http://www.nccn.org/profession als/physician_gls/f_guidelines.asp. Accessed June 7, 2011.

73. Roberts DL, Anstey AV, Barlow RJ, et al. U.K. guidelines for the management of cutaneous melanoma. Br J Dermatol 2002;146(1):7–17.

74. Cohn-Cedermark G, Rutqvist LE, Andersson R, et al. Long term results of a randomized study by the Swedish Melanoma Study Group on 2-cm versus 5-cm resection margins for patients with cutaneous melanoma with a tumor thickness of 0.8–2.0 mm. Cancer 2000;89(7):1495–501.

75. Khayat D, Rixe O, Martin G, et al. Surgical margins in cutaneous melanoma (2 cm vs 5 cm for lesions measuring less than 2.1-mm thick). Cancer 2003; 97(8):1941–6.

76. Lens MB, Dawes M, Goodacre T, et al. Excision margins in the treatment of primary cutaneous melanoma: a systematic review of randomized controlled trials comparing narrow vs wide excision. Arch Surg 2002;137(10):1101–5.

77. Thomas JM, Newton-Bishop J, A'Hern R, et al. Excision margins in high-risk malignant melanoma. N Engl J Med 2004;350(8):757–66.

78. Sladden MJ, Balch C, Barzilai DA, et al. Surgical excision margins for primary cutaneous melanoma. Cochrane Database Syst Rev 2009;4: CD004835.

79. Doherty V. Cutaneous melanoma. A national clinical guideline. 2007. Available at: http://www.guidelines. gov/content.aspx?id=3877. Accessed May 15, 2011.

80. DeFazio JL, Marghoob AA, Pan Y, et al. Variation in the depth of excision of melanoma: a survey of US physicians. Arch Dermatol 2010;146(9):995–9.

81. Dawn ME, Dawn AG, Miller SJ. Mohs surgery for the treatment of melanoma in situ: a review. Dermatol Surg 2007;33(4):395–402.

82. Emms SG. Anal sac tumours of the dog and their response to cytoreductive surgery and chemotherapy. Aust Vet J 2005;83(6):340–3.

83. Flanigan RC, Salmon SE, Blumenstein BA, et al. Nephrectomy followed by interferon alfa-2b compared with interferon alfa-2b alone for metastatic renal-cell cancer. N Engl J Med 2001; 345(23):1655–9.

84. Pascal RR, Hobby LW, Lattes R, et al. Prognosis of "incompletely excised" versus "completely excised" basal cell carcinoma. Plast Reconstr Surg 1968; 41(4):328–32.

85. Liu FF, Maki E, Warde P, et al. A management approach to incompletely excised basal cell carcinomas of skin. Int J Radiat Oncol Biol Phys 1991; 20(3):423–8.

86. Wolf DJ, Zitelli JA. Surgical margins for basal cell carcinoma. Arch Dermatol 1987;123(3):340–4.

87. Thomas DJ, King AR, Peat BG. Excision margins for nonmelanotic skin cancer. Plast Reconstr Surg 2003;112(1):57–63.

88. Brodland DG, Zitelli JA. Surgical margins for excision of primary cutaneous squamous cell carcinoma. J Am Acad Dermatol 1992;27(2 Pt 1):241–8.

89. Sarabi K, Selim A, Khachemoune A. Sporadic and syndromic keratoacanthomas: diagnosis and management. Dermatol Nurs 2007;19(2):166–70.

90. Cribier B, Asch P, Grosshans E. Differentiating squamous cell carcinoma from keratoacanthoma using histopathological criteria. Is it possible? A study of 296 cases. Dermatology 1999;199(3):208–12.

91. Ratner D. Keratoacanthoma. SKINmed 2004;3(1): 45–6.

92. Gloster HM. Dermatofibrosarcoma protuberans. J Am Acad Dermatol 1996;35(3 Pt 1):355–74 [quiz: 375–6].

93. Kimmel Z, Ratner D, Kim JY, et al. Peripheral excision margins for dermatofibrosarcoma protuberans: a meta-analysis of spatial data. Ann Surg Oncol 2007;14(7):2113–20.

94. Meguerditchian AN, Wang J, Lema B, et al. Wide excision or Mohs micrographic surgery for the treatment of primary dermatofibrosarcoma protuberans. Am J Clin Oncol 2010;33(3):300–3.

95. Miller S, Alam M, Anderson J, et al. Merkel cell carcinoma. 2011. Available at: http://www.nccn.org/professionals/physician_gls/f_guidelines.asp. Accessed June 7, 2011.

96. Medina-Franco H, Urist MM, Fiveash J, et al. Multimodality treatment of Merkel cell carcinoma: case series and literature review of 1024 cases. Ann Surg Oncol 2001;8(3):204–8.

97. Iorizzo LJ, Brown MD. Atypical fibroxanthoma: a review of the literature. Dermatol Surg 2011; 37(2):146–57.

98. Ang GC, Roenigk RK, Otley CC, et al. More than 2 decades of treating atypical fibroxanthoma at mayo clinic: what have we learned from 91 patients? Dermatol Surg 2009;35(5):765–72.

99. Davies RJ. Buffering the pain of local anaesthetics: a systematic review. Emerg Med (Fremantle) 2003; 15(1):81–8.

100. Whitcomb M, Drum M, Reader A, et al. A prospective, randomized, double-blind study of the anesthetic efficacy of sodium bicarbonate buffered 2% lidocaine with 1:100,000 epinephrine in inferior alveolar nerve blocks. Anesth Prog 2010;57(2):59–66.

101. Hochberg J, Meyer KM, Marion MD. Suture choice and other methods of skin closure. Surg Clin North Am 2009;89(3):627–41.

102. Adams B, Anwar J, Wrone DA, et al. Techniques for cutaneous sutured closures: variants and indications. Semin Cutan Med Surg 2003;22(4): 306–16.

103. Cho CY, Lo JS. Dressing the part. Dermatol Clin 1998;16(1):25–47.

104. O'Brien L, Pandit A. Silicon gel sheeting for preventing and treating hypertrophic and keloid scars. Cochrane Database Syst Rev 2006;1: CD003826.

105. Chung VQ, Kelley L, Marra D, et al. Onion extract gel versus petrolatum emollient on new surgical scars: prospective double-blinded study. Dermatol Surg 2006;32(2):193–7.

Needs Assessment for Mohs Micrographic Surgery

Maryam M. Asgari, MD, MPH[a,b,*], Jonathan M. Olson, MD[c],
Murad Alam, MD, MSCI[d,e,f]

KEYWORDS

- Mohs micrographic surgery • Needs assessment
- Skin cancers

Mohs micrographic surgery (MMS) is a surgical treatment of skin cancer that couples tissue conservation with complete microscopic margin control, allowing for superior cure rates and minimizing deformity.[1] The utility of MMS is based on the observation that skin cancers often grow contiguously, with fingerlike projections that can invade deeply or laterally from the clinically visible tumor. Unlike traditional methods of tumor excision, which involve removal of the clinically visible tumor along with an additional margin of normal-appearing tissue, the advantage of MMS is that it allows minimal removal of normal-appearing tissue. This situation is because MMS involves immediate histologic evaluation of excised tumor tissue using horizontal frozen sections, which allows for rapid visualization of 100% of the surgical margins, as opposed to the traditional bread-loaf technique, which reveals less than 1% of the interface between the specimen and the patient.[2] With MMS, the performing physician renders both the surgical and pathologic services, and the tissue is sampled until it is determined to be tumor-free. MMS has become the treatment of choice for nonmelanoma skin cancers (NMSCs), consisting of basal cell carcinomas (BCCs) and squamous cell carcinomas (SCCs) with a high risk for local recurrence.

INDICATIONS

MMS is often indicated for NMSCs at high risk for local recurrence or possible significant functional or cosmetic impairment. Clinical morphology, anatomic location and size, histology (including level of invasion), patient immunity, and recurrence after previous treatment are criteria that can be used to determine the appropriate use of MMS for treating a cutaneous neoplasm. The indications for MMS, as outlined in the clinical guidelines currently adapted by Medicare for reimbursement[3] include the following:

1. BCC in anatomic locations where they are prone to recur including the mask area of the face that are mainly embryonic fusion planes (central face, eyelids, eyebrows, periorbital areas, nose, lips, chin, mandible, periauricular

[a] Division of Research, Kaiser Permanente Northern California, 2000 Broadway, Oakland, CA 94612, USA
[b] Department of Dermatology, University of California at San Francisco, 1701 Divisadero Street, 3rd Floor, San Francisco, CA 94115, USA
[c] Division of Dermatology, Department of Medicine, University of Washington School of Medicine, 1959 NE Pacific Street, Room BB-1353, Box 356524, Seattle, WA 98195, USA
[d] Department of Dermatology, Northwestern University Feinberg School of Medicine, 676 North Saint Clair Street, Suite 1600, Chicago, IL 60611, USA
[e] Department of Otolaryngology-Head and Neck Surgery, Northwestern University Feinberg School of Medicine, 676 North Saint Clair Street, Suite 1325, Chicago, IL 60611, USA
[f] Department of Surgery, Northwestern University Feinberg School of Medicine, 251 East Huran Street, Chicago, IL 60611, USA
* Corresponding author. Division of Research, Kaiser Permanente Northern California, 2000 Broadway, Oakland, CA 94612.
E-mail address: maryam.m.asgari@kp.org

Dermatol Clin 30 (2012) 167–175
doi:10.1016/j.det.2011.08.010

areas, ear, temple), scalp, forehead, cheeks, and neck, genitalia, hands, and feet

2. NMSCs that have 1 or more of the following features: recurrent or positive margin on recent excision; aggressive pathology in the hands and feet, genitalia, and nail unit/periungual; large size (2.0 cm or greater); poorly defined borders; age less than 40 years; radiation-induced; immunocompromised host; arising in an old scar (eg, a Marjolin ulcer); associated with xeroderma pigmentosum; deeply infiltrating lesion or difficulty estimating depth of lesion; perineural invasion on biopsy

3. SCCs showing any of the following: undifferentiated to poorly differentiated, adenoid (acantholytic), adenosquamous, desmoplastic, infiltrative, perineural, periadnexal, or perivascular, and verrucous; subtypes including Bowen disease (BCC in situ), erythroplasia of Queryrat, and verrucous carcinoma; although tumors treated with excision have a cure rate of 80%, the reported cure rate with Mohs surgery approaches 98%[4]

4. Basal cell nevus syndrome

5. Other cutaneous neoplasms: aside from BCCs and SCC, MMS can successfully treat a variety of cutaneous tumors, as outlined later. Although its use and application is clear in most instances, its use for the some tumors is controversial because of tumor characteristics (multifocality, discontinuous growth patterns) or technique limitations (inherent disadvantages of frozen sections vs permanent sections).

Keratoacanthoma

Keratoacanthomas (KAs) are rapidly growing, solitary, cutaneous tumors that can often spontaneously regress, but can cause significant local tissue destruction before regressing.[5–7] Some KA subtypes, such as giant KA (>20–30 mm in diameter), KA centrifugum marginatum, and subungual KA, can be difficult to surgically treat with a standard excision. Furthermore, some KAs can show aggressive histologic features, such as perineural invasion.[5] Predicting which KAs will behave aggressively (grow rapidly, cause extensive local tissue damage, invade nerves) is not always possible. Because of the unpredictability of spontaneous regression and their potentially destructive nature, recurrent KAs and KAs near vital structures (where tissue conservation is warranted) are ideally treated with MMS.[6] As a cautionary note, eruptive KAs can sometimes arise as a complication of skin excision including Mohs,[7] and in the case of eruptive KAs after surgery, other treatment modalities, such as

intralesional methotrexate or oral retinoids, should also be considered.

Dermatofibrosarcoma Protuberans

Dermatofibrosarcoma protuberans (DFSP) is an uncommon, slow-growing, fibrohistiocytic tumor that can be locally aggressive, with distant subclinical extension.[8–10] It is often treated with wide local excision with a margin of at least 3 cm down to the fascia. Despite the wide surgical margins, multiple recurrences are frequently reported, with a recurrence rate of approximately 49%. Histologic identification of the tumor margin can be difficult using frozen sections, because malignant cells may resemble normal fibroblasts. The supplemental use of CD 34 immunostain or excision of a conservative additional margin for permanent section can be useful in helping to delineate tumor clearance. MMS is well established for the treatment of primary and recurrent DFSPs and is suggested as the treatment of choice for DFSP.

Microcystic Adnexal Carcinoma

Microcystic adnexal carcinoma (MAC)[11–15] also referred to as sclerosing sweat duct carcinoma, is a more recently described, uncommon, malignant eccrine tumor that is known for its aggressive local invasion of tissue. MAC rarely metastasizes; however, it usually involves deep soft tissue and dermis and has a propensity for perineural invasion.[16] Because MAC grows contiguously, it is well suited for removal with MMS. Local recurrences after traditional excisional surgery approach 47%, usually within the first 3 years.[12] Five-year recurrence rate for MMS is less (0%–22%).[11] MMS should be strongly considered as a first-line modality for the treatment of MAC.

Atypical Fibroxanthoma

Atypical fibroxanthoma (AFX) is a low-grade malignancy that is most often seen in actinically damaged skin on the head and neck of elderly patients.[17,18] Compared with excision, MMS has been shown to provide superior cure rates for AFX. On average, the available follow-up for AFX treated with MMS is approximately 30.7 months; the average recurrence rate is 3%.[18] Fewer recurrences are seen with MMS compared with excision, suggesting that MMS may have better cure rates for this rare tumor.

Melanoma

Use of MMS in melanoma is still controversial because of the inherent difficulty in distinguishing melanoma cells from benign melanocytic proliferations on frozen section, and its use is mostly limited to anatomic locations that preclude use of conventional excision with appropriate margins.[19-21] The use of melanoma-specific immunostains (including S-100, HMB-45, Mart-5, and Melan-A) has helped overcome this barrier, but the time and cost of immunostains have limited widespread adoption of MMS for treatment of melanoma.

Other Rare Tumors

Many other cutaneous neoplasms listed later are treated by using MMS either alone or as part of an overall treatment approach for these unusual neoplasms. However, the small number of such cases precludes any conclusions about the usefulness of this technique.

  i. Angiosarcoma[22]
  ii. Sebaceous gland carcinoma[23,24]
  iii. Extramammary Paget disease[25,26]
  iv. Malignant fibrous histiocytoma[27]
  v. Leiomyosarcoma or other spindle cell neoplasms of the skin[28]
  vi. Adenocystic carcinoma of the skin[29,30]
  vii. Apocrine or eccrine carcinoma of the skin[31]
  viii. Merkel cell carcinoma.[32,33]

UTILIZATION

Mohs surgery is performed on more than 876,000 tumors per year in the United States[34] and that rate is rapidly increasing.[35] Approximately half of all MMS cases are performed on Medicare beneficiaries.[35] Analysis of Medicare claims data can therefore yield useful information on time trends in MMS utilization. Although a few NMSCs in the Medicare population are treated with MMS, its utilization is increasing at a faster rate than the use of other treatment modalities, such as excision. The rate of Mohs surgery per 1000 Medicare beneficiaries increased by 236% between 1999 and 2009, whereas excisions and destructions of lesions increased by approximately 20%. It is unclear to what extent the increasing rate of Mohs surgery utilization is because of the epidemic increase in the incidence of NMSC over time, and to the increasing availability of Mohs surgeons, who were in short supply until 10 to 20 years ago. It has been suggested that previous lower utilization rates were associated with a lack of availability of Mohs surgery services. Mohs surgery was more likely than surgical excision on the face and less likely elsewhere. Tumor location was associated with MMS utilization, with 47% of facial lesions and 15% of lesions on the rest of the body treated with MMS. Patient age, race, and geographic region were also significantly associated with the likelihood of Mohs surgery. The use of Mohs for these cancers decreased with patient age (from 41% of patients aged 67 to 69 years to 34% of patients 85 years or older). Mohs was used in 37% of white patients, 23% of black patients, and 29% of patients of other races. Areas with high densities of Mohs surgeons were likely to have higher rates of MMS; however, some areas with low densities still had high rates of Mohs utilization.[35] There was wide variation in regional MMS utilization and geographic disparity that warrants further investigation.

USE OF CURETTAGE BEFORE MOHS

There is no standardized procedure for determining tumor margins before removing the first stage during MMS. Some Mohs surgeons perform light curettage of the tumor, which not only debulks the friable tumor tissue to facilitate tissue processing, but more importantly, can potentially help delineate its margins. Preoperative curettage has the potential to reduce the number of Mohs surgical stages required for tumor clearance, potentially increasing practice efficiency and decreasing cost of care.[36] Several studies have examined the effectiveness of curettage in delineating tumor margins before MMS and have yielded different conclusions.[37-39] Jih and colleagues[39] studied 150 previously biopsied BCCs and SCCs less than 1.5 cm in size, dividing the study into 3 parts: (1) a retrospective study of 50 tumors curetted before MMS by a surgeon who routinely curettes preoperatively; (2) a prospective study in which a surgeon who routinely does not curette preoperatively curetted 50 tumors before MMS; and (3) a comparative historical group of 50 noncuretted tumors treated with Mohs surgery by the latter surgeon. Histologic evaluation of the curetted tissue revealed that only 50% had tumor in the curettings, but in 76% of these, the curette left residual tumor at the surgical margins. Of the remaining 50% in which the curette removed only noncancer–containing skin, 34% had tumor present at the surgical margin. Overall, the curette removed tumor, leaving no residual tumor at the surgical margins in only 12% of lesions. Comparison with historical noncuretted tumors operated on by the same surgeon showed that curettage did not affect the mean number of stages or the proportion of tumors requiring more than 1 stage for histologic clearance.

A prospective evaluation of 599 patients with biopsy-proven BCCs treated with MMS examined preoperative tumor size, curetted dimensions before the first surgical stage, proposed excisional margins before each surgical stage, and the final defect dimensions after each surgical stage were measured.[37] Results showed that the curetted margin exceeded the observed extent of each tumor in most cases. A 1-mm excisional margin taken in the first stage of Mohs surgery without first performing curettage would have necessitated an extra surgical stage in 99.0% of the cases. These investigators concluded that careful presurgical curettage significantly reduces the number of Mohs surgical stages required for BCC treatment.[37]

A recent study[38] compared visual inspection, curettage, and dermoscopy in determining tumor extent before initial margins are taken for MMS. These investigators randomized 54 patients into 3 groups to delineate residual tumor (visual inspection, curettage, or dermoscopy) before MMS for BCCs on the nose and recorded the final number of stages and postoperative defect sizes. They found no statistically significant differences for the final number of stages ($P = .20$) or the final defect sizes ($P = .47$) among the 3 arms.

Part of the discrepancy between these studies lays in their design. In the study by Jih and colleagues,[39] 100 of the 150 tumors studied were from the practice of 1 Mohs surgeon who, in all likelihood, did not value the use of curettage before MMS because he did not routinely use it in his practice. Results from a single surgeon, or a study in which 1 surgeon dominates the findings, may be prone to bias because of different value on the use of curettage and variation in technique (eg, differential application of pressure during curettage, number of passes). Also, in all studies, the outcome measures were not recorded by blinded observers, leading to the potential for further bias. To better answer this question, a study design is needed in which Mohs surgeons (balanced among those who favor and do not favor preoperative curettage) are randomized to curettage or none a priori, and rigorous blinded methodologies are used to measure outcomes. Until then, the value of preoperative curettage for MMS is still to be determined.

USE OF PROPHYLACTIC ANTIBIOTICS

There is considerable practice variation in the use of prophylactic antibiotics for MMS. MMS is considered a clean surgical procedure (unless a tumor is secondarily colonized and infected), with an overall low rate of surgical site infection, estimated at around 0.7% to 2.5%.[40–42] Similarly, the rate of bacteremia during dermatologic procedures is low, estimated around 1.9%.[40] Yet prophylactic antibiotics may be administered to MMS patients despite a low risk of bacteremia and surgical site infections in most patients. There

are some indications for prophylactic antibiotics that are clear (including history of immunosuppression [solid organ transplant recipient, human immunodeficiency virus with low CD4 count, chronic lymphocytic leukemia]). However, some Mohs surgeons routinely use prophylactic antibiotics for patients with a history of prostheses (valves or joints), nonphysiologic heart murmurs or valvular disease, or repair type (skin graft or large flap) in which the data are not supportive.

With regard to cardiac indications, the American Heart Association (AHA) released updated guidelines for antibiotic prophylaxis in 2007[43] that recommend their use to prevent bacteremia in dental, oral, upper respiratory tract, and some genitourinary and gastrointestinal procedures, in patients with high-risk or moderate-risk cardiac conditions. MMS does not usually fall into any of the categories outlined earlier, unless oral or respiratory mucosa is breached during the procedure. However, if MMS is planned on the lip or on the nose where breach of the nasal mucosa is anticipated, antibiotic prophylaxis is indicated for the following cardiac conditions:

- Previous infective endocarditis
- Prosthetic cardiac valves
- Unrepaired cyanotic congenital heart defects, including palliative shunts and conduits
- Congenital heart defects completely repaired with prosthetic material or a device, whether placed by surgery or by catheter intervention, during the first 6 months after the procedure
- Repaired congenital defects with residual defects at the site or adjacent to the site of a prosthetic patch or prosthetic device
- Cardiac transplants and development of cardiac valvulopathy.

Patient groups that may have received routine antibiotic prophylaxis in the past but are no longer candidates for it include those with mitral and aortic valve disease, rheumatic heart disease, or structural disorders like ventricular or atrial septal defects or hypertrophic cardiomyopathy, according to the AHA statement. Thus, prophylactic antibiotics are rarely necessary for patients who have cardiac disease undergoing MMS.

In general, systemic prophylactic antibiotics are not indicated in patients undergoing MMS who have vascular grafts, or orthopedic prostheses. However, there are certain instances when their use may be warranted. A recently published Advisory Statement for antibiotic prophylaxis in dermatologic surgery[40] suggests their use in Mohs performed on the lower extremity/groin area in individuals with a total hip or knee replacement because of the documented increased risk of surgical site infection on the lower extremities. Mohs surgeons can use guidelines in formulating their approach based on individual patient characteristics and needs.

If antibiotic prophylaxis is deemed necessary, the most commonly used antibiotics for prophylaxis include dicloxacillin and cephalexin (2 g by mouth 1 hour before surgery). For patients who are allergic to penicillin, this author uses either cefdinir (600 mg by mouth 1 hour before surgery, unless the patient had an anaphylactic reaction to penicillin), azithromycin (500 mg by mouth 1 hour before surgery), or clindamycin (600 mg by mouth 1 hour before surgery). However, Mohs surgeons should strive to decrease unnecessary use of antimicrobials by avoiding them in situations in which good evidence indicates that they are ineffective.

MANAGING ANTICOAGULANTS

The use of anticoagulant medications such as aspirin, nonsteriodal antiinflammtory drugs (NSAIDs), warfarin, clopridogel, and dipyramidol, and supplements with anticoagulant effect such as vitamin E, ginger, and ginkgo, has increased in recent years. The risk of postoperative complications depends on the anticoagulant agent and regimen. Complication rates with aspirin seem to be low.[44,45] Numerous studies have compared the rate of hemorrhagic complications in patients using aspirin and other NSAIDs. A review of these published reports reveals that there is no increased risk of severe bleeding complications in patients using aspirin and other NSAIDS.[45]

In contrast, some anticoagulants clearly increase the risk of postoperative bleeding. Continuous treatment with clopridogel, a thienopyridine-class antiplatelet agent used to inhibit clotting, seems to increase risk of complications.[46] Postoperative bleeding complications seem to be increased 7-fold to-8-fold among patients taking warfarin[47,48] compared with controls. The risk of bleeding seems to be independent of their international normalized ratio at the time of surgery.[48]

Mohs surgeons must weigh the risk of postoperative complications against the risk of thrombotic complications when deciding how to manage perioperative anticoagulation. The trend in Mohs surgery has been to continue medically necessary anticoagulants while performing skin surgery,[49] but there is considerable variation in management of anticoagulants among Mohs surgeons. More adequately powered prospective studies are needed to better quantify the risk of postoperative bleeding and other complications attributable to anticoagulation therapy, especially examining the type, dose, and effect of combination anticoagulant therapy as well as herbal agents with anticoagulant properties on postoperative complications after MMS.

OUTCOMES
Recurrence

Observational studies have consistently shown that MMS has a low recurrence rate,[50,51] often lower than surgical excision, especially facial NMSCs.[52] The recurrence rate for MMS is estimated at between 1% and 3% for primary BCCs and 5% and 7% for recurrent BCCs. This rate compares favorably with reported rates for treatment with surgical excision, which are estimated at 3% to 10% in primary BCC and greater than 17% in recurrent BCCs.[53–55] The only randomized trial performed to date, which evaluated the rates of recurrence of 397 primary and 201 recurrent facial BCCs randomized to MMS versus excision, found that after 30 months of follow-up, 5 (3%) of the primary BCCs recurred after excision compared with 3 (2%) after MMS. For recurrent tumors, 3 (3%) recurred after excision compared with none after MMS during 18 months of follow-up.[51] After 5 years of follow-up, there were 7 (4·1%) recurrences in primary BCCs treated with surgical excision compared with 4 (2·5%) in patients treated with MSM, a statistically nonsignificant difference. However, for recurrent BCCs, only 2 (2·4%) treated with MMS recurred, versus 10 (12·1%) in the excision-treated patients. This difference significantly favored MMS for recurrent BCC.[56]

This trial has been criticized as having several methodologic issues including bias in treatment assignment (patients were not strictly randomized because of patient or physician preference) and possible misclassification (some patients who were randomized to excision crossed over to MMS but were analyzed with the excision group).[57] However, they are the only trial data available that directly compares MMS with surgical excision. For now, it is safe to say that MMS is the treatment of choice for recurrent facial BCCs. There is a need for more data from future randomized controlled trials for both BCCs and SCCs arising on the head and neck with sufficient follow-up in which the randomization process is more strictly enforced.

Patient Satisfaction

Patient satisfaction is an important outcome measure, especially for conditions such as skin cancer, in which multiple viable options are available. Patient satisfaction can be influenced by numerous variables, including sociodemographic factors, health status, tumor characteristics, and previous experience with the disease. For MMS, satisfaction may also be influenced by intraoperative variables (number of stages, defect diameter, repair type) as well as postoperative variables (complications, time lost for treatment, perceived involvement in care). As an outcome measure, patient satisfaction has been associated with several other important outcomes, including health status, quality of life (QOL), adherence to medical advice, and initiation of complaints.[58–61] To improve patient satisfaction, it is important for clinicians to understand the factors that affect it.

In a recently published prospective cohort study of 339 patients treated with Mohs, the relationship of preoperative, intraoperative, and postoperative variables that influence short-term (at 1 week) and long-term (at 1 year) satisfaction were explored.[62] Preoperative skin QOL and number of intraoperative Mohs stages were both found to be associated with short-term and long-term satisfaction. Some variables, such as postoperative bother from bleeding or perception of shared decision making, were significant predictors for short-term satisfaction, and others, such as marital status, were predictors of long-term satisfaction. The temporal changes in the variables that predict patient satisfaction suggest that attention should be paid to the time frame during which measures of satisfaction are ascertained.[63] For patients presenting for surgical treatment, questions about satisfaction asked at different time points may yield different outcomes. It may be important to measure skin-related QOL in patients undergoing MMS to help clinicians identify patients at risk for being unsatisfied. Further studies may help determine which skin-related QOL factors are amenable to intervention and possible improvement.

In comparing patient satisfaction across different treatments for NMSC, a recently published study examined short-term and long-term satisfaction among 834 consecutive patients at 2 centers before and after 3 treatments: electrodessication and curettage, excision, and MMS. In multivariable regression models adjusting for patient, tumor, and care characteristics, higher long-term satisfaction was independently associated with younger age, better pretreatment mental health and skin-related QOL, and treatment with Mohs surgery.[58] Thus, patients treated with Mohs compared with other treatments tend to be more satisfied long-term. This information, along with other outcome measures, such as QOL and risk of recurrence, may help guide clinicians in treatment selection.

Cost-effectiveness

MMS can be a cost-effective treatment in certain cutaneous malignancies in which there is high risk of incomplete tumor excision or recurrence. The cost of MMS is largely driven by the reconstruction method used for repair.[64] Cost may also be driven higher if reconstruction is performed by a different specialist, or if many Mohs stages per tumor are required for clearance. Many studies have compared costs across different treatments for NMSC, including MMS,[51,65–73] many with conflicting findings. Cook and Zitelli[67] found that taking into account treatment and 5-year follow-up MMS was 7% more expensive than excisions with permanent sections, but 11% cheaper than excisions with frozen sections. Their study did not include tumors that were treated with excision but relied on expert opinion to estimate resource utilization for excision from an MMS-treated sample. Using the older Medicare costing rules, Welch and colleagues[66] found for procedure costs only that MMS was about $130 more than for a like tumor treated with excision in a military population, and these investigators suggested that MMS could be cheaper than excision if differences in recurrence rates were factored into cost analysis. Bentkover and colleagues[71] examined the costs of the physician and facility fee using Medicare prevailing rates for BCC removal by MMS, compared with excision with rapid cross-sectional frozen section. They found that MMS cost $400 to $600 more than excision depending on number of stages or frozen sections performed. Bialy and colleagues[69] compared the costs for the treatment of facial and auricular NMSC, using a single MMS-treated sample of 98 patients. Excision costs for this same sample were estimated by an otolaryngologist based on a theoretic treatment plan. They used Current Procedural Technology codes and Connecticut Medicare reimbursement rates for 2002 and found that cost differences were sensitive to type of repair chosen and number of frozen sections and positive margins. Blázquez-Sánchez and colleagues[73] performed a cost-analysis study comparing MMS with excision in Spain and reported no difference in cost in patients with high-risk facial BCC. The differences in these observational study findings may be attributable to methodologic shortcomings (failure to account for treatment selection bias), differing costs depending on country of origin of the study, and different cost structures (microcosting vs total cost of care).

Using microcosting techniques, the randomized controlled trial conducted in the Netherlands of facial BCCs treated with MMS and excision[51]

List of Acronyms	
AFX	Atypical fibroxanthoma
AHA	American Heart Association
BCC	Basal cell carcinoma
DFSP	Dermatofibrosarcoma protuberans
KA	Keratoacanthoma
MAC	Microcystic adnexal carcinoma
MMS	Mohs micrographic surgery
NMSC	Nonmelanoma skin cancer
NSAID	Nonsteriodal antiinflammtory drugs
QOL	Quality of life
SCC	Squamous cell carcinoma

found that the surgical costs alone of MMS were almost twice that of excision. These costs included time spent by the staff directly involved in the procedures, the price of the materials used, and the price of processing and examination of histopathologic slides. There is a need for well-performed comparative effectiveness and cost-effectiveness studies to ascertain the relative value of MMS in treating subtypes of NMSCs.

SUMMARY

MMS is a unique technique that has the potential to offer the highest cure rates and maximum tissue conservation in the management of specific primary and recurrent skin cancers. Yet there are many areas of controversy that surround MMS, including appropriate indications for its use, technical quandaries (use of curretage, antibiotic prophylaxis, management of anticoagulants), and outcomes (recurrence, patient-oriented outcomes, cost). Recent efforts in these areas need to be assessed to identify research gaps in MMS to help fuel further work. The usefulness of MMS and its methods for delivery need more stringent, evidence-based, rigorous study.

REFERENCES

1. Shriner DL, McCoy DK, Goldberg DJ, et al. Mohs micrographic surgery. J Am Acad Dermatol 1998;39(1):79–97.
2. Otley CC, Salasche SJ. Mohs surgery: efficient and effective. Br J Ophthalmol 2004;88(9):1228.
3. Available at: http://www.medicarenhic.com/pa/policies/MOHS%20Micrographic%20Surgery%20(L26371).pdf. Accessed July 5, 2011.
4. Pugliano-Mauro M, Goldman G. Mohs surgery is effective for high-risk cutaneous squamous cell carcinoma. Dermatol Surg 2010;36(10):1544–53.
5. Petrie M, Eliezri Y, Campanelli C. Keratoacanthoma of the head and neck with perineural invasion: incidental finding or cause for concern? Dermatol Surg 2010;36(7):1209–13.
6. Garcia-Zuazaga J, Ke M, Lee P. Giant keratoacanthoma of the upper extremity treated with Mohs micrographic surgery: a case report and review of current treatment modalities. J Clin Aesthet Dermatol 2009;2(8):22–5.
7. Goldberg LH, Silapunt S, Beyrau KK, et al. Keratoacanthoma as a postoperative complication of skin cancer excision. J Am Acad Dermatol 2004;50(5):753–8.
8. Gloster HM, Harris KR, Roenigk RK. A comparison between Mohs micrographic surgery and wide surgical excision for the treatment of dermatofibrosarcoma protuberans. J Am Acad Dermatol 1996;35:82–7.
9. Ratner D, Thomas CO, Johnson TM, et al. Mohs micrographic surgery for the treatment of dermatofibrosarcoma protuberans. Results of a multiinstitutional series with an analysis of the extent of microscopic spread. J Am Acad Dermatol 1997;37(4):600–13.
10. Robinson JK. Dermatofibrosarcoma protuberans resected by Mohs' surgery (chemosurgery). A 5-year prospective study. J Am Acad Dermatol 1985;12(6):1093–8.
11. Diamantis SA, Marks VJ. Mohs micrographic surgery in the treatment of microcystic adnexal carcinoma. Dermatol Clin 2011;29(2):185–90, viii.
12. Friedman PM, Friedman RH, Jiang SB, et al. Microcystic adnexal carcinoma: collaborative series review and update. J Am Acad Dermatol 1999;41(2 Pt 1):225–31.
13. Chiller K, Passaro D, Scheuller M, et al. Microcystic adnexal carcinoma: forty-eight cases, their treatment, and their outcome. Arch Dermatol 2000;136(11):1355–9.
14. Thomas CJ, Wood GC, Marks VJ. Mohs micrographic surgery in the treatment of rare aggressive cutaneous tumors: the Geisinger experience. Dermatol Surg 2007;33(3):333–9.
15. Leibovitch I, Huilgol SC, Selva D, et al. Microcystic adnexal carcinoma: treatment with Mohs micrographic surgery. J Am Acad Dermatol 2005;52(2):295–300.
16. Wallace RD, Bernstein PE. Microcystic adnexal carcinoma. Ear Nose Throat J 1991;70(11):789–93.
17. Love WE, Schmitt AR, Bordeaux JS. Management of unusual cutaneous malignancies: atypical fibroxanthoma, malignant fibrous histiocytoma, sebaceous carcinoma, extramammary Paget disease. Dermatol Clin 2011;29(2):201–16, viii.
18. Seavolt M, McCall M. Atypical fibroxanthoma: review of the literature and summary of 13 patients treated with Mohs micrographic surgery. Dermatol Surg 2006;32:435–41.

19. Albertini JG, Elston DM, Libow LF, et al. Mohs micrographic surgery for melanoma: a case series, a comparative study of immunostains, an informative case report, and a unique mapping technique. Dermatol Surg 2002;28(8):656–65.

20. Snow SN, Mohs FE, Oriba HA, et al. Cutaneous malignant melanoma treated by Mohs surgery. Review of the treatment results of 179 cases from the Mohs Melanoma Registry. Dermatol Surg 1997; 23(11):1055–60.

21. Chang KH, Dufresne R Jr, Cruz A, et al. The operative management of melanoma: where does Mohs surgery fit in? Dermatol Surg 2011;37(8):1069–79.

22. Muscarella VA. Angiosarcoma treated by Mohs micrographic surgery. J Dermatol Surg Oncol 1993;19(12):1132–3.

23. Berlin AL, Amin SP, Goldberg DJ. Extraocular sebaceous carcinoma treated with Mohs micrographic surgery: report of a case and review of literature. Dermatol Surg 2008;34(2):254–7.

24. Snow SN, Larson PO, Lucarelli MJ, et al. Sebaceous carcinoma of the eyelids treated by Mohs micrographic surgery: report of nine cases with review of the literature. Dermatol Surg 2002;28(7): 623–31.

25. Lee KY, Roh MR, Chung WG, et al. Comparison of Mohs micrographic surgery and wide excision for extramammary Paget's disease: Korean experience. Dermatol Surg 2009;35(1):34–40.

26. Hendi A, Brodland DG, Zitelli JA. Extramammary Paget's disease: surgical treatment with Mohs micrographic surgery. J Am Acad Dermatol 2004; 51(5):767–73.

27. Brown MD, Swanson NA. Treatment of malignant fibrous histiocytoma and atypical fibrous xanthomas with micrographic surgery. J Dermatol Surg Oncol 1989;15(12):1287–92.

28. Starling J 3rd, Coldiron BM. Mohs micrographic surgery for the treatment of cutaneous leiomyosarcoma. J Am Acad Dermatol 2011;64(6):1119–22.

29. Krunic AL, Kim S, Medenica M, et al. Recurrent adenoid cystic carcinoma of the scalp treated with Mohs micrographic surgery. Dermatol Surg 2003; 29(6):647–9.

30. Chesser RS, Bertler DE, Fitzpatrick JE, et al. Primary cutaneous adenoid cystic carcinoma treated with Mohs micrographic surgery toluidine blue technique. J Dermatol Surg Oncol 1992;18(3):175–6.

31. Kim YJ, Kim AR, Yu DS. Mohs micrographic surgery for squamoid eccrine ductal carcinoma. Dermatol Surg 2005;31(11 Pt 1):1462–4.

32. Pathai S, Barlow R, Williams G, et al. Mohs' micrographic surgery for Merkel cell carcinomas of the eyelid. Orbit 2005;24(4):273–5.

33. Boyer JD, Zitelli JA, Brodland DG, et al. Local control of primary Merkel cell carcinoma: review of 45 cases treated with Mohs micrographic surgery

with and without adjuvant radiation. J Am Acad Dermatol 2002;47(6):885–92.

34. Available at: http://www.aad.org/pm/billing/medicare/_doc/ImpactofLossofMPRRExemptionforMohs.pdf. Accessed July 5, 2011.

35. Available at: http://www.globalacademycme.com/news/skin-allergy-news/single-view/mohs-surgery-in-medicare-patients-skyrocketing/ece6850424092bce 77258ed6573b9222.html. Accessed July 5, 2011.

36. Lee DA, Ratner D. Economic impact of preoperative curettage before Mohs micrographic surgery for basal cell carcinoma. Dermatol Surg 2006;32(7): 916–22 [discussion: 922–3].

37. Ratner D, Bagiella E. The efficacy of curettage in delineating margins of basal cell carcinoma before Mohs micrographic surgery. Dermatol Surg 2003; 29(9):899–903.

38. Guardiano RA, Grande DJ. A direct comparison of visual inspection, curettage, and epiluminescence microscopy in determining tumor extent before the initial margins are determined for Mohs micrographic surgery. Dermatol Surg 2010;36(8):1240–4.

39. Jih MH, Friedman PM, Goldberg LH, et al. Curettage prior to Mohs' micrographic surgery for previously biopsied nonmelanoma skin cancers: what are we curetting? Retrospective, prospective, and comparative study. Dermatol Surg 2005;31(1):10–5.

40. Wright TI, Baddour LM, Berbari EF, et al. Antibiotic prophylaxis in dermatologic surgery: advisory statement 2008. J Am Acad Dermatol 2008;59(3): 464–73.

41. Maragh SL, Brown MD. Prospective evaluation of surgical site infection rate among patients with Mohs micrographic surgery without the use of prophylactic antibiotics. J Am Acad Dermatol 2008;59(2):275–8.

42. Rogers HD, Desciak EB, Marcus RP, et al. Prospective study of wound infections in Mohs micrographic surgery using clean surgical technique in the absence of prophylactic antibiotics. J Am Acad Dermatol 2010;63(5):842–51.

43. Wilson W, Taubert KA, Gewitz M, et al. Prevention of infective endocarditis: guidelines from the American Heart Association: a guideline from the American Heart Association Rheumatic Fever, Endocarditis, and Kawasaki Disease Committee, Council on Cardiovascular Disease in the Young, and the Council on Clinical Cardiology, Council on Cardiovascular Surgery and Anesthesia, and the Quality of Care and Outcomes Research Interdisciplinary Working Group. Circulation. 2007 Oct 9;116(15): 1736–54. Epub 2007 Apr 19. Erratum in: Circulation. 2007 Oct 9;116(15):e376–7.

44. Alcalay J, Alkalay R. Controversies in perioperative management of blood thinners in dermatologic surgery: continue or discontinue? Dermatol Surg 2004;30(8):1091–4 [discussion: 1094].

45. Hurst EA, Yu SS, Grekin RC, et al. Bleeding complications in dermatologic surgery. Semin Cutan Med Surg 2007;26(4):189–95.

46. Cook-Norris RH, Michaels JD, Weaver AL, et al. Complications of cutaneous surgery in patients taking clopidogrel-containing anticoagulation. J Am Acad Dermatol 2011;65(3):584–91.

47. Lewis KG, Dufresne RG Jr. A meta-analysis of complications attributed to anticoagulation among patients following cutaneous surgery. Dermatol Surg 2008;34(2):160–4 [discussion: 164–5].

48. Blasdale C, Lawrence CM. Perioperative international normalized ratio level is a poor predictor of postoperative bleeding complications in dermatological surgery patients taking warfarin. Br J Dermatol 2008;158(3):522–6.

49. Kirkorian AY, Moore BL, Siskind J, et al. Perioperative management of anticoagulant therapy during cutaneous surgery: 2005 survey of Mohs surgeons. Dermatol Surg 2007;33(10):1189–97.

50. Leibovitch I, Huilgol SC, Selva D, et al. Basal cell carcinoma treated with Mohs surgery in Australia II. Outcome at 5-year follow-up. J Am Acad Dermatol 2005;53(3):452–7.

51. Smeets Nicole WJ, Krekels Gertruud AM, Ostertag Judith U, et al. Surgical excision vs Mohs' micrographic surgery for basal-cell carcinoma of the face: randomised controlled trial. Lancet 2004;364:1766–72.

52. Veronese F, Farinelli P, Zavattaro E, et al. Basal cell carcinoma of the head region: therapeutical results of 350 lesions treated with Mohs micrographic surgery. J Eur Acad Dermatol Venereol 2011. DOI:10.1111/j.1468-3083.2011.04165.x. [Epub ahead of print].

53. Rowe DE, Carroll RJ, Day CL Jr. Mohs surgery is the treatment of choice for recurrent (previously treated) basal cell carcinoma. J Dermatol Surg Oncol 1989;15(4):424–31.

54. Silverman MK, Kopf AW, Bart RS, et al. Recurrence rates of treated basal cell carcinomas. Part 3: surgical excision. J Dermatol Surg Oncol 1992;18(6):471–6.

55. Rowe DE, Carroll RJ, Day CL Jr. Long-term recurrence rates in previously untreated (primary) basal cell carcinoma: implications for patient follow-up. J Dermatol Surg Oncol 1989;15(3):315–28.

56. Mosterd K, Krekels GA, Nieman FH, et al. Surgical excision versus Mohs' micrographic surgery for primary and recurrent basal-cell carcinoma of the face: a prospective randomised controlled trial with 5-years' follow-up. Lancet Oncol 2008;9(12):1149–56.

57. Otley CC. Mohs' micrographic surgery for basal-cell carcinoma of the face. Lancet 2005;365(9466):1226–7 [author reply: 1227].

58. Asgari MM, Bertenthal D, Sen S, et al. Patient satisfaction after treatment of nonmelanoma skin cancer. Dermatol Surg 2009;35(7):1041–9.

59. Chren MM, Sahay AP, Bertenthal DS, et al. Quality-of-life outcomes of treatments for cutaneous basal cell carcinoma and squamous cell carcinoma. J Invest Dermatol 2007;127:1351–7.

60. Serup J, Lindblad AK, Maroti M, et al. To follow or not to follow dermatological treatment–a review of the literature. Acta Derm Venereol 2006;86:193–7.

61. Renzi C, Picardi A, Abeni D, et al. Association of dissatisfaction with care and psychiatric morbidity with poor treatment compliance. Arch Dermatol 2002;138(3):337–42.

62. Asgari MM, Warton EM, Neugabauer R, et al. Predictors of patient satisfaction in Mohs surgery: analysis of pre-, intra- and postoperative factors in a large prospective cohort. Arch Dermatol, in press.

63. Jackson JL, Chamberlin J, Kroenke K. Predictors of patient satisfaction. Soc Sci Med 2001;52(4):609–20.

64. Wilson LS, Pregenzer M, Bertenthal D, et al. Costs of non melanoma skin cancer treatments. Derm Surg, in press.

65. Smeets NW, Kuijpers DI, Nelemans P, et al. Mohs' micrographic surgery for treatment of basal cell carcinoma of the face–results of a retrospective study and review of the literature. Br J Dermatol 2004;151:141–7.

66. Welch ML, Anderson LL, Grabski WJ. Evaluation and management of nonmelanoma skin cancer: the military perspective. Dermatol Clin 1999;17(1):19–28.

67. Cook J, Zitelli JA. Mohs micrographic surgery: a cost analysis. J Am Acad Dermatol 1998;39(5 Pt 1):698–703.

68. Higashi MK, Veenstra DL, Langley PC. Health economic evaluation of non-melanoma skin cancer and actinic keratosis. Pharmacoeconomics 2004;22:83–94.

69. Bialy TL, Whalen J, Veledar E, et al. Mohs micrographic surgery vs traditional surgical excision: a cost comparison analysis. Arch Dermatol 2004;140:736–42.

70. Lear W, Mittmann N, Barnes E, et al. Cost comparisons of managing complex facial basal cell carcinoma: Canadian study. J Cutan Med Surg 2008;12:82–7.

71. Bentkover SH, Grande DM, Soto H, et al. Excision of head and neck basal cell carcinoma with a rapid, cross-sectional, frozen-section technique. Arch Facial Plast Surg 2002;4:114–9.

72. Essers Brigitte AB, Dirksen Carmen D, Nieman Fred HM, et al. Cost-effectiveness of Mohs micrographic surgery vs surgical excision for basal cell carcinoma of the face. Arch Dermatol 2006;142:187–94.

73. Blázquez-Sánchez N, de Troya-Martín M, Frieyro-Elicegui M, et al. [Cost analysis of Mohs micrographic surgery in high-risk facial basal cell carcinoma]. Actas Dermosifiliogr 2010;101(7):622–8 [in Spanish].

Needs Assessment for Cosmetic Dermatologic Surgery

Murad Alam, MD, MSCI[a,b,c,]*, Jonathan M. Olson, MD[d],
Maryam M. Asgari, MD, MPH[e,f]

KEYWORDS

- Cosmetic procedures • Needs assessment
- Cosmetic dermatologic surgery
- Comparative effectiveness

Key Points

- Serious adverse events resulting from cosmetic dermatologic procedures are exceedingly rare. Dermatologists safely perform a range of noninvasive and minimally invasive cosmetic procedures in an outpatient, in-office setting under minimal or local anesthesia.
- Sequelae after cosmetic dermatology procedures are typically mild, transient erythema and edema.
- There are few unbiased, objective outcome measures for evaluating the effects of cosmetic dermatology procedures.

Most important recommendation

- There is a need for more prospective comparative studies of cosmetic dermatologic procedures and devices.

Cosmetic dermatologic surgery has been a rapidly expanding area within dermatologic surgery, comprising a projected $3 billion market segment in the United States by 2017.[1] The purpose of such surgery is to improve the appearance of the skin by reducing dyschromias, textural irregularities, contour irregularities, and skin sagging. The main procedural subcategories within this area include cutaneous laser and energy treatments, fillers and neurotoxins, and the treatment of leg veins. Other procedures include liposuction, hair transplantation, and surgical lifting. Possible instigating factors that have led to rapid growth in demand for cosmetic

---

[a] Department of Dermatology, Northwestern University Feinberg School of Medicine, 676 North Saint Clair Street, Suite 1600, Chicago, IL 60611, USA
[b] Department of Otolaryngology-Head and Neck Surgery, Northwestern University Feinberg School of Medicine, 676 North Saint Clair Street, Suite 1325, Chicago, IL 60611, USA
[c] Department of Surgery, Northwestern University Feinberg School of Medicine, 251 East Huran Street, Chicago, IL 60611, USA
[d] Division of Dermatology, Department of Medicine, University of Washington School of Medicine, 1959 NE Pacific Street, Room BB-1353, Box 356524, Seattle, WA 98195, USA
[e] Division of Research, Kaiser Permanente Northern California, 2000 Broadway, Oakland, CA 94612, USA
[f] Department of Dermatology, University of California at San Francisco, 1701 Divisadero Street, 3rd Floor, San Francisco, CA 94115, USA
* Corresponding author. Department of Dermatology, Northwestern University Feinberg School of Medicine, 676 North Saint Clair Street, Suite 1600, Chicago, IL 60611.
E-mail address: m-alam@northwestern.edu

Dermatol Clin 30 (2012) 177–187
doi:10.1016/j.det.2011.08.009

dermatologic surgery include media portrayals of physical beauty, increased personal disposable income, concerns about ageism in a recessionary economy, and increasing social acceptance of cosmetic procedures. Since 2003, training in cosmetic dermatologic surgery has been a major part of the curriculum of the Accreditation Council for Graduate Medical Education (ACGME)-approved clinical fellowships in procedural dermatology; there is also increased emphasis on such training in dermatology residency programs.

Dermatologists have been active in the realm of cosmetic dermatology for many decades. They have been responsible for the development of most cutaneous lasers and energy devices, the popularization of prepackaged soft-tissue augmentation materials (ie, fillers), the adaptation of botulinum toxin to treat rhytids, the development of tumescent liposuction, the discovery of hair transplantation, and other advances. In recent years, many new devices and procedures have been introduced. Further research is needed to optimize the effectiveness of these procedures and to assess the comparative effectiveness and safety of procedures for similar indications.

DEFINITIONS AND BOUNDARIES

This area of cosmetic dermatologic surgery is poorly defined but can be equated with elective outpatient procedures typically performed under local anesthesia or conscious sedation that are designed to improve physical appearance or decrease the visible signs of aging[1] and that are not reimbursed by public or private insurers and, therefore, are an out-of-pocket expense for patients. During the past several decades, areas have been incrementally added to this category. Although most practicing dermatologists deliver some cosmetic procedures, for most dermatologists, cosmetic procedures compose a minority of their practice, as little as 10% for most general dermatologists.

COMMON INDICATIONS

Cosmetic dermatologic surgery may be performed to reduce scars, including acne-associated scarring, traumatic scars, striae and stretch marks; the visible manifestations of skin aging, including skin color (eg, erythema, lentigines, melasma, hyperpigmentation, hypopigmentation), texture (eg, fine surface irregularity, deeper rhytids, cellulite), and sagging (eg, jowls, abdominal sagging); and excess fat and lipoatrophy.

COMPARATIVE EFFECTIVENESS AND SAFETY

There is a trend toward the use of noninvasive[2-4] (eg, no de-epithelialization or skin incision or excision: nonablative lasers,[5-7] injectable toxins and fillers[8-13]) and minimally invasive procedures (eg, partially ablative fractional lasers that leave part of the epidermis intact and liposuction with small puncture incisions) that additively provide esthetic improvements approaching those of invasive procedures (eg, face-lift or abdominoplasty) while reducing the duration of recovery time and the risk of serious adverse events relative to those associated with such invasive procedures. Several noninvasive or minimally invasive procedures for the same indication may be used additively to yield a desired cosmetic outcome. Cosmetic dermatologic procedures may be performed sequentially, and each procedure type may entail up to several component treatments spaced weeks or months apart. Typical postprocedure sequelae include mild erythema and edema and in some cases ecchymoses and crusting/erosions that need to re-epithelialize. It has been suggested that reduction of adverse events associated with minimally invasive and noninvasive cosmetic procedures may be associated with a commensurate reduction in efficacy. There are few comparative studies of safety and efficacy of minimally invasive/noninvasive procedures versus invasive procedures for the same indications. Likewise, there are few studies comparing different minimally invasive or noninvasive procedures for similar indications. Serious adverse events are rare even with so-called major cosmetic dermatology procedures, such as liposuction, blepharoplasty, rhytidectomy, and ablative facial resurfacing. The most frequent unexpected and concerning adverse event is unwanted scarring. Illness requiring hospitalization or death is exceedingly rare.

SITE OF SERVICE

Cosmetic dermatologic surgery procedures are usually performed in an outpatient clinic setting under local anesthesia. Minimal oral sedation or intravenous conscious sedation may be used. It has been suggested that outpatient surgeries are less safe than surgeries in hospital-based operating rooms, but the data on procedures, such as liposuction, has shown the reverse to be true. Deaths reported secondary to liposuction tend to occur in hospital-based operating rooms and under the care of nondermatologists.[14-20] Comparative studies are difficult to perform because of the absence of national or state-based registries of adverse events associated with cosmetic procedures. Additionally, because payers do not reimburse these services, health insurers and health maintenance organizations typically do not retain this information in a centralized manner. In general, the provision of cosmetic dermatologic procedures is highly fragmented, with hundreds of private practices consisting of one or a few dermatologists each collectively providing the bulk of such services. Although a small minority of US dermatologic practices devote most of their time and derive most of their revenue from cosmetic dermatologic surgery, there is no specific accreditation for such practices. Postresidency fellowship training in cosmetic dermatologic surgery is available but not ACGME-approved or eligible for the American Board of Medical Specialties subspecialty certification or vetted by some other generally accepted accrediting body. Some noninvasive cosmetic procedures are performed by estheticians or other nonphysician providers in a spa setting with no or minimal physician oversight.[21–23] It is unclear where complaints and adverse events associated with such procedures are reported because state medical boards are not the repositories for complaints associated with nonphysician providers.

Patient Selection

Because cosmetic dermatologic surgeries are by definition elective, patient selection is considered important to maximize effectiveness and minimize adverse events. Risk factors that may result in exclusion include body dysmorphic disorder or other significant psychiatric comorbidity, skin of color (eg, Fitzpatrick skin types IV to VI), tanned skin, history of keloids or hypertrophic scarring, connective tissue disease, degree of photodamage, or patient age. Limited data is available regarding the incidence of body dysmorphic disorder in patients presenting for cosmetic dermatologic surgery, and most surgeons do not use any formal screening tool beyond general clinical acumen to detect this.[24,25] Skin of color is at risk of hyperpigmentation and other pigmentary abnormalities after cosmetic procedures, particularly skin resurfacing procedures and incisional or excisional procedures.[26–28] A greater proportion of cosmetic dermatologic surgery procedures are being performed on Latino, African American, and Asian patients than were a decade ago, and this group continues to be poorly studied. The long-pulsed Nd:YAG laser is perhaps the most successful device developed specifically for skin-of-color patients and this reduces the risk of hyperpigmentation during hair removal in such patients. Milder resurfacing procedures

fractionated across a larger number of treatments may be necessary to minimize the risk in the skin-of-color cohort. Tanned patients are generally excluded from receiving laser treatments to avoid hyperpigmentation. Treatment of patients with connective tissue disease, especially scleroderma, is controversial and no prospective studies exist. It is generally thought that noninvasive skin tightening devices, such as radiofrequency, infrared light, and ultrasound devices, are less effective in elderly patients with significant skin sagging. However, attempts to accurately predict patient response to nonablative tightening devices based on specific skin characteristics or demographic variables have been unsuccessful, with a proportion of unexpected treatment failures.

Limitations in Clinical Research

Clinical research on cosmetic dermatologic surgical procedures is particularly challenging. First, funding for such research is precarious. Federal funding for clinical research tends to be disease based, and aging and the visible manifestations thereof are not widely considered a disease process. Similarly, given the safety of cosmetic dermatologic procedures, research on safety and monitoring of associated serious adverse events is not compelling. The funding that is available includes seed funding from some professional societies. Industry funding is primarily for multicenter trials to support US Food and Drug Administration (FDA) applications for new drug or device clearance/approval or new indications for previously approved drugs or devices. There is additional research required to support or repudiate the contention that cosmetic procedures have a significant beneficial effect on patient quality of life.[29]

Regarding patient selection and recruitment, there are inherent difficulties in recruiting large numbers of patients or a population-based sample. Individual cosmetic practices are staffed by one or a few physicians and see small numbers of patients; most cosmetic practices are not located in academic medical centers or in academically oriented private practices, and the leadership of these other practices may not be interested in facilitating clinical research; cosmetic patients may value privacy and discretion and be unwilling to enroll in clinical trials. As a consequence, investigator-initiated randomized control trials are uncommon and, when performed, these may be underpowered[30] and susceptible to a type II error given their limited capacity to detect small effects.

There is a dearth of validated, objective, or unbiased outcome measures to assess the effects of cosmetic interventions. The most commonly used measures are ratings of pretreatment and posttreatment photographs by experienced clinicians and questionnaire or survey instruments. Photographic raters may be blinded or not but, even when blinded, may be hobbled by the lack of objective criteria beyond global appearance, which may be improved or worsened. Questionnaire and survey instruments are seldom validated, and although several new photographic scales have been developed in the past decade, these have only been psychometrically tested at a rudimentary level and are not routinely used by investigators in this area.[31–38] An emerging movement to assess patient satisfaction through self-report survey instruments[39] seems theoretically sound (ie, patients receive cosmetic procedures to improve their appearance in their own eyes, not to please investigators) but is vulnerable to potential biases: patients may be prone to overestimate esthetic improvements to please their treating physicians, to think better about themselves, and because the frequent mild to moderate discomfort associated with such procedures may induce a placebo effect.

Interpretation of clinical research results is limited by the well-documented problem of potential bias among investigators with industry ties.[40–43] This potential bias is exacerbated in cosmetic dermatologic surgery because virtually all funding is from industry sponsors. Possibly as a consequence, there are few comparative trials of different devices in the same class or different methods to treat similar clinical problems. That being said, it is difficult, impractical, and potentially counterproductive to exclude investigators with industry ties because these are some of the most experienced and skilled physicians available and the ones with the greatest working knowledge of novel technologies.

The lack of postmarketing data is troubling because many cosmetic dermatologic procedures are device based rather than drug based, and many of the relevant devices are cleared through the FDA 510K process, which requires little demonstration of treatment effectiveness.

TOPIC AREAS

For each topic area in cosmetic dermatologic surgery, there is limited information regarding overall safety and efficacy, and it is difficult to offer generalizations about specific indications, patient selection, and numbers of treatments. As noted before, within and across categories, there is limited comparative effectiveness data. There are few randomized control studies of comparative effectiveness and many of these are compared with placebo or with combination therapies (eg, therapy A vs therapy A plus B) rather than between 2 discrete standard-of-care approaches. Further, devices using similar technology, such as lasers with similar wavelengths or different hyaluronic acid-based fillers, are difficult to differentiate based on treatment efficacy or safety.

Some major topic areas are subsequently outlined. Comparative effectiveness findings from significant randomized control trials are briefly summarized.

Lasers, Light Sources, and Energy Devices

In general, there is a lack of evidence regarding optimal laser treatment of specific indications (frequency, pulse size, pulse duration, number of treatments, and so forth for a given condition).

1. Modification of erythema and pigmentation (eg, pulse dye laser [PDL], intense pulsed light [IPL], pottasium-titanyl-phosphate [KTP] laser, Nd:YAG lasers; Q-switched alexandrite, ruby; superficial fractionated devices)
   a. Several lasers and light sources have been used to reduce skin redness and telangiectasia and brownish or pigmented discoloration, such as lentigines and tattoo. Such selective lasers are usually optimized to treat either erythema or pigmentation and seldom cause any epidermal injury or induce sequelae beyond transient minimal erythema and edema. IPL devices and some lasers, such as some modified pulsed-dye lasers in which special handpieces allow for the treatment of pigmentation, can treat both effectively.
   b. Long-pulsed pulsed-dye laser and intense pulsed-light devices are both safe and effective for treatment of facial telangiectasia,[44] but a long-pulse pulsed-dye laser may be more effective.[45] The 532-nm KTP laser may be more effective but may cause more redness and swelling.[46] Fine telangiectasia may respond to treatment with the nonpurpuragenic long-pulse pulsed-dye laser but thicker telangiectasia respond better to purpuragenic treatment[47] or stacking of pulses.[48]
   c. The nonablative fractional laser seems more effective in the treatment of surgical scars than the pulsed-dye laser.[49] When the pulsed-dye laser is used, treatment can be safely commenced on the day of suture removal and the variation of pulse

duration has minimal impact on effectiveness.[50] Intralesional corticosteroid, topical 5-fluorouracil, intralesional 5-fluorouracil, and pulsed-dye laser are each effective for the treatment of keloidal and hypertrophic scars, but the risk of adverse events is greatest with intralesional corticosteroid.[51]

   d. Pulsed-dye laser is more effective than IPL in the treatment of port-wine stains.[52] Pulsed-dye laser treatment of port-wine stains at 2- versus 6-week intervals is equally well tolerated and more effective.[53] Childhood hemangiomas are more safely treated with long-pulsed than short-pulsed pulsed-dye lasers.[54]

   e. Cherry angiomata treated with electrodessication are less improved than those treated with KTP or pulsed-dye laser.[55] Similarly, KTP laser is slightly more effective and less painful than electrodessication for treatment of spider angiomata.[56] Dermatosis papulosa nigra is treated effectively with either electrodessication or KTP laser, but KTP laser is less painful.[57]

   f. Nanosecond (ie, Q-switched) 532-nm laser is more effective and less associated with adverse effects for the treatment of lentigines than the microsecond (long-pulse) 532-nm laser.[58] Separately, the Q-switched alexandrite laser or pulsed-dye laser with compression handpiece is more effective for the treatment of facial lentigines and dyschromia than IPL.[59,60]

2. Nonablative and partially ablative resurfacing (eg, lasers and light devices, including 1550 nm, 1927 nm, YSGG, other similar non-CO2 fractionated devices, and superficial chemical peels)

   a. So-called nonablative fractional resurfacing devices use technologies other than carbon dioxide laser to remove a small fraction of the treated epidermis and partial thickness dermis in each treatment. So multiple treatments are required, but the healing time from each is brief. Superficial chemical peels provide many of the same effects. Posttreatment sequelae are usually intense erythema and possibly some erosion, with these remitting within 2 to 5 days.

   b. Glycolic acid peels and salicylic acid peels both have efficacy against acne vulgaris.[61] The 1% tretinoin peel and the 70% glycolic acid peels have similar efficacy in the treatment of melasma.[62] The 1550-nm fractional laser therapy is as effective as triple topical therapy for the treatment of melasma,

although both treatments are associated with discomfort and a high risk of recurrence.[63] A series of glycolic acid peels and microdermabrasion treatments are associated with similar minimal efficacy for facial skin rejuvenation.[64]

3. Ablative resurfacing (eg, fractional CO2, dermabrasion, moderate to deep chemical peels)

   a. Ablative resurfacing is associated with fractional or full-face carbon dioxide laser, dermabrasion, or moderate to deep chemical peels. In all of these cases, there is a significant epidermal and dermal injury mediated by heat, friction, or chemical activity, respectively. Re-epithelialization times may be 4 to 5 days to several weeks.

   b. There are no side-by-side studies of fractional carbon dioxide laser, dermabrasion, and moderate to deep chemical peels for the treatment of photodamage. Cryotherapy is more effective than 33% to 35% trichloroacetic acid (TCA) solution in the treatment of lentigines but is more painful and takes longer to heal.[65,66] A single 35% trichloroacetic acid peel causes more improvement of photoaging than a series of 30% glycolic acid peels but is associated with more discomfort.[67]

4. Skin tightening

   a. Noninvasive (eg, monopolar, bipolar, and unipolar radiofrequency [RF]; ultrasound; infrared light/laser)

      i. So-called noninvasive skin tightening is induced by energy devices that deploy heat to cause immediate collagen contraction, collagen remodeling, and contraction of the fibrous septa of the subcutaneous fat. Heat is delivered into the dermis and subcutis while sparing the epidermis. The major modalities in this arena are radiofrequency, broadband light, ultrasound, and combinations of these technologies.

      ii. The 1064-nm and 1320-nm lasers are about equally effective for the treatment of acne scars.[68] The 1320-nm and 1450-nm lasers are both effective for the treatment of atrophic scarring.[69] Efficacy of infrared and radiofrequency devices for modest temporary improvement in the appearance of cellulite is similar.[70] Fractional radiofrequency treatment induces less reduction in facial laxity than facelift.[71]

   b. *Invasive (eg, resections of excess skin, blepharoplasty, facelift)

      i. Invasive skin-tightening procedures are those that resect skin, possibly also with underlying muscle, or with plicating the fascia, as in the case of facelift. Dermatologists perform these procedures in an office setting, using local or tumescent anesthesia, and sometimes conscious sedation. There are no large cohort or comparative studies on these procedures in the dermatology literature except for one comparing fractional radiofrequency tightening to facelift.[71] In this study, fractional radiofrequency tightening provided about one-third the benefit of facelift.

5. Fat reduction
   a. Liposuction, tumescent
   b. Cryolipolysis
   c. Low-level laser light
   d. Ultrasound
   e. Radiofrequency

There are novel methods for fat reduction that use energy devices in a manner similar to noninvasive skin-tightening devices. Fat-reduction devices deliver energy even deeper than skin-tightening devices. At present, no radiofrequency or ultrasound devices are cleared by the US FDA for fat reduction. A single low-level laser device is, thus, cleared but is controversial regarding its approval process. Cryolipolysis uses a method similar to popsicle panniculitis, to destroy fat, and has been shown to reduce lateral abdominal fat, including love handles. Tumescent liposuction is used by dermatologists to remove large quantities of fat, up to several liters at a time, through small puncture incisions; at present, none of the minimally invasive or noninvasive modalities for fat reduction make claims for comparable effectiveness, although there are no comparative studies.

Injectables

6. Soft tissue augmentation (eg, hyaluronic acid derivatives, calcium hydroxylapatite, poly-L-lactate)
   a. Prepackaged soft tissue augmentation materials have proliferated since the introduction of bovine collagen in 1983. These newer materials do not require skin testing and are typically injected into the subcutaneous fat just below the dermis. The purpose is to correct soft tissue atrophy, depressions, and rhytids. Persistence of the filling effect may be several months to several years, depending on the material type, the anatomic site, and the patient characteristics. Most materials used in the United States are temporary and metabolized.

   b. Laser, radiofrequency, and IPL treatments can be safely administered immediately after hyaluronic acid derivative injections for soft tissue augmentation.[72]
   c. Separately, hyaluronic acid derivative fillers, injectable poly-L-lactic acid, or injectable calcium hydroxylapatite provides a longer-lasting correction than bovine collagen.[73-75] Mixing calcium hydroxylapatite or hyaluronic acid derivative fillers with lidocaine reduces injection pain but not efficacy.[76-80] Retreatment intervals for hyaluronic acid fillers do not seem to impact the overall persistence of effect.[81]

7. Neurotoxins (eg, onabotulinumtoxinA, abobotulinumtoxinA, incobotulinumtoxinA)
   a. In dermatologic surgery, neurotoxins are used for the reduction of dynamic facial creases caused by muscle motion, treatment of hyperhidrosis or headache, and off-label to facilitate scar healing. The transient result lasts about 3 to 6 months for a facial cosmetic effect. There are no reports of serious adverse events from the cosmetic use of approved botulinum toxins in the United States.
   b. Injectable botulinum toxin A is more effective than topical 20% aluminum chloride for primary focal axillary hyperhidrosis.[82] For the treatment of axillary hyperhidrosis, injectable botulinum toxin A reconstituted in lidocaine is as effective and less painful than that reconstituted in saline.[83] For the treatment of axillary hyperhidrosis or crow's feet rhytids, lower doses of botulinum toxin A are as safe and effective.[84,85] Botulinum toxin A is less painful on injection when reconstituted with saline with preservative than without.[86] Botulinum toxin A reconstituted 2 weeks before injection can be used safely and effectively.[87,88] Varying dilution of botulinum toxin A may have limited effect on efficacy.[89]
   c. Clinical effectiveness of onabotulinumtoxinA and abobotulinumtoxinA for facial rhytids is difficult to compare because the comparable dose ratio is unclear.[90] OnabotulinumtoxinA has a wider radius of action than abobotulinumtoxinA.[91,92] The injection of more dilute solutions of botulinum toxin A results in a wider radius of action.[93]

Other Procedures

8. Treatment of leg veins
   a. Leg veins include fine red telangiectatic veins, blue thicker reticular veins, and

bulging varicose veins. Smaller and medium caliber veins are typically treated with injections of sclerosing agents. Veins can also be surgically removed (phlebectomy). Deeper venous incompetence, like greater saphenous regurgitation associated with reflux on Doppler ultrasound and possibly physical discomfort, can be corrected by minimally invasive means like endovenous ablation. In this technique laser or radiofrequency catheters are inserted into the vein and used to seal it with thermal energy.

    i. Sclerotherapy (eg, saline, sotradecol, polidocanol, with or without foam)

       1. Foamed and liquid polidocanol and sodium tetradecyl sulfate are similarly safe and effective for the treatment of varicose and telangiectatic leg veins.[94]

    ii. Endovenous ablation (eg, laser, radiofrequency)

    iii. Ambulatory phlebectomy

9. Hair removal and hair transplantation

  a. Several laser devices can induce prolonged remission of hair growth after several treatments. Dark, coarse hairs are most responsive.

  b. Hair transplantation uses the concept of donor-site dominance to transplant hairs from the existing reservoir, usually the back of the head, to areas where male or female pattern baldness has occurred.

10. Liposuction, tumescent (and autologous fat transplantation)

  a. Tumescent liposuction entails the use of a dilute anesthetic solution combined with epinephrine to anesthetize the area to be treated in a manner that provides hemostatic control. Tumescent liposuction is usually performed in an outpatient setting under no to minimal sedation. Autologous fat transfer is the reverse of liposuction and entails reinjecting harvested fat into patients at a site of tissue atrophy. For instance, liposuction aspirate may be used to correct facial cheek atrophy.

  b. Laser-assisted and suction-assisted lipoplasty have similar efficacy and safety.[95] Tumescent anesthesia used on the head and neck is more rapidly absorbed systemically than truncal anesthesia and can result in the rapid rise in plasma lidocaine level.[96] Centrifuged fat may have greater longevity for dorsal hand augmentation than noncentrifuged fat.[97] Autologous frozen fat and fresh fat are similarly effective for fat augmentation of the hands.[98]

11. Skin and subcutaneous tissue resection

  a. Removal of excess skin associated with aging or weight loss is a surgical procedure. Using tumescent anesthesia, excisions of skin both on and off the face are feasible in the office.

    i. Facelift

    ii. Blepharoplasty

    iii. Resection of excess skin after weight loss

*Invasive procedures for similar indications, also listed separately.

SUMMARY

Cosmetic dermatologic procedures are proliferating in the United States. Many of these are novel techniques that use complex devices, such as lasers and energy devices. To the extent that cosmetic procedures rarely elicit the scrutiny of the FDA drug division, they are less studied with regard to safety and efficacy. Although such procedures are mostly safe, with minimal associated risks, further research is needed to document these risks and suggest methods for their minimization. Additionally, more comparative effectiveness research is needed to identify highly effective treatment strategies and develop standard treatment protocols. One of the many challenges in this regard is that many of the devices required in such procedures are proprietary and continually undergoing changes. More significantly, at present, there is no primary funding source for ongoing research beyond industry support.

List of Acronyms	
ACGME	Accreditation Council for Graduate Medical Education
FDA	US Food and Drug Administration
IPL	Intense pulsed light
KTP	Potassium-titanyl-phosphate
PDL	Pulse dye laser
RF	Radiofrequency
TCA	Trichloroacetic acid

REFERENCES

1. Draelos ZD. What defines aging? J Cosmet Dermatol 2009;8:237–8.

Minimally Invasive Cosmetic Procedures

2. Tierney EP, Hanke CW. Recent advances in combination treatments for photoaging: review of the literature. Dermatol Surg 2010;36:829–40.
3. Ogden S, Griffiths TW. A review of minimally invasive cosmetic procedures. Br J Dermatol 2008;159: 1036–50.
4. Hirsch R, Stier M. Complications and their management in cosmetic dermatology. Dermatol Clin 2009; 27:507–20, vii.

Safety of Nonablative Lasers and Energy Devices

5. Anolik R, Chapas AM, Brightman LA, et al. Radiofrequency devices for body shaping: a review and study of 12 patients. Semin Cutan Med Surg 2009;28: 236–43.
6. Avram MM, Harry RS. Cryolipolysis for subcutaneous fat layer reduction. Lasers Surg Med 2009;41:703–8.
7. Sadick NS. Overview of ultrasound-assisted liposuction, and body contouring with cellulite reduction. Semin Cutan Med Surg 2009;28:250–6.

Safety of Fillers and Injectables

8. Hanke CW, Rohrich RJ, Busso M, et al. Facial soft-tissue fillers conference: assessing the state of the science. J Am Acad Dermatol 2011;64(Suppl 4): S66–85.
9. Hanke CW, Rohrich RJ, Busso M, et al. Facial soft-tissue fillers: assessing the state of the science conference—proceedings report. J Am Acad Dermatol 2011;64(Suppl 4):S53–65.
10. Babamiri K, Nassab R. The evidence for reducing the pain of administration of local anesthesia and cosmetic injectables. J Cosmet Dermatol 2010;9:242–5.
11. Alam M, Dover JS. Management of complications and sequelae with temporary injectable fillers. Plast Reconstr Surg 2007;120(Suppl 6):98S–105S.
12. Alam M, Gladstone H, Kramer EM, et al. American Society for Dermatologic Surgery. ASDS guidelines of care: injectable fillers. Dermatol Surg 2008; 34(Suppl 1):S115–48.
13. Alam M, Dover JS, Klein AW, et al. Botulinum a exotoxin for hyperfunctional facial lines: where not to inject. Arch Dermatol 2002;138:1180–5.

Liposuction Safety

14. Habbema L. Safety of liposuction using exclusively tumescent local anesthesia in 3,240 consecutive cases. Dermatol Surg 2009;35:1728–36.

15. Coldiron BM, Healy C, Bene NI. Office surgery incidents: what seven years of Florida data show us. Dermatol Surg 2008;34:285–91 [discussion: 291–2].
16. Coldiron B, Fisher AH, Adelman E, et al. Adverse event reporting: lessons learned from 4 years of Florida office data. Dermatol Surg 2005;31(9 Pt 1): 1079–92 [discussion: 1093].
17. Schnur P, Penn J, Fodor PB. Deaths related to liposuction. N Engl J Med 1999;341:1002–3.
18. Klein JA. Deaths related to liposuction. N Engl J Med 1999;341:1001.
19. Rigel DS, Wheeland RG. Deaths related to liposuction. N Engl J Med 1999;341:1001–2.
20. Hanke CW, Coleman WP 3rd. Morbidity and mortality related to liposuction. Questions and answers. Dermatol Clin 1999;17:899–902.

Nonphysician, Non-office-based Practice of Cosmetic Dermatology

21. Friedman PM, Jih MH, Burns AJ, et al. Nonphysician practice of dermatologic surgery: the Texas perspective. Dermatol Surg 2004;30:857–63.
22. Brody HJ, Geronemus RG, Farris PK. Beauty versus medicine: the nonphysician practice of dermatologic surgery. Dermatol Surg 2003;29:319–24.
23. Alam M. Who is qualified to perform laser surgery and in what setting? Semin Plast Surg 2007;21: 193–200.

Body Dysmorphic Disorder

24. Conrado LA, Hounie AG, Diniz JB, et al. Body dysmorphic disorder among dermatologic patients: prevalence and clinical features. J Am Acad Dermatol 2010;63:235–43.
25. Malick F, Howard J, Koo J. Understanding the psychology of the cosmetic patients. Dermatol Ther 2008;21:47–53.

Cosmetic Procedures in Skin of Color

26. Davis EC, Callender VD. Aesthetic dermatology for aging ethnic skin. Dermatol Surg 2011 May 17. DOI:10.1111/j.1524-4725.2011.02007.x.[Epub ahead of print].
27. Battle EF Jr. Cosmetic laser treatments for skin of color: a focus on safety and efficacy. J Drugs Dermatol 2011;10:35–8.
28. Alam M, Bhatia A, Kundu R, et al. Cosmetic dermatology of skin of color. China: The McGraw-Hill Companies, Inc; 2009.

Limitations in Clinical Research in Cosmetic Dermatologic Surgery

29. Sadick NS. The impact of cosmetic interventions on quality of life. Dermatol Online J 2008;14:2.

30. Alam M, Barzilai DA, Wrone DA. Power and sample size of therapeutic trials in procedural dermatology: how many patients are enough? Dermatol Surg 2005;31:201–5.

Ordinal Measurement Scales for Esthetic Outcomes

31. Carruthers A, Carruthers J. A validated facial grading scale: the future of facial ageing measurement tools? J Cosmet Laser Ther 2010;12:235–41.

32. Carruthers A, Carruthers J, Hardas B, et al. A validated brow positioning grading scale. Dermatol Surg 2008;34(Suppl 2):S150–4.

33. Carruthers A, Carruthers J, Hardas B, et al. A validated hand grading scale. Dermatol Surg 2008;34(Suppl 2):S179–83.

34. Carruthers A, Carruthers J, Hardas B, et al. A validated grading scale for crow's feet. Dermatol Surg 2008;34(Suppl 2):S173–8.

35. Carruthers A, Carruthers J, Hardas B, et al. A validated grading scale for marionette lines. Dermatol Surg 2008;34(Suppl 2):S167–72.

36. Carruthers A, Carruthers J, Hardas B, et al. A validated lip fullness grading scale. Dermatol Surg 2008;34(Suppl 2):S161–6.

37. Carruthers A, Carruthers J, Hardas B, et al. A validated grading scale for forehead lines. Dermatol Surg 2008;34(Suppl 2):S155–60.

38. Verhaegen PD, van der Wal MB, Middelkoop E, et al. Objective scar assessment tools: a clinimetric appraisal. Plast Reconstr Surg 2011;127:1561–70.

Patient-Reported Outcomes for Cosmetic Procedures

39. Pusic AL, Lemaine V, Klassen AF, et al. Patient-reported outcome measures in plastic surgery: use and interpretation in evidence-based medicine. Plast Reconstr Surg 2011;127:1361–7.

Conflicts of Interest

40. Alam M, Kim NA, Havey J, et al. Blinded versus unblinded peer review of manuscripts submitted to a dermatology journal: a randomized multi-rater study. Br J Dermatol 2011. DOI:10.1111/j.1365-2133.2011.10432.x. [Epub ahead of print].

41. Smith Begolka W, Elston DM, Beutner KR. American Academy of Dermatology evidence-based guideline development process: responding to new challenges and establishing transparency. J Am Acad Dermatol 2011;64:e105–12.

42. American Academy of Dermatology Board of Directors. Position statement on contemporary issues: conflict of interest. J Am Acad Dermatol 2008;59:1005–8.

43. Stossel TP. Conflicts of interest in dermatology: more than skin deep? J Invest Dermatol 2007;127:1829–30.

Topic Areas

44. Neuhaus IM, Zane LT, Tope WD. Comparative efficacy of nonpurpuragenic pulsed dye laser and intense pulsed light for erythematotelangiectatic rosacea. Dermatol Surg 2009;35:920–8.

45. Nymann P, Hedelund L, Haedersdal M. Long-pulsed dye laser vs. intense pulsed light for the treatment of facial telangiectasias: a randomized controlled trial. J Eur Acad Dermatol Venereol 2010;24:143–6.

46. Uebelhoer NS, Bogle MA, Stewart B, et al. A split-face comparison study of pulsed 532-nm KTP laser and 595-nm pulsed dye laser in the treatment of facial telangiectasias and diffuse telangiectatic facial erythema. Dermatol Surg 2007;33:441–8.

47. Alam M, Dover JS, Arndt KA. Treatment of facial telangiectasia with variable-pulse high-fluence pulsed-dye laser: comparison of efficacy with fluences immediately above and below the purpura threshold. Dermatol Surg 2003;29:681–4 [discussion: 685].

48. Rohrer TE, Chatrath V, Iyengar V. Does pulse stacking improve the results of treatment with variable-pulse pulsed-dye lasers? Dermatol Surg 2004;30(2 Pt 1):163–7 [discussion: 167].

49. Tierney E, Mahmoud BH, Srivastava D, et al. Treatment of surgical scars with nonablative fractional laser versus pulsed dye laser: a randomized controlled trial. Dermatol Surg 2009;35:1172–80.

50. Nouri K, Elsaie ML, Vejjabhinanta V, et al. Comparison of the effects of short- and long-pulse durations when using a 585-nm pulsed dye laser in the treatment of new surgical scars. Lasers Med Sci 2010;25:121–6, 51.

51. Manuskiatti W, Fitzpatrick RE. Treatment response of keloidal and hypertrophic sternotomy scars: comparison among intralesional corticosteroid, 5-fluorouracil, and 585-nm flashlamp-pumped pulsed-dye laser treatments. Arch Dermatol 2002;138:1149–55.

52. Faurschou A, Togsverd-Bo K, Zachariae C, et al. Pulsed dye laser vs. intense pulsed light for port-wine stains: a randomized side-by-side trial with blinded response evaluation. Br J Dermatol 2009;160:359–64.

53. Tomson N, Lim SP, Abdullah A, et al. The treatment of port-wine stains with the pulsed-dye laser at 2-week and 6-week intervals: a comparative study. Br J Dermatol 2006;154:676–9.

54. Kono T, Sakurai H, Groff WF, et al. Comparison study of a traditional pulsed dye laser versus a long-pulsed dye laser in the treatment of early childhood hemangiomas. Lasers Surg Med 2006;38:112–5.

55. Collyer J, Boone SL, White LE, et al. Comparison of treatment of cherry angiomata with pulsed-dye laser, potassium titanyl phosphate laser, and electrodesiccation: a randomized controlled trial. Arch Dermatol 2010;146:33–7.

56. Erceg A, Greebe RJ, Bovenschen HJ, et al. A comparative study of pulsed 532-nm potassium titanyl phosphate laser and electrocoagulation in the treatment of spider nevi. Dermatol Surg 2010;36:630–5.

57. Kundu RV, Joshi SS, Suh KY, et al. Comparison of electrodesiccation and potassium-titanyl-phosphate laser for treatment of dermatosis papulosa nigra. Dermatol Surg 2009;35:1079–83.

58. Vejjabhinanta V, Elsaie ML, Patel SS, et al. Comparison of short-pulsed and long-pulsed 532 nm lasers in the removal of freckles. Lasers Med Sci 2010;25:901–6.

59. Galeckas KJ, Collins M, Ross EV, et al. Split-face treatment of facial dyschromia: pulsed dye laser with a compression handpiece versus intense pulsed light. Dermatol Surg 2008;34:672–80.

60. Wang CC, Sue YM, Yang CH, et al. A comparison of Q-switched alexandrite laser and intense pulsed light for the treatment of freckles and lentigines in Asian persons: a randomized, physician-blinded, split-face comparative trial. J Am Acad Dermatol 2006;54:804–10.

61. Kessler E, Flanagan K, Chia C, et al. Comparison of alpha- and beta-hydroxy acid chemical peels in the treatment of mild to moderately severe facial acne vulgaris. Dermatol Surg 2008;34:45–50 [discussion: 51].

62. Khunger N, Sarkar R, Jain RK. Tretinoin peels versus glycolic acid peels in the treatment of melasma in dark-skinned patients. Dermatol Surg 2004;30:756–60 [discussion: 760].

63. Kroon MW, Wind BS, Beek JF, et al. Nonablative 1550-nm fractional laser therapy versus triple topical therapy for the treatment of melasma: a randomized controlled pilot study. J Am Acad Dermatol 2011;64:516–23.

64. Alam M, Omura NE, Dover JS, et al. Glycolic acid peels compared to microdermabrasion: a right-left controlled trial of efficacy and patient satisfaction. Dermatol Surg 2002;28:475–9.

65. Raziee M, Balighi K, Shabanzadeh-Dehkordi H, et al. Efficacy and safety of cryotherapy vs. trichloroacetic acid in the treatment of solar lentigo. J Eur Acad Dermatol Venereol 2008;22:316–9.

66. Sezer E, Erbil H, Kurumlu Z, et al. A comparative study of focal medium-depth chemical peel versus cryosurgery for the treatment of solar lentigo. Eur J Dermatol 2007;17:26–9.

67. Kitzmiller WJ, Visscher MO, Maclennan S, et al. Comparison of a series of superficial chemical peels with a single midlevel chemical peel for the correction of facial actinic damage. Aesthet Surg J 2003;23:339–44.

68. Yaghmai D, Garden JM, Bakus AD, et al. Comparison of a 1,064 nm laser and a 1,320 nm laser for the nonablative treatment of acne scars. Dermatol Surg 2005;31(8 Pt 1):903–9.

69. Tanzi EL, Alster TS. Comparison of a 1450-nm diode laser and a 1320-nm Nd:YAG laser in the treatment of atrophic facial scars: a prospective clinical and histologic study. Dermatol Surg 2004;30(2 Pt 1):152–7.

70. Nootheti PK, Magpantay A, Yosowitz G, et al. A single center, randomized, comparative, prospective clinical study to determine the efficacy of the VelaSmooth system versus the Triactive system for the treatment of cellulite. Lasers Surg Med 2006;38:908–12.

71. Alexiades-Armenakas M, Rosenberg D, Renton B, et al. Blinded, randomized, quantitative grading comparison of minimally invasive, fractional radiofrequency and surgical face-lift to treat skin laxity. Arch Dermatol 2010;146:396–405.

72. Goldman MP, Alster TS, Weiss R. A randomized trial to determine the influence of laser therapy, monopolar radiofrequency treatment, and intense pulsed light therapy administered immediately after hyaluronic acid gel implantation. Dermatol Surg 2007;33:535–42.

73. Narins RS, Brandt F, Leyden J, et al. A randomized, double-blind, multicenter comparison of the efficacy and tolerability of Restylane versus Zyplast for the correction of nasolabial folds. Dermatol Surg 2003;29:588–95.

74. Narins RS, Baumann L, Brandt FS, et al. A randomized study of the efficacy and safety of injectable poly-L-lactic acid versus human-based collagen implant in the treatment of nasolabial fold wrinkles. J Am Acad Dermatol 2010;62:448–62.

75. Moers-Carpi MM, Tufet JO. Calcium hydroxylapatite versus nonanimal stabilized hyaluronic acid for the correction of nasolabial folds: a 12-month, multicenter, prospective, randomized, controlled, split-face trial. Dermatol Surg 2008;34:210–5.

76. Marmur E, Green L, Busso M. Controlled, randomized study of pain levels in subjects treated with calcium hydroxylapatite premixed with lidocaine for correction of nasolabial folds. Dermatol Surg 2010;36:309–15.

77. Monheit GD, Campbell RM, Neugent H, et al. Reduced pain with use of proprietary hyaluronic acid with lidocaine for correction of nasolabial folds: a patient-blinded, prospective, randomized controlled trial. Dermatol Surg 2010;36:94–101.

78. Weinkle SH, Bank DE, Boyd CM, et al. A multicenter, double-blind, randomized controlled study of the safety and effectiveness of Juvéderm injectable gel with and without lidocaine. J Cosmet Dermatol 2009;8:205–10.

79. Baumann LS, Shamban AT, Lupo MP, et al. Comparison of smooth-gel hyaluronic acid dermal fillers with cross-linked bovine collagen: a multicenter, double-masked, randomized, within-subject study. Dermatol Surg 2007;33(Suppl 2):S128–35.

80. Smith S, Busso M, McClaren M, et al. A randomized, bilateral, prospective comparison of calcium hydroxylapatite microspheres versus human-based collagen for the correction of nasolabial folds. Dermatol Surg 2007;33(Suppl 2):S112–21 [discussion: S121].

81. Narins RS, Dayan SH, Brandt FS, et al. Persistence and improvement of nasolabial fold correction with nonanimal-stabilized hyaluronic acid 100,000 gel particles/mL filler on two retreatment schedules: results up to 18 months on two retreatment schedules. Dermatol Surg 2008;34(Suppl 1):S2–8 [discussion: S8].

82. Flanagan KH, King R, Glaser DA. Botulinum toxin type a versus topical 20% aluminum chloride for the treatment of moderate to severe primary focal axillary hyperhidrosis. J Drugs Dermatol 2008;7:221–7.

83. Vadoud-Seyedi J, Simonart T. Treatment of axillary hyperhidrosis with botulinum toxin type A reconstituted in lidocaine or in normal saline: a randomized, side-by-side, double-blind study. Br J Dermatol 2007;156:986–9.

84. Heckmann M, Plewig G. Hyperhidrosis study group. Low-dose efficacy of botulinum toxin A for axillary hyperhidrosis: a randomized, side-by-side, open-label study. Arch Dermatol 2005;141:1255–9.

85. Lowe NJ, Lask G, Yamauchi P, et al. Bilateral, double-blind, randomized comparison of 3 doses of botulinum toxin type A and placebo in patients with crow's feet. J Am Acad Dermatol 2002;47:834–40.

86. Alam M, Dover JS, Arndt KA. Pain associated with injection of botulinum A exotoxin reconstituted using isotonic sodium chloride with and without preservative: a double-blind, randomized controlled trial. Arch Dermatol 2002;138:510–4.

87. Hexsel D, Rutowitsch MS, de Castro LC, et al. Blind multicenter study of the efficacy and safety of injections of a commercial preparation of botulinum toxin type A reconstituted up to 15 days before injection. Dermatol Surg 2009;35:933–9 [discussion: 940].

88. Yang GC, Chiu RJ, Gillman GS. Questioning the need to use Botox within 4 hours of reconstitution: a study of fresh vs 2-week-old Botox. Arch Facial Plast Surg 2008;10:273–9.

89. Carruthers A, Bogle M, Carruthers JD, et al. A randomized, evaluator-blinded, two-center study of the safety and effect of volume on the diffusion and efficacy of botulinum toxin type A in the treatment of lateral orbital rhytides. Dermatol Surg 2007;33:567–71.

90. Lowe P, Patnaik R, Lowe N. Comparison of two formulations of botulinum toxin type A for the treatment of glabellar lines: a double-blind, randomized study. J Am Acad Dermatol 2006;55:975–80.

91. Hexsel D, Dal'Forno T, Hexsel C, et al. A randomized pilot study comparing the action halos of two commercial preparations of botulinum toxin type A. Dermatol Surg 2008;34:52–9.

92. Trindade de Almeida AR, Marques E, de Almeida J, et al. Pilot study comparing the diffusion of two formulations of botulinum toxin type A in patients with forehead hyperhidrosis. Dermatol Surg 2007; 33(Spec No 1):S37–43.

93. Hsu TS, Dover JS, Arndt KA. Effect of volume and concentration on the diffusion of botulinum exotoxin A. Arch Dermatol 2004;140:1351–4.

94. Rao J, Wildemore JK, Goldman MP. Double-blind prospective comparative trial between foamed and liquid polidocanol and sodium tetradecyl sulfate in the treatment of varicose and telangiectatic leg veins. Dermatol Surg 2005;31:631–5 [discussion: 635].

95. Prado A, Andrades P, Danilla S, et al. A prospective, randomized, double-blind, controlled clinical trial comparing laser-assisted lipoplasty with suction-assisted lipoplasty. Plast Reconstr Surg 2006;118: 1032–45.

96. Rubin JP, Xie Z, Davidson C, et al. Rapid absorption of tumescent lidocaine above the clavicles: a prospective clinical study. Plast Reconstr Surg 2005;115:1744–51.

97. Butterwick KJ. Lipoaugmentation for aging hands: a comparison of the longevity and aesthetic results of centrifuged versus noncentrifuged fat. Dermatol Surg 2002;28:987–91.

98. Butterwick KJ, Bevin AA, Iyer S. Fat transplantation using fresh versus frozen fat: a side-by-side two-hand comparison pilot study. Dermatol Surg 2006; 32:640–4.

Conclusions and Recommendations: United States Dermatologic Health Care Need Assessment

Laura Huff, MD[a], Lauren McLaughlin, BS[b],
Ryan Gamble, MD[a], Robert P. Dellavalle, MD, PhD, MSPH[c],*

KEYWORDS

- Health care needs • Skin disease • Supply • Demand
- Reform • Recommendation • Workforce

This needs assessment attempted to identify gaps between current and desired outcomes for skin diseases in the United States. The authors address these 3 questions: (1) What is the burden of a skin disease in the United States? (2) What impact does the disease burden have on quality of life, the economy, and the health care system as a whole? and (3) How can the health care system best address the burden to reduce the impact of skin disease?

Defining health care need can be challenging. The authors used the model presented in the recently published UK dermatologic health care needs assessment, where need, supply, and demand overlap.[1] Supply is defined as all health care provided to society and demand is defined as what patients ask for.[2] Supply and demand encompass both health care needs and health care wants because not all dermatologic care is medically necessary. The authors emphasize skin conditions determined to be health care needs. An article on cosmetic dermatology, which the

authors consider a health care want, is also provided due to the high demand in society for elective procedures. This publication provides health care providers and policy makers an evidence-based, up-to-date tool during this important era of health care reform in the United States.

SUMMARY

Presented here are summary points from each article, written by the authors of each respective section. For a more thorough discussion, readers should refer to the corresponding full-length articles.

The Burden of Skin Disease in the United States and Canada

- Skin conditions are frequently cited among the most common health problems in the United States and Canada.
- The burden of skin disease has avoided accurate estimation because of many

Funding/Support: None.

[a] Department of Dermatology Research Labs, University of Colorado School of Medicine, Mail Stop F-8127, PO Box 6511, Aurora, CO 80045, USA

[b] Rocky Vista University College of Osteopathic Medicine, 8401 South Chambers Road, Parker, CO 80134, USA

[c] Dermatology Service, Denver Department of Veterans Affairs Medical Center, University of Colorado School of Medicine, Colorado School of Public Health, 1055 Clermont Street, Mail Code #165, Denver, CO 80220, USA

* Corresponding author.

E-mail address: robert.dellavalle@ucdenver.edu

Dermatol Clin 30 (2012) 189–194

doi:10.1016/j.det.2011.09.003

0733-8635/12/$ – see front matter Published by Elsevier Inc.

derm.theclinics.com

obstacles, including defining skin disease, *International Classification of Diseases* version 9 codes being unreliable, and lack of epidemiologic data on skin disease as well as difficulty in calculating total costs of skin disease.
- Improved collaboration focusing on the burden of skin disease at an international level has allowed for better estimation of the burden of skin disease during the past decade.

Services Available and Their Effectiveness

- The benefits of dermatologists' expertise include greater cost-effectiveness and more training and experience treating common skin conditions. Patients increasingly recognize the benefits of specialist care, and the demand for dermatologists' services continues to rise. The supply of dermatologists has not kept up with the demand despite increases in use of nonphysician clinicians.
- The role of self-care and primary care in skin disease remains significant. Efficacy of self-care depends on patients' ability to understand and carry out appropriate self-treatment regimens. Primary care doctors are frequently called on to treat common skin problems, so a solid grounding in basic dermatology topics for all primary care trainees is essential.

Models of Care

- Patients enrolled in a health maintenance organization are more likely to see a nondermatologist and less likely to see a dermatologist for a skin complaint than those enrolled in a preferred provider organization.
- Dermatologist supply has been shown to positively correlate with improved skin disease outcomes. The increasing wait times and shortage in the dermatology workforce have created the need for physician extenders in dermatology practices.
- The Department of Veterans Affairs health care system's nationwide centralization allows for comprehensive comparative effectiveness research and has recently undertaken a mission to evaluate teledermatology.

Dermatologic Health Disparities

- Although racial and socioeconomic disparities are evident in diseases, such as melanoma, nonmelanoma skin cancer (NMSC), and atopic dermatitis, a paucity of data exists on the overall impact of health disparities on dermatologic diseases.
- The recent passage of health care reform and the impending increased patient load may exacerbate dermatologic health disparities given the dermatology workforce shortage.
- Additional investigations exploring disparities in dermatologic education and research are needed.

A Review of Health Outcomes in Patients with Psoriasis

- Health outcomes unique to psoriasis includes major impacts on health-related quality of life due to physical discomfort, impaired emotional functioning, and negative body image and self-image as well as limitations in daily activities, social contacts, and work. Furthermore, there is growing literature on the association between psoriasis and cardiovascular, rheumatologic, endocrine, malignancy, and psychiatric comorbidities.
- The costs of health care maintenance and medications for the treatment of psoriasis continue to increase. Research in developing novel agents to treat psoriasis remains one of the greatest areas of future need because access and affordability is a main prohibitive treatment factor for the uninsured or underinsured.

Health Outcomes in Atopic Dermatitis

- Multiple disease-severity and quality-of-life instruments exist to assess atopic dermatitis, but only selected instruments have been validated.
- Treatment of atopic dermatitis includes a variety of therapies, from medications to nutritional supplements to psychotherapy. Large randomized controlled trials are needed for the treatment categories of oral antihistamines, probiotics, and psychological counseling.

Contact Dermatitis in the United States: Epidemiology, Economic Impact, and Workplace Prevention

- Contact dermatitis is the most common work-related skin disorder and hands are the most frequently affected site.
- Occupation is a key factor in the development of contact dermatitis.
- Occupational contact dermatitis is more likely to be allergic than irritant in nature.

Acne Vulgaris: Pathogenesis, Treatment, and Needs Assessment

- Acne is one of the most common dermatologic conditions. The disease burden results in high cost and physician burden in the United States.
- Current treatment of acne focuses on the evidence-based recommendations of topical retinoids and avoidance of antibiotic monotherapy. Other treatments oral contraceptive therapy for female patients and systemic treatments such as isotretinoin. Further research is required to establish best practice guidelines.
- To better meet the treatment needs of acne, physicians should pursue more innovative technologic means. These include, but are not limited to, more extensive education in medical school for primary care providers, teledermatology, and further education of midlevel providers.

US Skin Disease Assessment: Ulcers and Wound Care

- Chronic ulcers are a growing cause of patient morbidity and health care cost in the United States.
- Most common causes of chronic ulcers include venous leg ulcers, pressure ulcers, diabetic neuropathic foot ulcers, and leg ulcers of arterial insufficiency.
- Chronic wounds account for an estimated $6 billion to $15 billion annually in US health care costs.

Melanoma: Epidemiology, Diagnosis, Treatment, and Outcomes

- Melanoma incidence and mortality have risen in the past few decades. Despite increased surveillance and improvements in screening, these trends emphasize the continued need for better screening tests that assist patients and general practitioners in the early detection of melanoma.
- Many factors are associated with an increased risk for melanoma, including personal and family history of melanoma, nevi count, and certain medical conditions. Additionally, risk behaviors, such as indoor tanning, can serve as targets for the melanoma prevention efforts of public health practitioners and health providers.
- Although the tumorigenesis of melanoma has not been completely elucidated, genes, such as p16/ARF and BRAF, have been implicated as serving a role. Efforts to understand melanoma pathogenesis have infomred and will continue to inform the discovery of new adjuvant systemic therapies for melanoma.

Epidemiology, Health Outcomes, and Treatments of NMSCs

- Without a national tumor registry, epidemiologic studies regarding accurate incidence and mortality rates continue to be challenging. Nonetheless, trend analyses suggest that NMSC incidence in the United States is increasing, which emphasizes the need for continued vigilance and surveillance of the population.
- Health outcomes unique to NMSCs include quality-of-life assessments that incorporate appearance and emotional domains. Furthermore, treatment modality seems to have effects on all aspects of health outcomes, such as rates of recurrence, quality of life, and costs.
- Few long-term randomized controlled trials comparing the efficacies of alternative therapies for primary NMSCs exist. This is, perhaps, one of the greatest areas of research needs because cost, cosmesis, and efficacy are all considerations when determining the type of treatment, particularly for low-risk tumors.

Infectious Skin Diseases: A Review and Needs Assessment

- Bacterial, fungal, and viral skin infections represent broad categories of disease that range in severity from benign to life threatening.
- Infectious skin diseases are highly prevalent and can be difficult to treat given the emergence of several highly virulent pathogens as well as the limited therapeutic efficacy of available treatments in some cases.
- Future research in infectious skin disease may emphasize increased disease surveillance and cost analyses, evaluation of existing therapies, and ongoing development of superior treatment modalities.

General Dermatology Surgery Needs Assessment

- There are several effective treatment modalities for actinic keratoses, including cryotherapy and photodynamic therapy, and for small, low-risk, NMSCs, including electrodessication and curettage, and excision.

- For invasive skin cancers and other higher-risk skin cancers, surgical excision is the most effective treatment.
- Surgical excision with appropriate margins remains the treatment of choice of melanoma.

Cosmetic Dermatology

- Serious adverse events resulting from cosmetic dermatologic procedures are rare. Dermatologists safely perform a range of noninvasive and minimally invasive cosmetic procedures in an outpatient, in-office setting under minimal or local anesthesia.
- Sequelae after cosmetic dermatology procedures are typically mild transient erythema and edema.
- There are few unbiased objective outcome measures for evaluating the effects of cosmetic dermatology procedures.

Mohs Micrographic Surgery

- Utilization rates of Mohs micrographic surgery (MMS) are rapidly increasing with a paucity of data to support its cost-effectiveness compared with other surgical modalities in treating a wide variety of cutaneous malignancies.

- Evidence-based guidelines for the use of antibiotic prophylaxis for MMS suggest limited indications.
- More adequately powered prospective studies are needed to better quantify the risk of postoperative bleeding and other complications attributable to various anticoagulation therapies to help develop guidelines for their management in the MMS perioperative period.

EXPERT RECOMMENDATIONS

The purpose of this issue of *Dermatologic Clinics* is to evaluate whether the dermatologic infrastructure in the United States is using its resources appropriately to improve the health of the population. The authors wrote this article especially for policy makers to concisely highlight the areas viewed as most imperative for health care reform. The following is a discussion of dermatology recommendations recently published from other health care experts, such as the Institute of Medicine, UK needs assessment, and the Lewin Group as well as from this US skin disease needs assessment. These collective recommendations offer a framework for dermatologic policy making that is both feasible and affordable.

Table 1
Dermatology-related priority research areas from the Institute of Medicine, 2009

Area	Priority	Quartile
Psoriatic arthritis	Compare the effectiveness of different strategies of introducing biologics into the treatment algorithm for inflammatory diseases, including Crohn's disease, ulcerative colitis, rheumatoid arthritis, and psoriatic arthritis.	First
Infectious disease	Compare the effectiveness of various screening, prophylaxis, and treatment interventions in eradicating MRSA in communities, institutions, and hospitals.	First
Workforce	Compare the effectiveness (including resource use, workforce needs, net health care expenditures, and requirements for large-scale deployment) of new remote patient monitoring and management technologies (eg, telemedicine, Internet, remote sensing) and usual care in managing chronic disease, especially in rural settings.	Second
Psoriasis	Compare the effectiveness (including effects on quality of life) of treatment strategies (eg, topical steroids, ultraviolet light, methotrexate, biologic response modifiers) for psoriasis.	Second
Chronic wounds	Compare the effectiveness of topical treatments (eg, antibiotics platelet-derived growth factor) and systemic therapies (eg, negative pressure wound therapy, hyperbaric oxygen) in managing chronic lower extremity wounds.	Third
Acne	Compare the effectiveness of long-term treatments for acne.	Fourth

Data from Ratner R, Eden J, Wolman D. Initial national priorities for comparative effectiveness research. Institute of Medicine. 2009 [cited 2011 Jul 14]. Available at: http://www.iom.edu/Reports/2009/ComparativeEffectivenessResearchPriorities.aspx.

In 2009, the Institute of Medicine published a report, the *Initial National Priorities for Comparative Effectiveness Research*, which was a list of the top 100 priority areas for comparative effectiveness research.[3] This list was in response to the American Recovery and Reinvestment Act (ARRA) of 2009, when Congress asked the Institute of Medicine to determine national priorities for ARRA-funded comparative effectiveness research. The Institute of Medicine, through stakeholder input, started with a list of more than 2600 topics and narrowed it to a list of the top 100 priority topics for research

funding. This list is ranked by quartile, with the first quartile the most important. Of this list, there are 4 topics specific to dermatology and 2 others that are indirectly related (shown in **Table 1**). In the first quartile are psoriatic arthritis and methicillin-resistant *Staphylococcus aureus* (MRSA). In the second quartile are psoriasis and workforce needs. The third quartile lists chronic lower-extremity wounds and the fourth quartile lists acne.

The UK skin conditions needs assessment also took on the task of making recommendations for the future of dermatology. Their report provided

Table 2
Expert recommendations

Area	Recommendation
Workforce and models of care	Tackle the workforce shortage by increasing the number of dermatologists and access to dermatologists and midlevel providers, while improving dermatology training for primary care providers and using novel economical approaches like teledermatology.
Health disparities	Explore the overall impact of health disparities, with a focus on unknown areas in addition to addressing the documented disparities in melanoma, NMSC, and atopic dermatitis.
Psoriasis	Make available all treatment options to patients with moderate-to-severe psoriasis, with emphasis on increasing access and affordability of biologic agents.
Atopic dermatitis	Develop effective and safe treatment for moderate-to-severe atopic dermatitis.
Contact dermatitis	Improve surveillance methods of occupational contact dermatitis and address unmet need for national dermatitis prevention programs.
Acne	Address the extremely high burden by creating best practice guidelines, improving education for primary care and midlevel providers, and using teledermatology.
Ulcers and wound care	Identification of ulcers, with accurate documentation of therapeutic response, is crucial to prevent and heal chronic ulcers with the added potential of saving health care dollars.
Melanoma	Implement better screening and early detection; focus on prevention by decreasing indoor tanning.
Nonmelanoma skin cancer and general dermatology surgery	Increase education for prevention of NMSCs and explore randomized controlled trials with long follow-up to better delineate the comparative effectiveness of different nonexcisional treatments of NMSC.
Infectious skin disease	Increase disease surveillance and research cost analysis; evaluate current therapies and develop new superior treatments.
Mohs micrographic surgery	More clinical trial data are needed to assess outcomes for MMS, including tumor recurrence rates, patient-centered outcomes, and cost-effectiveness.
Cosmetic dermatology	There is need for more prospective comparative studies of cosmetic dermatologic procedures and devices.

List of Acronyms	
ARRA	American Recovery and Reinvestment Act
DFU	Diabetic neuropathic foot ulcers
HCNA	Health Care Needs Assessment
ICD	International Classification of Diseases
MMS	Mohs micrographic surgery
MRSA	Methicillin-resistant *Staphylococcus aureus*
NMSC	Non-melanoma skin cancer
PrU	Pressure ulcers
UK	United Kingdom
VLU	Venous leg ulcers

10 key recommendations for dermatologic reform in the United Kingdom. One of the 10 recommendations is to improve self-care by providing better patient information and improving pharmacist's knowledge. Another recommendation is to use tools to measure patient-reported outcomes and quality of life. The other 8 recommendations involve service structure topics, such as better training for general practitioners and nurses, more appropriate referrals to specialists, and rearranging the service structure into a pyramidal approach where there are multiple layers of providers with varying degrees of specialized knowledge.[1]

In 2005, the Lewin Group conducted a thorough investigation of the cost of skin disease in the United States. They identified the 5 most costly skin diseases as skin ulcers and wounds, acne, cutaneous fungal infections, NMSC, and atopic dermatitis. These 5 diseases cost a total of $16 billion in direct medical costs, which is 60% of the total costs associated with the 21 dermatologic diseases included in their study.[4] Because these diseases account for the majority of health care spending, it is important to focus reform in these areas.

The collaborative recommendations from the expert authors of this issue of *Dermatologic Clinics* are shown in **Table 2**. The authors offer a recommendation for service structure to address the workforce shortage and recommendations to address each skin disease based on health care need.

In comparing these recommendations to those of the Institute of Medicine, UK needs assessment, and the Lewin Group, many similarities are evident. The disease topics for which recommendations are made are similar to the diseases highlighted by both the Institute of Medicine (psoriasis, wounds, acne, and infectious disease)[3] and the Lewin Group (ulcers and wounds, acne, cutaneous fungal infections, NMSC, and atopic dermatitis).[4] The UK needs assessment focuses much attention on service structure improvements. This recommendation to address the workforce shortage by increasing midlevel providers, improving training for primary care providers, and using teledermatology is in line with the UK's recommendation.[1] The Institute of Medicine similarly highlighted the importance of workforce needs and telemedicine in the second quartile of their top 100 areas that need research.[3]

These need-based recommendations, in conjunction with the recommendations from the Institute of Medicine, the UK skin conditions needs assessment, and the Lewin Group, provide thorough evidence-based recommendations for dermatology. These collective recommendations should provide future directions for policy makers, so that the United States can more effectively and efficiently use the allotted resources.

REFERENCES

1. Schofield JK, Grindley D, Williams HC. Skin conditions in the UK: a health care needs assessment. 2011. Available at: http://www.nottingham.ac.uk/scs/documents/documentsdivisions/documentsdermatology/hcnaskinconditionsuk2009.pdf. Accessed September 24, 2011.

2. Wright J, Williams R, Wilkinson JR. Development and importance of health needs assessment. BMJ 1998; 316:1310–3.

3. Ratner R, Eden J, Wolman D. Initial national priorities for comparative effectiveness research. Institute of Medicine; 2009. Available at: http://www.iom.edu/Reports/2009/ComparativeEffectivenessResearchPriorities.aspx. Accessed September 24, 2011.

4. The Lewin Group. The burden of skin diseases. 2005. Available at: http://www.lewin.com/content/publications/april2005skindisease.pdf. Accessed September 24, 2011.

Index

Note: Page numbers of article titles are in **boldface** type.

A

ABCDE criteria
   and atypical nevi, 158
   for melanoma identification, 116
Ablative resurfacing
   and cosmetic dermatologic surgery, 181
ACD. See *Allergic contact dermatitis.*
Acne vulgaris
   and age of onset, 99, 100
   antibiotics for, 101
   antimicrobials for, 101
   and burdens of treatment, 102
   and combined oral contraceptives, 101, 102
   costs associated with, 102
   and diet, 100, 101
   epidemiology of, 99, 100
   oral isotretinoin for, 102
   pathogenesis of, 100
   and photodynamic therapy, 158
   and physician assistants, 103
   and physician demands, 102
   prevention of, 100, 101
   and *Propionibacterium acnes,* 100
   risk factors for, 100
   scarring from, 102
   services available for, 102, 103
   and smoking, 100
   and sun exposure, 100
   topical retinoids for, 102
   treatment of, 101, 102
Acne vulgaris: pathogenesis, treatment, and needs assessment, **99–106**
Acral lentiginous melanoma, 118
Actinic keratoses
   and cryosurgery, 154
   and photodynamic therapy, 157
Acyclovir
   for herpes simplex virus, 147
AD. see *Atopic dermatitis.*
Adalimumab
   for psoriasis, 66
Adjuvant systemic therapies
   for melanoma, 120
AFX. See *Atypical fibroxanthoma.*
Age
   and incidence of nonmelanoma skin cancer, 127
AK. See *Actinic keratoses.*
ALA. See *5-Aminolevulinic acid.*

Alcohol abuse
   and psoriasis, 64
Alefacept
   for psoriasis, 67
Allergic contact dermatitis, 87–95
Ambulatory phlebectomy
   and cosmetic dermatologic surgery, 183
5-Aminolevulinic acid
   and photodynamic therapy, 157
Anti-tumor necrosis factor
   for psoriasis, 66
Antibiotics
   for acne vulgaris, 101
   and Mohs micrographic surgery, 170, 171
   and surgical dressings, 161, 162
Anticoagulants
   and Mohs micrographic surgery, 171
Antihistamines
   for atopic dermatitis, 78, 79
Antimicrobials
   for acne vulgaris, 101
Asymmetry
   and melanoma, 116
Atopic dermatitis, 90, 94
   and assessment of health outcomes, 73–75
   and the Children's Dermatology Life Quality Index, 74, 75, 77, 80
   and the Dermatitis Family Impact scale, 74–76, 79, 80
   and dermatologic health disparities, 54
   disease severity scales for, 73–75
   and the Eczema Area and Severity Index, 73, 74, 77, 78
   educational interventions for, 80
   emollients for, 76
   and the Infants' Dermatitis Quality of Life Index, 74, 76, 80
   oral antihistamines for, 78, 79
   phototherapy for, 79
   pimecrolimus for, 78
   prevalence and incidence of, 73
   probiotics for, 79, 80
   psychological interventions for, 80
   and quality of life, 73–80
   and results of health outcomes, 75, 76
   and the Severity Scoring of Atopic Dermatitis scale, 73, 74, 76–79
   topical calcineurin inhibitors for, 77, 78
   topical corticosteroids for, 76, 77

Dermatol Clin 30 (2012) 195–203
doi:10.1016/S0733-8635(11)00187-2
0733-8635/12/$ – see front matter © 2012 Elsevier Inc. All rights reserved.

Atopic (*continued*)
    topical tacrolimus for, 77, 78
    treatment of, 76–80
Atopy
    and contact dermatitis, 90, 91
Atypical fibroxanthoma
    and Mohs micrographic surgery, 168
    and surgical excision, 161
Atypical nevi
    and ABCDE criteria, 158
    and surgical excision, 158, 159

B

Bacterial skin diseases, 141–143
Basal cell carcinoma, 125–135
    and cryosurgery, 154, 155
    and electrosurgery, 155, 156
    and Mohs micrographic surgery, 167–173
    and photodynamic therapy, 157
    and surgical excision, 159, 160
BCC. See *Basal cell carcinoma.*
Bevacizumab
    for melanoma, 120
Biologic therapy
    for psoriasis, 66, 67
Border irregularity
    and melanoma, 116
Botulinum toxin A
    and cosmetic dermatologic surgery, 182
Bowen disease
    and photodynamic therapy, 158
BRAF inhibitors
    for melanoma, 120
Buffering anesthesia, 161
The burden of skin disease in the United States and
    Canada, **5–18**

C

Calcineurin inhibitors
    for atopic dermatitis, 77, 78
Canada
    mortality of skin disease in, 8, 9
    prevalence and incidence of skin disease in, 8
    skin disease in, 5–15
Candida albicans
    and fungal infections, 144, 145
Cardiovascular comorbidities
    and psoriasis, 63, 64
CDLQI. See *Children's Dermatology Life Quality
    Index.*
Cellulitis
    and cost of treatment, 143
    incidence of, 142
    treatment of, 142, 143
Children's Dermatology Life Quality Index

and atopic dermatitis, 74, 75, 77, 80
Chronic ulcers
    care for, 110
    management team for, 110
Clinical triage assistants
    and skin disease, 20, 21, 29
COC. See *Combined oral contraceptives.*
Color variegation
    and melanoma, 116
Combined oral contraceptives
    and acne vulgaris, 101, 102
Conclusions and recommendations: United States
    dermatologic health care need assessment,
    189–194
Contact dermatitis
    and age, 90
    allergic, 87–95
    and atopy, 90, 91
    avoidance of, 94
    and burdens on the patient, 93, 94
    and common allergens, 89
    and common irritants, 88
    costs of, 92, 93
    and environment, 89, 90
    incidence and prevalence of, 91, 92
    irritant, 87, 89–91, 95
    and occupation, 89
    occupational, 89–96
    and patch testing, 95
    and patient education, 94, 95
    prevention of, 94, 95
    and quality of life, 93, 94
    and race and ethnicity, 90
    risk factors for, 89–91
    and sex, 90
Contact dermatitis in the United States:
    epidemiology, economic impact, and workplace
    prevention, **87–98**
Corticosteroids
    for atopic dermatitis, 76, 77
    for psoriasis, 65
Cosmetic dermatologic surgery
    and ablative resurfacing, 181
    and ambulatory phlebectomy, 183
    and botulinum toxin A, 182
    definitions and boundaries of, 178
    effectiveness of, 178
    and endovenous ablation, 183
    and energy devices, 180
    and erythema, 180, 181
    and fat reduction, 182
    and hair removal, 183
    and hair transplantation, 183
    indications for, 178
    and injectables, 180–182
    and lasers, 180
    and leg veins, 182, 183

and light sources, 180
and limitations in clinical research, 179, 180
and liposuction, 183
and neurotoxins, 182
and nonablative resurfacing, 181
patient selection for, 179
and pigmentation, 180, 181
safety of, 178
and sclerotherapy, 183
and site of service, 178–180
and skin and subcutaneous tissue
    resection, 183
and skin tightening, 181, 182
and soft tissue augmentation, 182
and topic areas, 180–183
Cryosurgery
    for actinic keratoses, 154
    background of, 154
    for basal cell carcinoma, 154, 155
    indications for, 154
    for squamous cell carcinoma, 154, 155
    technique of, 154
CTA. See Clinical triage assistants.
Curettage
    before Mohs micrographic surgery, 169, 170

D

Debulking
    and surgical excision, 159
Dermatitis Family Impact scale
    and atopic dermatitis, 74–76, 79, 80
Dermatofibrosarcoma protuberans
    and Mohs micrographic surgery, 168
    and surgical excision, 160, 161
Dermatologic health care needs
    expert recommendations for, 192
Dermatologic health disparities, 53–59
    and atopic dermatitis, 54
    and dermatology education, 55, 56
    and the dermatology workforce, 54, 55
    and health care reform, 54, 55
    and nonmelanoma skin cancer, 54
    and Patient Protection and Affordability Care
        Act, 55
    and race and ethnicity, 53, 54
    and research, 56
    and skin cancer, 54
    and socioeconomic status, 54
Dermatology education
    and health disparities, 55, 56
Dermatology Life Quality Index, 10, 11
Dermatology workforce
    and dermatologic health disparities, 54, 55
DFI. See Dermatitis Family Impact scale.
DFSP. See Dermatofibrosarcoma protuberans.
DFU. See Diabetic neuropathic foot ulcers.

Diabetes
    and neuropathic foot ulcers, 108, 109
Diabetic neuropathic foot ulcers
    and hyperbaric oxygen therapy, 109
    and living skin equivalents, 109
    and negative pressure wound therapies, 109
    prevention of, 109
    and total contact casting, 109
    treatment of, 109
Diameter
    and melanoma, 116
Diet
    and acne vulgaris, 100, 101
Disease severity scales
    for atopic dermatitis, 73–75
DLQI. See Dermatology Life Quality Index.

E

EASI. See Eczema Area and Severity Index.
Eczema Area and Severity Index
    and atopic dermatitis, 73, 74, 77, 78
ED&C. See Electrodesiccation and curettage.
Electrodesiccation and curettage, 155, 156
Electrosurgery
    advantages of, 155
    background of, 155
    and basal cell carcinoma, 155, 156
    and electrodesiccation and curettage, 155, 156
    indications for, 155
    and lentigo maligna melanoma, 156
    and squamous cell carcinoma, 156
    technique of, 155
Emollients
    for atopic dermatitis, 76
Endovenous ablation
    and cosmetic dermatologic surgery, 183
Energy devices
    and cosmetic dermatologic surgery, 180
Erythema
    and cosmetic dermatologic surgery, 180, 181
Evolution
    and melanoma, 116, 117
Exercise
    and psoriasis, 64

F

Fat reduction
    and cosmetic dermatologic surgery, 182
Fee-for-service
    and models of care, 39–41, 44, 45
FFS. See Fee-for-service.
Fungal infections
    and Candida albicans, 144, 145
    and tinea capitis, 144
    and tinea corporis, 144

Fungal (*continued*)
   and tinea cruris, 144
   and tinea pedis, 144
   and tinea unguium, 144
   and *Trichophyton rubrum,* 144
Fungal skin diseases, 143–145
   and cost of treatment, 145
   incidence of, 145
   superficial, 144–145
   treatment of, 145

G

Geographic location
   and incidence of nonmelanoma skin cancer,
      126, 127

H

Hair removal
   and cosmetic dermatologic surgery, 183
Hair transplantation
   and cosmetic dermatologic surgery, 183
HBOT. See *Hyperbaric oxygen therapy.*
HCNA. See *Health care needs assessment.*
Health care needs assessment
   dermatologic, 1, 2
   and skin disease, 1, 2
   in the United Kingdom, 2
   in the United States, 1, 2
Health care reform
   and dermatologic health disparities, 54, 55
Health maintenance organizations
   vs. preferred provider organizations, 44, 45
Health outcomes in atopic dermatitis, **73–86**
Herpes simplex virus
   acyclovir for, 147
   and cost of treatment, 147, 148
   incidence of, 146
   treatment of, 147
   and treatment resistance, 147
HMO. See *Health maintenance organizations.*
HSV. See *Herpes simplex virus.*
Hyperbaric oxygen therapy
   for diabetic neuropathic foot ulcers, 109

I

ICD. See *Irritant contact dermatitis.*
IDQOL. See *Infants' Dermatitis Quality of Life Index.*
Infants' Dermatitis Quality of Life Index
   and atopic dermatitis, 74, 76, 80
Infectious skin diseases: a review and needs
      assessment, **141–151**
Infliximab
   for psoriasis, 66
Injectables
   and cosmetic dermatologic surgery, 180–182

Inpatient dermatology services, 23, 24
Institute of Medicine
   dermatology-related priority research areas
      from, 192
Interferon-α
   for melanoma, 120
Interleukin-2
   for melanoma, 120
Introduction: US dermatologic health care needs
      assessment, **1–3**
Ipilimumab
   for melanoma, 120
Irritant contact dermatitis, 87, 89–91, 95
Isotretinoin
   for acne vulgaris, 102

K

Keratoacanthoma
   and Mohs micrographic surgery, 168
   and surgical excision, 160

L

Lasers
   and cosmetic dermatologic surgery, 180
Leg veins
   and cosmetic dermatologic surgery, 182, 183
Lentigo maligna melanoma, 118
   and electrosurgery, 156
Lifestyle changes
   and psoriasis comorbidities, 64
Light sources
   and cosmetic dermatologic surgery, 180
Liposuction
   and cosmetic dermatologic surgery, 183
Living skin equivalents
   for diabetic neuropathic foot ulcers, 109
LSE. See *Living skin equivalents.*

M

MAC. See *Microcystic adnexal carcinoma.*
MAL. See *Methylaminolevulinate.*
Malignancy
   and psoriasis comorbidities, 63, 64
Malpractice
   and models of care, 48
Margin assessment
   and surgical excision, 159
MCC. See *Merkel cell carcinoma.*
Medicare
   and models of care, 39, 40, 42–45, 47
Melanoma
   and ABCDE criteria, 116
   acral lentiginous, 118
   adjuvant systemic therapies for, 120

and anatomic distribution, 117
and asymmetry, 116
bevacizumab for, 120
biopsy of, 117
and border irregularity, 116
BRAF inhibitors for, 120
and clinical morphology, 116, 117
clinical presentation of, 116, 117
and color variegation, 116
diagnosis of, 117–119
and diameter, 116
and distant metastasis, 119
epidemiology of, 113, 114
etiology of, 114–116
and evolution, 116, 117
and family and personal history, 115, 116
genetic mechanisms of, 114, 115
incidence of, 113, 114
interferon-α for, 120
interleukin-2 for, 120
ipilimumab for, 120
lentigo maligna, 118
and Mohs micrographic surgery, 168, 169
mortality for, 114
needs in detection and care, 120, 121
and nevus count, 116
nodular, 118
and the p16/ARF locus, 115
pathogenesis of, 114
prevention of, 119
and primary tumors, 118, 119
prognosis for, 120
radiotherapy for, 120
and regional lymph nodes, 119
and relative tumor density, 117
risk factors for, 115, 116
sorafenib for, 120
staging of, 118, 119
subtypes of, 117, 118
superficial spreading, 117, 118
and surgical excision, 159
surgical excision for, 119
treatment of, 119, 120
and tumor progression, 114
and ultraviolet light exposure, 119
and ultraviolet radiation exposure, 115
Melanoma: epidemiology, diagnosis, treatment, and
outcomes, **113–124**
Merkel cell carcinoma
and surgical excision, 161
Metastasis
and melanoma, 119
Methicillin-resistant *Staphylococcus aureus*, 141–143
Methotrexate
for psoriasis, 66
Methylaminolevulinate
and photodynamic therapy, 157

Microcystic adnexal carcinoma
and Mohs micrographic surgery, 168
MMS. See *Mohs micrographic surgery.*
Models of care
and access to dermatology care, 44
fee-for-service, 39–41, 44, 45
health maintenance organizations, 39, 44, 45
and improving dermatology care, 45
and increasing patient awareness, 46
and increasing training of nondermatologists, 46
and malpractice, 48
and Medicare, 39, 40, 42–45, 47
and physician extenders, 46, 47
preferred provider organizations, 41, 42
and role of pharmaceuticals, 48
and supply and demand, 45, 46
Veterans Health Administration, 42–44
and wait times, 47, 48
Models of care and organization of services,
39–51
Mohs micrographic surgery
and atypical fibroxanthoma, 168
and basal cell carcinoma, 167–173
cost-effectiveness of, 172, 173
curettage before, 169, 170
and dermatofibrosarcoma protuberans, 168
and general dermatologic surgery needs
assessment, 153, 155–157, 159–162
indications for, 167–169
and keratoacanthoma, 168
and managing anticoagulants, 171
and melanoma, 168, 169
and microcystic adnexal carcinoma, 168
and nonmelanoma skin cancer, 167–173
outcomes of, 171–173
and patient satisfaction, 172
and prophylactic antibiotics, 170, 171
and recurrences, 171
and squamous cell carcinoma, 167–169, 171
utilization of, 169
MRSA. See *Methicillin-resistant* Staphylococcus
aureus.

N

Needle types
and suturing, 161
Needs assessment for cosmetic dermatologic
surgery, **177–187**
Needs assessment for general dermatologic surgery,
153–166
Needs assessment for Mohs micrographic surgery,
167–175
Negative pressure wound therapies
for diabetic neuropathic foot ulcers, 109
Neurotoxins
and cosmetic dermatologic surgery, 182

Nevus count
    and melanoma, 116
NMSC. See *Nonmelanoma skin cancer.*
Nodular melanoma, 118
Nonablative resurfacing
    and cosmetic dermatologic surgery, 181
Nondermatologists
    increasing training of, 46
Nonmelanoma skin cancer, **125–139**
    costs of, 132, 133
    and dermatologic health disparities, 54
    and disease mortality, 8, 15
    epidemiology of, 125–130
    and estimation of incidence, 127–130
    health outcomes of, 130–133
    and incidence by age, 127
    and incidence by geographic location, 126, 127
    and incidence by race and ethnicity, 127
    and incidence by skin cancer type, 126
    and incidence in the United States, 125, 126
    increasing incidence of, 126, 128, 129
    and Mohs micrographic surgery, 167–173
    and morbidity and mortality, 130, 131
    and quality of life, 131, 132
    radiation for, 134
    and research needs, 134–136
    superficial therapy for, 134
    and surgical excision, 159
    surgical treatment for, 133, 134
    treatment of, 133, 134
    and ultraviolet light exposure, 125–127, 126, 131
Nonphysician clinicians
    and skin disease, 28, 29
NP. See *Nurse practitioners.*
NPC. See *Nonphysician clinicians.*
NPWT. See *Negative pressure wound therapies.*
Nurse practitioners
    and skin disease, 20–22, 28

O

Occlusion
    and surgical dressings, 161, 162
Occupational contact dermatitis, 89–96
OCD. See *Occupational contact dermatitis.*
Oral systemic agents
    for psoriasis, 66
OTC. See *Over-the-counter.*
Outpatient dermatology services, 23
Over-the-counter products
    skin disease and, 24–26, 31, 32
Overeating
    and psoriasis, 64

P

p16/ARF locus
    and melanoma, 115

PA. See *Physician assistants.*
PASI. See *Psoriasis Area and Severity Index.*
Patch testing
    and contact dermatitis, 95
Patient awareness
    and models of care, 46
Patient Protection and Affordability Care Act
    and dermatologic health disparities, 55
PCP. See *Primary care physicians.*
PDT. See *Photodynamic therapy.*
Pharmaceuticals
    and models of care, 48
Photodynamic therapy
    and acne, 158
    and actinic keratoses, 157
    and 5-aminolevulinic acid, 157
    background of, 156, 157
    and basal cell carcinoma, 157
    and Bowen disease, 158
    indications for, 157
    and methylaminolevulinate, 157
    and squamous cell carcinoma, 158
Phototherapy
    for atopic dermatitis, 79
    for psoriasis, 65, 66
Physician assistants
    and acne vulgaris treatment, 103
    and skin disease, 20–22, 28, 29
Physician extenders
    and models of care, 46, 47
Pigmentation
    and cosmetic dermatologic surgery, 180, 181
Pimecrolimus
    and atopic dermatitis, 78
PPACA. See *Patient Protection and Affordability Care Act.*
PPO. See *Preferred provider organizations.*
Preferred provider organizations
    vs. health maintenance organizations, 44, 45
Pressure ulcers
    prevention of, 109, 110
    treatment of, 109, 110
Primary care physicians
    and psoriasis, 68
    and skin disease, 20, 25, 26, 32, 33
Probiotics
    for atopic dermatitis, 79, 80
Propionibacterium acnes
    and acne vulgaris, 100
PrU. See *Pressure ulcers.*
Psoralen plus ultraviolet A
    for psoriasis, 63–65, 67, 68
Psoriasis
    adalimumab for, 66
    and alcohol abuse, 64
    alefacept for, 67
    and anti-tumor necrosis factor, 66

biologic therapy for, 66, 67
burdens of, 62
combination therapy for, 67
and comorbidities, 62–64
corticosteroids for, 65
and costs of treatment, 67, 68
and defining treatment goals, 64
and disease severity, 61
economic burden of, 62
and exercise, 64
infliximab for, 66
methotrexate for, 66
and national resources, 68
oral systemic agents for, 66
and overeating, 64
phototherapy for, 65, 66
prevalence and incidence of, 61, 62
and primary care physicians, 68
psoralen plus ultraviolet A for, 63–65, 67, 68
and Psoriasis Area and Severity Index, 61, 66, 67
psychological burden of, 62
and quality of life, 62
retinoids for, 65, 66
and smoking, 64
and specialty care, 68
subtypes of, 61, 62
topical treatments for, 65
treatment of, 64–68
ustekinumab for, 67
Psoriasis Area and Severity Index, 61, 66, 67
Psoriasis comorbidities
    assessment of, 64
    cardiovascular, 63, 64
    and lifestyle changes, 64
    malignancy, 63, 64
    psychiatric, 63
    rheumatologic, 63, 64
    and risk modification, 64
    and shared mechanisms, 62, 63
Psychiatric comorbidities
    and psoriasis, 63
PUVA. See Psoralen plus ultraviolet A.

Q

QOL. See Quality of life.
Quality of life
    and atopic dermatitis, 73–80
    and contact dermatitis, 93, 94
    and Dermatology Life Quality Index, 10, 11
    and nonmelanoma skin cancer, 131, 132
    and psoriasis, 62
    and skin disease, 10–15

R

Race and ethnicity
    and contact dermatitis, 90

and dermatologic health disparities, 53, 54
and incidence of nonmelanoma skin cancer, 127
Radiation
    for nonmelanoma skin cancer, 134
Radiotherapy
    for melanoma, 120
Relative tumor density
    and melanoma, 117
Research
    and dermatologic health disparities, 56
Retinoids
    for acne vulgaris, 102
    for psoriasis, 65, 66
A review of health outcomes in patients with
    psoriasis, **61–72**
Rheumatologic comorbidities
    and psoriasis, 63, 64
Risk modification
    and psoriasis comorbidities, 64
RTD. See Relative tumor density.

S

Scarring
    from acne vulgaris, 102
    optimization of, 162
SCC. See Squamous cell carcinoma.
Sclerotherapy
    and cosmetic dermatologic surgery, 183
SCORAD. See Severity Scoring of Atopic Dermatitis
    scale.
Self-care
    efficacy of, 30–32
    and skin disease, 20, 24, 25, 30, 32
Services available and their effectiveness, **19–37**
SES. See Socioeconomic status.
Severity Scoring of Atopic Dermatitis scale, 73, 74,
    76–79
Skin and subcutaneous tissue resection
    and cosmetic dermatologic surgery, 183
Skin cancer
    deaths from, 8–11, 15
    and dermatologic health disparities, 54
Skin-care products
    costs of, 15
Skin disease
    in Canada, 5–15
    classification of, 5, 6
    and clinical triage assistants, 20, 21, 29
    costs in the workplace, 14, 15
    costs of, 11–15
    costs of skin-care products, 15
    and deaths from cancer, 8–11, 15
    and effectiveness of care by primary care
        physicians, 32, 33
    and effectiveness of specialist care, 32, 33
    and effectiveness of subspecialist care, 33, 34

Skin (*continued*)
  and effectiveness of teledermatology care, 33
  and efficacy complications, 34, 35
  and efficacy of self-care, 30–32
  and efficacy of treatment, 30–35
  epidemiology of, 6–9
  and health care needs assessment, 1, 2
  and inpatient dermatology services, 23, 24
  intangible costs of, 15
  and levels of health care providers, 20–23
  and location of services, 23, 24
  mortality of, 8, 9
  most common, 7
  and non-melanoma skin cancer, 8, 15
  and nurse practitioners, 20–22, 28
  and outpatient dermatology services, 23
  and over-the-counter products, 24–26, 31, 32
  and physician assistants, 20–22, 28, 29
  prevalence and incidence of, 6–8
  and primary care physician services, 25, 26
  and primary care physicians, 20, 25, 26, 32, 33
  and quality of life, 10–15
  and self-care, 20, 24, 25, 30, 32
  and specialist care, 20–22, 26–29, 32, 33
  and specialist nonphysician clinicians, 28, 29
  and subspecialist care, 22, 23, 29, 30, 33, 34
  and teledermatology services, 24, 33
  and unique services, 26–28
  in the United States, 5–15
  and willingness to pay, 11, 15
Skin tightening
  and cosmetic dermatologic surgery, 181, 182
Smoking
  and acne vulgaris, 100
  and psoriasis, 64
Socioeconomic status
  and dermatologic health disparities, 54
Soft tissue augmentation
  and cosmetic dermatologic surgery, 182
Sorafenib
  for melanoma, 120
Specialist care
  and skin disease, 20–22, 26–29, 32, 33
Specialty care
  for psoriasis, 68
Squamous cell carcinoma, 125–136
  and cryosurgery, 154, 155
  and electrosurgery, 156
  and Mohs micrographic surgery,
    167–169, 171
  and photodynamic therapy, 158
  and surgical excision, 160
Subspecialist care
  and skin disease, 22, 23, 29, 30, 33, 34
Sun exposure
  and acne vulgaris, 100
Superficial spreading melanoma, 117, 118

Superficial therapy
  for nonmelanoma skin cancer, 134
Supply and demand
  of dermatologic health care needs, 2
  and models of care, 45, 46
Surgical dressings
  and antibiotics, 161, 162
  and occlusion, 161, 162
Surgical excision
  and atypical fibroxanthoma, 161
  and atypical nevi, 158, 159
  and basal cell carcinoma, 159, 160
  and debulking, 159
  and dermatofibrosarcoma protuberans,
    160, 161
  and keratoacanthoma, 160
  and margin assessment, 159
  and melanoma, 159
  for melanoma, 119
  and Merkel cell carcinoma, 161
  and nonmelanoma skin cancer, 159
  for nonmelanoma skin cancer, 133, 134
  and rare tumors, 160, 161
  and squamous cell carcinoma, 160
Suturing
  materials for, 161
  and needle types, 161
  techniques for, 161

T

Tacrolimus
  and atopic dermatitis, 77, 78
TCC. See *Total contact casting*.
Teledermatology
  and skin disease, 24, 33
Tinea capitis, 144
Tinea corporis, 144
Tinea cruris, 144
Tinea pedis, 144
Tinea unguium, 144
TNM staging
  of melanoma, 118, 119
Total contact casting
  for diabetic neuropathic foot ulcers, 109
Trichophyton rubrum
  and fungal infections, 144
Tumor progression
  and melanoma, 114

U

Ulcers
  chronic, 110
  diabetic neuropathic foot, 108, 109
  pressure, 109, 110
  venous leg, 107, 108

Ultraviolet light exposure
    and melanoma, 119
    and nonmelanoma skin cancer, 125–127, 126, 131
Ultraviolet radiation exposure
    and melanoma, 115
United Kingdom
    health care needs assessment in, 2
United States
    contact dermatitis in, 87–96
    health care needs assessment in, 1, 2
    incidence of nonmelanoma skin cancer in,
        125, 126
    mortality of skin disease in, 8
    prevalence and incidence of skin disease in, 6–8
    skin disease in, 5–15
    ulcer and wound care in, 107–110
US skin disease assessment: ulcer and wound care,
    107–111
Ustekinumab
    for psoriasis, 67

V

Venous leg ulcers
    prevention of, 107, 108
    treatment of, 107, 108
Veterans Health Administration
    and models of care, 42–44
VHA. See *Veterans Health Administration.*
Viral skin diseases, 146–148
VLU. See *Venous leg ulcers.*

W

Wait times
    and models of care, 47, 48
Willingness to pay
    and skin disease, 11, 15
Workplace
    and costs of skin disease, 14, 15
WTP. See *Willingness to pay.*

Moving?

Make sure your subscription moves with you!

To notify us of your new address, find your **Clinics Account Number** (located on your mailing label above your name), and contact customer service at:

Email: journalscustomerservice-usa@elsevier.com

800-654-2452 (subscribers in the U.S. & Canada)
314-447-8871 (subscribers outside of the U.S. & Canada)

Fax number: 314-447-8029

Elsevier Health Sciences Division
Subscription Customer Service
3251 Riverport Lane
Maryland Heights, MO 63043

*To ensure uninterrupted delivery of your subscription, please notify us at least 4 weeks in advance of move.

Moving?

Make sure your subscription moves with you!

To notify us of your new address, find your Clinics Account Number (located on your mailing label above your name), and contact customer service at:

Email: journalscustomerservice-usa@elsevier.com

800-654-2452 (subscribers in the U.S. & Canada)
314-447-8871 (subscribers outside of the U.S. & Canada)

Fax number: 314-447-8029

Elsevier Health Sciences Division
Subscription Customer Service
3251 Riverport Lane
Maryland Heights, MO 63043

Printed and bound by CPI Group (UK) Ltd, Croydon, CR0 4YY

03/10/2024

01040350-0002